THE ANATOMY OF MADNESS

Essays in the History of Psychiatry

VOLUME III

THE ANATOMY OF MADNESS

Essays in the History of Psychiatry

VOLUME III

The Asylum and its Psychiatry

EDITED BY

W.F. Bynum, Roy Porter,
and Michael Shepherd

Routledge
LONDON AND NEW YORK

First published in 1988 by
Routledge
11 *New Fetter Lane, London EC4P 4EE*
Published in the USA by
Routledge
in association with Routledge, Chapman and Hall, Inc.
29 *West 35th Street, New York, NY* 10001

Typeset by Graphicraft Typesetters Ltd. Hong Kong

Printed in Great Britain at The University Press, Cambridge

British Library Cataloguing in Publication Data

The anatomy of madness: essays in the history of psychiatry.
Vol. 3: The Asylum and its psychiatry
1. *Medicine. Psychiatry, to* 1985
I. Porter, Roy, 1946– *II. Bynum, W.F. (William Frederick),* 1943– *III. Shepherd, Michael,* 1923–
616.89'009
ISBN 0–415–00859–*x*

Library of Congress Cataloging in Publication Data

(Revised for Vol. 3)

The Anatomy of madness.
"Most of the papers in these volumes arose from a seminar series on the history of psychiatry and a one-day seminar on the same theme held at the Wellcome Institute for the History of Medicine, London, during the academic year 1982–83*"–V.* 1, *acknowledgements.*
Includes bibliographies and indexes.
Contents: v. 1. *People and ideas.– –v.* 3. *The asylum and its psychiatry.*
1. *Psychiatry–Europe–History–19th century–Collected works.* 2. *Psychiatric hospitals–Europe–History–19th century–Collected works. I. Porter, Roy,* 1946- . *II. Shepherd, Michael,* 1923– *III. Wellcome Institute for the History of Medicine.*
RC450.A1A53 1985 362.2'094 85–9824
ISBN 0–4227–9340–9 *(v.* 1*)*
ISBN 0–4227–9440–6 *(v.* 2*)*

Contents

Contributors

MICHAEL J. CLARK was formerly a graduate student of Nuffield and Linacre Colleges, Oxford, where his D.Phil thesis 'The data of alienism ...' examined the relations between evolutionary physiological psychology, neurology, and the development of British psychiatry during the latter part of the nineteenth century. Since 1984 he has been a Wellcome Research Fellow in the Department of History at Lancaster University, where he has been working with Dr Roger Smith on a history of English legal medicine between the mid-nineteenth and mid-twentieth centuries. He has published several articles and reviews on the history of psychiatry, and is currently revising his thesis for publication alongside his work on the history of legal medicine.

DAVID COCHRANE is a Planning Administrator with South West Thames Regional Health Authority where his functions include policy analysis and the planning of new capital projects. His primary research interests are the process of change in health policy and the problems of planning and implementing community care. He is currently completing a PhD dissertation on the political impact of mental hospital scandals in the 1960s and 1970s.

JAMES G. DONAT completed his PhD thesis in 1986, in the history of medicine, at University College London. Previous to this he had trained at the C.G. Jung Institute in Zurich, and is also a graduate of McCormick Theological Seminary in Chicago.

WALTRAUD ERNST was a student of psychology and political science at the University of Konstanz and a post-graduate student of the history of South Asia at the School of Oriental and African Studies, London where she completed her PhD thesis on European psychiatry and the development of lunatic asylums in nineteenth-century India, in September 1986. She is currently expanding this research to the period 1800–1947 at the Wellcome Institute for the History of Medicine, London.

PATRIZIA GUARNIERI graduated in philosophy from the University of Florence in 1977, followed two years later by the award of Perfezionamento from the University of Urbino for her published thesis 'La Rivista Filosophica. Conoscenza e valori nel neokantismo italiano'. In 1981 she was awarded a Fulbright Visiting Scholarship to Harvard University and in 1984 a NATO-Cnr Fellowship to the Wellcome Institute for the History of Medicine, London. Her research is in positivist culture and the nineteenth century, and books published include *Introduzione a James* and *Individualità difformi: La psichiatria antropologica di E. Morselli.* She is currently a lecturer at Stanford University in Florence.

ANNE HARRINGTON is an Alexander von Humboldt Fellow, based at the University of Freiburg (West Germany). She is currently pursuing research into the wider cultural significance of the holistic, neo-vitalistic movement in German neuro-biology from the *fin de siècle* to the rise of the Third Reich. Her book *Medicine, Mind and the Double Brain: A study in nineteenth-century thought* has recently been published by Princeton University Press.

RICHARD RUSSELL studied history at Lancaster as a mature student, where he was introduced to the topic of Victorian lunatic asylums by Dr Roger Smith. He went on to Sheffield University to write his PhD thesis on the relationship between medical specialists in insanity and their patients and subsequently worked for a time in one of the mental hospitals where he researched.

JANET SAUNDERS studied at Birmingham University and the Centre for the Study of Social History at the University of Warwick, completing a doctoral thesis on Victorian institutions and their inmates, in 1983. She is currently employed as a software developer in the computer industry but continues a research interest in social history, presently working on the institutional care of the mentally handicapped in Warwickshire in the 1930s.

CHRISTINE STEVENSON studied the history of art and architecture at the University of Victoria, Canada, the Universities of Helsinki and Copenhagen, and the Courtauld Institute of Art, London, where she completed her PhD in 1986. She currently studies hospital iconography and is writing a book about the history of hospital architecture and works as Publications Officer at the Wellcome Institute for the History of Medicine.

MARGARET S. THOMPSON graduated BA from the University of Washington, MA from the University of Stockholm, and completed her PhD at Boston University in 1984. Her doctoral dissertation *The Mad, the Bad and the Sad: Psychiatric care in the Royal Edinburgh Asylum (Morningside)* is to be published by the Scottish Academic Press. She is a lecturer in social, political, and medical history at Bentley College, Waltham, Massachusetts and currently lectures at the History of Medicine and Science Unit at Edinburgh University where she is also working on the Statistical Package for the Social Sciences project examining mental health in Scotland.

NANCY TOMES is an Associate Professor at the State University of New York at Stony Brook. She received a PhD in history from the University of Pennsylvania in 1978, where she worked primarily on the social history of nineteenth-century American asylums. Since the publication of her first book, *A Generous Confidence: Thomas Story Kirkbride and the Art of Asylum-Keeping, 1840–1883*, in 1984, she has written on the evolution of psychiatry and the mental health professions in the twentieth century, and the comparative history of Anglo-American psychiatry in the nineteenth century.

TREVOR TURNER obtained a Classics degree at Bristol and trained in medicine at St Bartholomew's Hospital, London, qualifying in 1976. Subsequently specializing in psychiatry at the Maudsley Hospital, he was lecturer at St Bartholomew's 1982–5, where he is now a Consultant Psychiatrist. He obtained the Diploma in the History of Medicine, Society of Apothecaries in 1980 and MRC Psych. in 1981. Published papers include studies on psychiatric aspects of endocrine illness, prisons, and adolescence, and the role of asylum care. He is currently completing an MD thesis on the Ticehurst Asylum case books using modern diagnostic criteria.

The editors

W.F. Bynum is Head of the joint Academic Unit for the History of Medicine at the Wellcome Institute for the History of Medicine and University College London. He is the editor (with Roy Porter and E.J. Browne) of *A Dictionary of the History of Science*, and the author of a number of articles on the history of psychiatry. His study of the relationship between basic science and clinical medicine in the nineteenth century will be published by Cambridge University Press.

Roy Porter is Senior Lecturer at the Wellcome Institute for the History of Medicine, London. After working early on the history of the earth sciences, and writing *The Making of Geology*, he has subsequently researched in parallel into social history (*English Society in the Eighteenth Century*), and the social dimensions of the history of medicine. He is currently working on the early history of psychiatry in Britain, on quackery and on the lay experience of illness and doctors.

Michael Shepherd is Professor of Epidemiological Psychiatry and Honorary Director, General Practice Research Unit at the Institute of Psychiatry, University of London. He is the author of several monographs and many research papers; a bibliography of his publications may be found in a volume of his selected papers, *The Psychosocial Matrix of Psychiatry*. In 1970 he founded the distinguished journal *Psychological Medicine*, which he still edits. He is also general editor of the multivolume *Handbook of Psychiatry*.

Acknowledgements

This book has come together because the editorial staff at Tavistock (now Routledge) showed such faith in the publication of the first two volumes of this series of research studies into the history of insanity and psychiatry. That faith was repaid by the favourable reception those volumes met with from reviewers and readers alike; and believing that there was much further unpublished work in this field which could be advantageously gathered between the covers of a book, the editors have chosen to commission the present volume. We believe it helps fulfil the aim of the earlier volumes, in showing that our vision of the history of psychiatry is one which will be modified and amplified in many ways by new strands of empirical research and conceptual analysis. Our thanks thus to Routledge, and especially, as always, to Gill Davies, for being such an encouraging editor. We should also like to thank – also as ever – the Wellcome Trust for its continuing generous support of research into the history of medicine, and the staff of the Wellcome Institute for the History of Medicine, whose services have made the physical tasks of organizing and editing this book so pleasant.

Introduction

Leading currents of scholarship over the last couple of decades have made it tempting to identify the history of psychiatry with the history of the asylum.[1] Michel Foucault designated as the great foundation act the 'great confinement' launched above all in France, but more generally across Europe, in the mid-seventeenth century.[2] Andrew Scull saw the treatment of the mad in England as focusing upon the growth of *Museums of Madness* and, in a roughly comparable way, David Rothman highlighted *The Discovery of the Asylum* as the turning-point in the treatment of the insane in the United States.[3] And, discussing more recent developments in handling the insane, Scull has focused attention on *Decarceration*.[4] These works, and a growing body of first-rate scholarship operating within similar assumptions, have argued that the key response of emergent modern society to the threats and anxieties posed by madness was institutionalization (and that post-industrial society has typically been involved in acts of dismantling).

There is a danger that the attention given to madhouses, mental hospitals, or (as they have more recently been called) psychiatric units has been excessive, resulting in certain distortions. If the scale and, indeed, horrors of 'the great confinement', of old Bethlem, of the madhouse trade in lunacy dominate our view, we easily forget that, at least before the second half of the nineteenth century, a very large percentage of people commonly regarded as psychiatrically abnormal were not confined in lunatic asylums at all. Many were held in other non-specialist institutions, such as workhouses or gaols, and very substantial numbers remained more or less within the community, under family or parochial care (a word which may or may not warrant being encased in inverted commas). It was still common in the mid-nineteenth century for the well-off to have crazy relatives supervised by domestic servants or by attendants employed by specialist physicians. Moreover, the eighteenth century saw the flourishing of what we might call 'neurotic conditions' ('the English malady' and so forth) and office psychiatry became substantial business during the nineteenth century.[5]

All in all, therefore, it would be foolish to view the rise of psychiatry and the emergence of the asylum as coterminous, indeed synonymous, with each other. As Peter Miller and Nickolas Rose have rightly stressed, the medical and professional care of the insane always extended far beyond the madhouse walls. (In that sense, recent deinstitutionalization may be seen not so much as a blow against psychiatry but as a correct admission that psychiatry is in no way confined to the asylum, but pervades the whole of society.)[6]

Yet, despite these reservations, it would be historically wilful not to give a certain pride of place in the annals of madness to the defining role played by the asylum. From the late eighteenth century in particular, there was a proliferation of all types of special receptacles for the insane: private asylums run on a profit-making basis, retreats run by monks and nuns within Catholic Europe, charitable and subscription foundations, city and state-owned institutions, wards and wings attached to general hospitals, and so forth. Aggregate numbers of the confined insane steadily increased, rising to almost 100,000 in Britain by 1900, and to nearly 40,000 even in Italy. Legislation – concerning licensing, certification, inspection, and so forth – boldly inscribed confinement within the framework of the administrative, paternalistic state. And not least, the asylum became the seedbed for the rise of the psychiatric profession. It is no accident that the first professional organization for psychiatrists in Britain was called the Association of Asylum and Medical Officers for the Insane, and one of the first professional journals was known as the *Asylum Journal*.[7]

The reasons for the rise of the asylum are manifold, and they have been fiercely debated.[8] This is not the place to reopen these controversies. What should be emphasized here is the enormous attractiveness of the promise of the asylum to the idealistic late-eighteenth- or early-nineteenth-century mind. Properly reformed or newly founded, the asylum could be the antithesis of the 'hell on earth' stereotype of the old madhouse, of 'unreformed Bedlam'. It would be clean, sanitary, tranquil, humane, protective, a retreat from the cares of the world, 'far from the madding crowd'. Above all, it would be therapeutic.[9]

What strikes us most powerfully, indeed poignantly, when we listen to the chorus of advocates of the asylum in the age of Thomas Arnold, Joseph Mason Cox, Chiarugi, Pinel, the Tukes, Reil, down to the early years of John Conolly, is their benevolent expectation that the asylum could realistically be an engine for working cures. At some level, this was not a new hope (after all, traditional madhouses such as Bethlem had refused to take 'incurables', on the grounds that such would prove a waste of resources). What was new, however, was an optimism. Traditionally the rationales for confining the mad were largely negative (to protect both the madman and society from harm). Now they became positive – working a cure.

This was based upon the firm conviction that new philosophies and techniques had been evolved (what we may successively call 'moral management' and 'moral therapy') facilitating therapeutic success. These involved many strategies, including behavioural conditioning, work therapy, internal classification, and not least, as Christine Stevenson's essay in this volume shows, a powerful emergent notion that precisely tailoring asylum architecture to the real needs of the mad and their doctors, (rather than to external goals such as palatial design, or, indeed, mere economy) would prove efficacious. Light, ventilation, visibility, and not least a pleasant rural environment were all argued to be therapeutic desiderata.[10]

The asylum solution had its honest doubters and swingeing critics. But, around the turn of the nineteenth century, they formed a small minority. Overall, the asylum took on for a time a status as panacea equivalent to the steam engine, the rights of man, or the spread of universal knowledge. Madness could after all be cured, reason could be restored. The asylum was the magic machine in which this could be achieved. The asylum superintendent or doctor was the new exorcist for a scientific society. Those visiting institutions such as the York Retreat might have been pardoned for exclaiming that they had seen the future and it worked.[11]

All this forms a background which the contributors to this volume essentially take as established. What specifically concerns them – and what gives this collection its thematic unity – was the denting, even shattering of this noble dream. It was one thing to advocate new model asylums, one thing indeed to set them up. It was quite another to make them deliver the goods, effect the much-touted cures. In fact, given that miracle cures did not instantly appear, it was no easy matter for their theorists and practitioners to agree on either day-to-day or wider philosophies of management. Two essays below illustrate this fact particularly clearly.

Waltraud Ernst probes what happened to British administrators, traders, and soldiers who went mad in India in the early days of the Raj. Given that in certain respects India was used as a kind of laboratory for experiments in administration, we might expect to find a coherent and unified lunacy policy. Far from it! For one thing, quite distinctive sorts of institutions emerged in Bombay, Madras, and Calcutta. For another, there seems to have been an oscillation between preferring private solutions (the entrepreneurial madhouse) and attempting to establish rather more public asylums under direct control of the governors. Nor was there even agreement as to whether there was something intrinsic to the Indian climate which precipitated insanity amongst Europeans (thus perhaps pointing to siting asylums among the cooler hill-stations).

In a broadly comparable study, Nancy Tomes examines one of the crucial divergences between British and North American psychiatry during the first three-quarters of the nineteenth century. A powerful current within British psychiatry sought to push 'moral therapy' to its logical extreme: the doctrine and practice of total 'non-restraint', the abolition of all forms of mechanical restraint and physical coercion whatsoever, even for therapeutic ends.[12] Advocates such as Robert Gardiner Hill contended that the rationale for non-restraint was not dogmatic liberalism but therapeutic effectiveness. Free to move, patients would in fact become more tractable and receptive to treatment.

Many American psychiatrists (perhaps ironically for the land of the free) condemned this as doctrinaire. They argued that certain modes of restraint on certain patients were therapeutically indicated. It was vital that there should be no restraint upon clinical judgement – doctors must be free to use the treatments which they saw as appropriate. What is significant (as Tomes points out) is that the English experience was demonstrating, by around the 1850s and 1860s, that non-restraint was not indeed the panacea it had been claimed to be; and hence, for practical reasons, a greater element of overt or covert restraint was reintroduced. In the USA meanwhile, the effective ideology underpinning an increased use of restraint was not therapeutic optimism but the need to solve the problem of the confinement, often long term, of boisterous and unruly patients. Towards the close of the nineteenth century, as Tomes has demonstrated elsewhere, custodialism was once more becoming the order of the day in many American asylums.[13]

A similar situation came to obtain in Britain. Recent in-depth studies of nineteenth-century asylums have certainly helped to dispel the myth of the madhouse simply as warehouse, and the related notion that once admitted to the Victorian asylum, patients rarely left except in a hearse.[14] Stays often remained short, and John Walton above all has stressed how families would commonly have mad relatives confined only during their worst bouts, later resuming care over them.[15] Nevertheless, studies of even the best asylums, such as Ticehurst, have confirmed that there was indeed a significant increase of long-stay patients and a shift from expectations of cure to an emphasis rather on care and management.[16] As Richard Russell's essay below emphasizes, for an increasingly vocal band of late Victorian commentators, all this amounted to the 'failure' of the asylum. By 1876, the Lunacy Commissioners – so staunch in their earlier advocacy of the therapeutic benefits of non-restraint – were suggesting that only some 7 per cent of the mad were actually, after all, curable.[17]

What was then to be done? Was there a fundamental crisis of confidence in the asylum? Clearly not. There was, perhaps, a tacit agreement to view the institution in a new light (or rather in an old) – as custodial rather than curative. But that hardly halted its juggernaut growth. Two essays in this collection in fact underline just how rapid the expansion of institutional care for the intellectually abnormal continued to be towards the close of the nineteenth century. In his examination of the policy of the London County Council in the generation before the First World War, David Cochrane documents an extraordinary expansion in facilities. In 1891, a staggering 15,000 pauper lunatics were confined in asylums in the London region; by 1909, that figure had leapt to just under 26,000. The London County Council accepted its obligation to build facilities for the mentally disturbed and defective, and build it did – a whole series of large, barrack-like premises, from Claybury to Epsom, many capable of housing a couple of thousand patients, and amounting primarily to a triumph of bureaucratic social engineering rather than to a therapeutic blueprint. The official architects got rich, but only a small percentage of the patients got better.

But expansionism in the latter part of the nineteenth century was not merely confined to numbers. The qualitative as well as the quantitative dimension underwent growth, as though the whole dynamic of institutionalization had taken on a dynamism of its own, quite independent of the expectation of curing. For one thing, an increasing proportion of those being admitted to insane asylums as the Victorian age went on were not from the classes of people classically considered lunatics – were not, in other words, people who would necessarily have been admitted to an equivalent asylum in 1750 or 1800. Notably these included a statistically significant percentage of habitual drunkards.

Chronic drunkenness had traditionally been regarded chiefly as a vice or a sin, and the hopeless drunk had often found himself punished by the courts. During the first half of the nineteenth century, however, the condition was successively medicalized and psychiatrized, the notion of 'alcoholism' as a disease, indeed a mental disease, gained a purchase, and the asylums began to acquire a goodly complement of old drunks.[18] As Margaret Thompson shows in her investigation of the Edinburgh asylum population in the last part of the nineteenth century, certain sections of the Morningside Asylum commonly comprised more than 10 per cent of alcoholics (the figure was so high partly because the superintendent, Dr Thomas Clouston, was particularly willing to admit such patients).

Another category appearing in increasing abundance in the later-nineteenth-century asylum were patients suffering from a whole range of neurological defects, sensory-motor disorders, ataxias, paralyses. Epileptics were common, as were the victims of tertiary syphilis, though the relationship between those displaying the characteristic symptoms of general paresis of the insane (GPI) and earlier bouts of syphilis remained an open medical question (it was a link, for example, on which Thomas Clouston kept an open mind, while admitting to Morningside many who suffered from the condition).

How far the late Victorian asylum had thus become a general dumping ground for 'sinners' – or at least for those whom high-minded Victorian moral idealists were glad to be able to exclude from normal society – is a contentious question weighed up in several of the contributions below.[19] As has often been pointed out, if traditional vices now newly received the stigma of mental illness, admission to the asylum certainly was not seen as 'punitive' – the Victorians undoubtedly had more unpleasant ways of showing their displeasure against unregenerates than by confinement to the lunatic asylum. At Morningside, for example, alcoholics received rather privileged treatment, being regaled with a lavish, fattening diet of egg custards and given some of the more interesting work. Moreover, admission to the asylum was by no means a 'life sentence' for what J.C. Prichard would have called the 'morally insane'. As Thompson demonstrates, although a percentage of the women admitted to Morningside were placed there essentially because they were unruly and difficult prostitutes, their very unruliness ensured that they were typically rather quickly released.[20]

These issues – the status of the asylum and its regime within a total social system of control, punishment, and regeneration – were ones which greatly exercised contemporary psychiatrists, as Tomes's essay demonstrates. Asylum superintendents sought to exonerate themselves from all possibility of allegations that their practices – such as the use of physical confinement and mechanical constraint – were punitive (after all, if mental disorder really were a medical condition, punishment would have been a categorical mistake). Seclusion, wet packs, and heavy sedation were always justified (one might say rationalized) upon medical rather than penal grounds, though patients' own accounts clearly show that, within the asylum context, this might be known to be a pious fiction. Foucault wrote of the gigantic moral imprisonment which followed in the wake of the notion of 'moral therapy', and the phrase 'social control' has been widely touted by recent historians and sociologists to capture the essence of this trend.[21] This term inevitably carries conspiratorial overtones, however, whose question-begging nature renders it a less helpful term than the more contemporary idea of 'paternalism'. What cannot be in doubt is that the moral mission of paternalism continued to swell the numbers of those confined.

This is particularly conspicuous in the case of those metaphorical siblings of the insane, the mentally defective (those traditionally known as idiots or fools, and increasingly labelled by such categories as imbecile, feeble-minded, or, mainly in America, moron). Time had been when doctors and administrators had fought to keep such classes out of the institutions (on the grounds that being essentially incurable, they would constitute an unacceptable drain on precious resources). By the last decades of the nineteenth century, however, as Janet Saunders's paper demonstrates, the 'weak-minded' were indeed being 'quarantined' in ever larger numbers, to some extent within the classic lunatic asylum (though in separate wings wherever possible), but increasingly also in distinctive institutions or special schools for the mentally retarded or educationally subnormal.

Paternalist aspirations of protecting those who could not help themselves, by placing them in a sheltered environment, formed the ideals behind this further twist to the confinement spiral. The reality, as Saunders shows, was often rather messier. For the mills of the Victorian system of justice and the expanding administrative state did their grinding work thoroughly, and came up with large populations of social flotsam and jetsam – not least hordes of simple-minded petty criminals and law-breakers – who could not be subjected by Victorian sensibilities to the age-old remedy of being given a good whipping and being booted into the next parish. Prison too seemed inappropriate (prison governors had no desire for such nuisances); many typically gravitated into institutions for imbeciles.

A fundamental transformation has been suggested in the last few pages. There was something satisfyingly neat about the scenario of the asylum in 1796 when the York Retreat was opened, or in 1828 when the Lunacy Commission first undertook its mission of bringing hope, purpose, and ideals to the asylums. Lunatic asylums were for those who had temporarily gone out of their minds, according to the Lockean concept of insanity as the misassociation of ideas. The asylum was there to restore reason to such victims. It would work cures. By 1870 or the outbreak of the First World War this was no longer a realistic description or prescription. The asylums had filled up (or had *been* filled up) with an extraordinarily heterogeneous population.[22] Many such people might be somewhat relieved, cared for, or protected via the asylum. But the dream that all but a small proportion might actually be cured had essentially been abandoned. Exposure to the realities of the asylum had forced a major transformation in the expectations of psychiatry itself. This forms the common core of several of the discussions in this volume.

At one level, the implicit goals and aspirations of psychiatry began to change. In the flood tide of early-nineteenth-century optimism, the mark of psychiatric success was plain to see: it was the cure rate. Increasingly, psychiatry ceased to define its prime mission in terms of the short-term criterion of restoration to rationality. The asylum came to be thought of not as an engine for cures but more as a territory over which the alienist held suzerainty, an imperial colony or fiefdom to be managed with justice, economy, and administrative flair.

Importantly, it came to be seen as a research laboratory, as a source of valuable statistics of insanity (Richard Russell suggests that publishing asylum statistics almost degenerated into a mindless end in itself in the Victorian psychiatric journals), as a kind of zoo ripe for the meticulous observation of animal behaviour. (One is perhaps reminded of Charcot in Paris, concentrating his attentions on a small, hand-picked sample of prize hysterics, or the development of university-based psychiatric clinics in Germany, where the exceptional rather than the run-of-the-mill patient took pride of place.) Rather more worryingly, there are signs of the equivalent of 'absentee management' becoming more common as the nineteenth century wore on. Charlotte Mackenzie's forthcoming book on Ticehurst Asylum indicates that the Newington family, so assiduous in cultivating personal ties with their charges earlier in the century, grew more aloof and remote,[23] lavishing more attention on the gardens than on the patients; and Russell detects a tendency for a psychiatric élite, led by Henry Maudsley, to withdraw from asylum management altogether, preferring to cultivate private practice and careers in psychiatric writing.

These matters require further investigation; but if the career pattern followed by Maudsley is in any way representative, it offers some interesting pointers. There can be little doubt that Maudsley, perhaps the biggest name in British psychiatry in the post-1870 generation, grew ever more disillusioned with the prospects of the large public asylum. His monument – his setting up of the Maudsley Hospital in 1907 via a personal donation of £30,000 – was significantly intended not as a general receptacle for the insane but specifically as a clinic designed for psychiatric research. Maudsley had come to believe that the classic vast public asylum, centred on the system of compulsory confinement, was good neither for patients nor for psychiatry.

It is surely not insignificant that so much of Maudsley's vast oeuvre had little to do with practical psychiatry as it would have been understood by Pinel or Esquirol, or even by his own father-in-law, John Conolly. Its concerns were more theoretical, abstract, cosmic. Maudsley had less concern with techniques of cure, with evaluating therapies, than with the study of mind itself, viewed in the context of Victorian metaphysics and science. How consciousness was connected to the body, how the progress of evolution developed ever higher faculties, but how that process of evolutionary development itself taxed the mental and physical constitution, creating in its train tendencies to weakness and degeneracy, how the mechanics of action incorporated both a physical-organic component, yet the freedom of the will – these, as Trevor Turner demonstrates in his essay, were the great issues which preoccupied Maudsley. One might almost say that Maudsley escaped from psychiatry into a general philosophical psychology.

In cultivating these wider concerns he was not alone. Patrizia Guarnieri's biographical study of the man who, alongside Lombroso, was Italy's premier psychiatrist, Enrico Morselli, shows very similar patterns at work. For with Morselli too, the immediate problems of patient cure and patient care began to take a back seat in the agenda of psychiatry. In the context of wider evolutionary and anthropological concerns – ones of pressing relevance in a newly united Kingdom of Italy deeply preoccupied with its own internal 'racial' divides, with the problem of relating the feudal south to the industrial north – Morselli devoted his attentions to the wider questions of the historico-social pathology of mind. What sort of a theory of mental evolution and mental regression would explain the differential incidence of mental disorder amongst rich and poor, male and female, rural and urban populations? How could rational policies for improvement be devised?[24]

Michael Clark's study of morbid introspection shows just how common was this wider reflective dimension in late-nineteenth-century psychiatry. Doctors of the mind had always been perturbed over self-absorption (it was one of the classic features of Burtonian melancholy, prompting Democritus Junior's practical advice: 'be not solitary; be not idle'). The worry assumed increasingly metaphysical proportions in the High Victorian age. For could morbidly solipsistical self-preoccupation truly be differentiated from that cultivation of an intense individualism, of a highly developed introspective reflective moral self, which constituted the pride and glory of the Victorian character?[25] And if too much thinking was a sign of mental pathology, maybe psychiatry itself (the scientific equivalent of contemplating one's own navel, or, as the Victorians might have said, a mode of mental masturbation) was the paradigm case of the condition (thus prompting Maurice Craig's *aperçu* that psychiatry might essentially be an introspective science).

In other words, in many different ways the movement of psychiatry during the nineteenth century was away from the irrational man in the asylum (pure specimens of this kind had proved too few) and rather in the direction of the study of the aberrations and pathology of the mind in general, within the normal relations of society. In some ways, this reflected long-established preoccupations. As James Donat demonstrates in his study of the Ulster Revival of 1859, there were many features of the psychiatric response to this outbreak of religious convulsionism which could have come out of the mouths of seventeenth- or eighteenth-century doctors, terrified of 'enthusiasm'.[26] But alongside the general accounts of 'hysteria' there were new undercurrents as well – fears of psychic throwbacks, of recidivism, and suggestions of racial diatheses – which dovetailed with wider Victorian concerns.

And these naturally lead us on to the overwhelming late-nineteenth-century preoccupation with the enigmas of the divided consciousness, the phenomenon, manifest so clearly in spiritualism, in hypnotic suggestion, and in related occurrences such as *déjà vu*, of the mind operating at different levels, mutually exclusive from each other.[27] In its extreme forms it led to the psychiatric concern with the divided self and multiple personality, an individual ontogeny sometimes understood within a phylogenic perspective which thought in terms of differential rates of evolution, or of evolution and retrogression proceeding alongside each other. Less luridly, as Anne Harrington demonstrates in her account of *fin-de-siècle* French neo-mesmerism, it could generate the analysis of a whole range of mysteries of mind-body interactions, above all the peculiar 'transference' of sensation by suggestion from mind to body, from one body region to another, indeed from one person to another. So multifarious, so common did these manifestations become that psychiatrists began to doubt whether any such thing as normality or rationality remained. Experimental subjects seemed to replicate all the phenomena of early modern witchcraft, evoking an uncanny alliance between new psychiatric science and exploded occultism. The progress of psychiatry seemed to reveal that the human mind was hopelessly adrift in oceans of the irrational. This has been studied of late as the phenomenon of 'degeneration'; but the concerns ran deeper than that.[28] By a diabolical dialectic of the cunning of reason, the aspiration, widely entertained in 1800, of curing a relatively small population of lunatics, seemed by 1900 in danger of revealing the fundamental craziness of the human mind itself.

The essays in this volume thus coalesce around not so much the rise and fall of psychiatry as its successive hopes and fears. The institution of the asylum concentrated the new discipline, but necessarily led to the emergence of a wider psycho-politics concerned with the very place of abnormality within society and confined by it. And in turn institutional psychiatry generated new insights into the general functioning of the human mind which broke down the very divide between the normal and the insane which the asylum had originally helped to institute. All these essays represent major new research initiatives, indicating that subtle integration of wider intellectual perspectives with in-depth investigation into primary sources which marks the scholarly temper of the times. They follow naturally from the contributions printed in the *Anatomy of Madness* volumes I and II, and demonstrate the liveliness of continuing research into the field of the history of psychiatry.

Notes

1 See discussion in 'Introduction' to W.F. Bynum, Roy Porter, and Michael Shepherd (eds) (1985) *The Anatomy of Madness*, 2 vols, London: Tavistock, vol. I, pp. 1–24.

2 Michel Foucault (1965) *Madness and Civilization*, trans. Richard Howard, New York: Random House; cf. K. Doerner (1981) *Madmen and the Bourgeoisie*, trans. J. Neugroschel and J. Steinberg, Oxford: Basil Blackwell.

3 A. Scull (1979) *Museums of Madness*, London: Allen Lane; David Rothman (1971) *The Discovery of the Asylum*, Boston: Little, Brown & Co.

4 A. Scull (1984) *Decarceration* revised edn, Cambridge: Polity Press.

5 For discussion, see Roy Porter (1987) *Mind Forg'd Manacles*, London: Athlone Press, chapters 3 and 4 and 'Conclusion'.

6 P. Miller and N. Rose (1986) *The Power of Psychiatry*, Cambridge: Polity Press.

7 D.J. Mellett (1982) *The Prerogative of Asylumdom*, New York: Garland; J. Goldstein (1987) *Console and Classify: The French Psychiatric Profession in the Nineteenth Century*, Cambridge: Cambridge University Press.

8 See 'Introduction' in Bynum, Porter, and Shepherd (eds), *The Anatomy of Madness*, vol. I, pp. 1–24, and A. Scull (1977) 'Madness and segregative control: the rise of the insane asylum', *Social Problems* 24: 338–51; A. Scull (1981) 'The discovery of the asylum revisited: lunacy reform in the new American republic', in A. Scull (ed.) *Madhouses, Mad-Doctors and Madmen*, London: Athlone Press, pp. 144–65; A. Scull (1980) 'A convenient place to get rid of inconvenient people: the Victorian lunatic asylum', in A.D. King (ed.) *Buildings and Society*, London: Routledge & Kegan Paul, pp. 37–60; A. Scull (1981) 'Humanitarianism or control? Some observations on the historiography of Anglo-American psychiatry', *Rice University Studies* 67: 35–7.

9 W.F. Bynum (1974) 'Rationales for therapy in British psychiatry: 1780–1835', *Medical History* 18: 317–34; M. Donnelly (1983) *Managing the Mind*, London: Tavistock; M. Fears (1977) 'Therapeutic optimism and the treatment of the insane', in R. Dingwall (ed.) *Health Care and Health Knowledge*, London: Croom Helm, pp. 66–81; M. Fears (1978) 'The "moral treatment" of insanity: a study in the social construction of human nature', University of Edinburgh PhD thesis. On Bedlam see P. Allderidge (1985) 'Bedlam: fact or fantasy?', in Bynum, Porter, and Shepherd (eds), *The Anatomy of Madness*, vol. II, pp. 17–33.

10 Thomas A. Markus (ed.) (1982) *Order in Space and Society*, Edinburgh: Mainstream Publishing; Robin Evans (1982) *The Fabrication of Virtue: English Prison Architecture, 1750–1840*, Cambridge: Cambridge University Press.

11 Anne Digby (1985) 'Moral treatment at the York Retreat', in Bynum, Porter, and Shepherd (eds), *The Anatomy of Madness* vol. II, pp. 52–72; Anne Digby (1985) *Madness, Morality and Medicine*, Cambridge: Cambridge University Press.

12 W.F. Bynum (1982) 'Theory and practice in British psychiatry from J.C. Prichard (1786–1848) to Henry Maudsley (1835–1918)', in T. Ogawa (ed.) *History of Psychiatry*, Osaka: Taniguchi Foundation, pp. 196–216.

13 N. Tomes (1984) *A Generous Confidence: Thomas Story Kirkbride and the Art of Asylum-Keeping, 1840–1883*, Cambridge: Cambridge University Press; S.E.D. Shortt (1986) *Victorian Lunacy: Richard M. Bucke and the Practice of Late Nineteenth-Century Psychiatry*, Cambridge: Cambridge University Press.

14 R. Russell (1983) 'Mental physicians and their patients; psychological medicine in the English pauper lunatic asylums of the later nineteenth century', Sheffield University PhD thesis.

15 John K. Walton (1979) 'Lunacy in the Industrial Revolution: a study of asylum admissions in Lancashire, 1848–1850', *Journal of Social History* 13: 1–22; John K. Walton (1981) 'The treatment of pauper lunatics in Victorian England: the case of Lancaster Asylum, 1816–1870', in Scull (ed.), *Madhouses, Mad-Doctors and Madmen*, pp. 166–200; John K. Walton (1985) 'Casting out and bringing back in Victorian England', in Bynum, Porter, and Shepherd (eds), *The Anatomy of Madness*, vol. II, pp. 132–46.

16 Charlotte MacKenzie (1985) 'Social factors in the admission, discharge and continuing stay of patients at Ticehurst Asylum, 1845–1917', in Bynum, Porter, and Shepherd (eds), *The Anatomy of Madness*, vol. II, pp. 147–74.

17 N. Hervey (1987) 'The Lunacy Commission 1845–60 with special reference to the implementation of policy in Kent and Surrey', University of Bristol PhD thesis; N. Hervey (1985) 'A slavish bowing down', in Bynum, Porter, and Shepherd (eds), *The Anatomy of Madness*, vol. II, pp. 98–131.

18 P. McCandless (1984) 'Curses of civilization; insanity and drunkenness in Victorian Britain', *British Journal of Addiction* 79: 49–58; W.F. Bynum (1968) 'Chronic alcoholism in the first half of the nineteenth century', *Bulletin of the History of Medicine* 42: 160–85; Roy Porter (1985) 'The drinking-man's disease: the pre-history of alcoholism in Georgian Britain', *British Journal of Addiction* 80: 385–96.

19 See also Michael J. Clark (1981) 'The rejection of psychological approaches to mental disorder in late nineteenth-century British psychiatry', in Scull (ed.), *Madhouses, Mad-Doctors and Madmen*, pp. 271–312; Bonnie Ellen Blustein (1981) '"A hollow square of psychological science": American neurologists and psychiatrists in conflict', in Scull (ed.), *Madhouses, Mad-Doctors and Madmen*, pp. 241–70.

20 For attitudes toward women see Elaine Showalter (1981) 'Victorian women and insanity', in Scull (ed.), *Madhouses, Mad-Doctors and Madmen*, pp. 313–38; Elaine Showalter (1986) *The Female Malady*, New York: Pantheon.

21 For discussion see 'Introduction', Bynum, Porter, and Shepherd (eds), *The Anatomy of Madness*, Vol. II, pp. 1–16; F. and R. Castel and A. Lovell (1981) *The Psychiatric Society*, New York: Columbia University Press.

22 Cf. Richard Hunter and Ida Macalpine (1974) *Psychiatry for the Poor, 1851: Colney Hatch Asylum, Friern Hospital 1973: A Medical and Social History*, London: Dawsons; Ruth Hodgkinson (1966) 'Provision for pauper lunatics, 1834–1871', *Medical History* 10: 138–54.

23 Charlotte MacKenzie (1987) 'A family asylum: a history of the private madhouse at Ticehurst in Sussex, 1792–1917', University of London PhD thesis.

24 For the wider background see Annamaria Tagliavini (1985) 'Aspects of the history of psychiatry in Italy in the second half of the nineteenth century', in Bynum, Porter, and Shepherd (eds), *The Anatomy of Madness*, vol. II, pp. 175–96; D. Pick (Spring 1986) 'The faces of anarchy: Lombroso and the politics of criminal science in post-unification Italy', *History Workshop* 21: 60–86.

25 Cf. H. Maudsley (1870) *Body and Mind: An Inquiry into their Connection and Mutual Influence, Especially in Reference to Mental Disorders*, London: Macmillan; Clark, 'The rejection of psychological approaches', in Scull (ed.), *Madhouses, Mad-doctors and Madmen.*

26 M. Heyd (1981) 'The reaction to enthusiasm', *Journal of Modern History* 53: 258–80; Michael MacDonald (1981) *Mystical Bedlam: Madness, Anxiety and Healing in Seventeenth-Century England*, Cambridge: Cambridge University Press; George Rosen (1968) *Madness in Society: Chapters in the Historical Sociology of Mental Illness*, London: Routledge & Kegan Paul. For Irish background see Mark Finnane (1981) *Insanity and the Insane in Post-Famine Ireland*, London: Croom Helm.

27 Henri F. Ellenberger (1971) *The Discovery of the Unconscious: The History and Evolution of Dynamic Psychiatry*, New York: Basic Books; Vieda Skultans (1975) *Madness and Morals*, London: Routledge & Kegan Paul; S.P. Fullinwider (1975) 'Insanity and the loss of self: the moral insanity controversy revisited', *Bulletin of the History of Medicine* 49: 87–101; Ruth Harris (1985) 'Murder under hypnosis in the case of Gabrielle Bompard: psychiatry in the courtroom in Belle Époque Paris', in Bynum, Porter, and Shepherd (eds), *The Anatomy of Madness*, vol. II, pp. 196–241; J.P. Williams (1985) 'Psychical research and psychiatry in late Victorian Britain: trance as ecstasy or trance as insanity', in Bynum, Porter, and Shepherd (eds), *The Anatomy of Madness*, vol. I, pp. 233–54.

28 For an introduction to degenerationism and a lead into the bibliography see Ian Dowbiggin (1985) 'Degeneration and hereditarianism in French mental medicine 1840–90', in Bynum, Porter, and Shepherd (eds), *The Anatomy of Madness*, vol. I, pp. 188–232; J.E. Chamberlin and S.L. Gilman (eds) (1985) *Degeneration: The Dark Side of Progress*, New York: Columbia University Press.

CHAPTER ONE

Madness and the picturesque in the Kingdom of Denmark

Christine Stevenson

Between 1792 and 1804, four architects prepared increasingly elaborate projects for the rehousing of Copenhagen's St Hans Hospital, whose inmates included the largest collection of lunatics to be found in the kingdom which then embraced Denmark, Norway, Iceland, the German duchies of Schleswig and Holstein, and territories in the East and West Indies. Three of these architects were members of a commission founded in 1794 to supervise the rebuilding of the hospital. Nothing happened until 1808, the year after the old buildings on the fortification line were damaged during Copenhagen's siege and bombardment by the British. St Hans was then finally moved to Bistrupsgaard Manor, 30 kilometres (18½ miles) west of the city. There, new construction was slow and far less ambitious than the projects the rebuilding commission had sponsored. Ten years later C.F. Hansen, Denmark's Chief Inspector of Buildings, designed an asylum which opened in the town of Schleswig in 1820. Hansen based the hospital's plan on the last of the designs prepared for the St Hans rebuilding commission, and the Schleswig Asylum, the first purpose-built mental hospital in Germany,[1] represents the real fruit of the Copenhagen commissioners' activity.

In Copenhagen, the lunatics had shared St Hans Hospital with the venereally diseased and 'incurable', the other classes of inmate there; elsewhere, notably in the German duchies, lunatics were still in the prisons. Appeals for decent shelter for lunatics, segregated so that they would no longer inconvenience the honest poor, nor felons and their gaolers, had long been made. The recognition of the insane as a group crossing all social boundaries (and which might therefore provide a source of income) and whose study and cure would be promoted by special buildings became a new theme in Danish social journalism and government protocols.

So far, so predictable. The early history of Danish institutional psychiatry does no violence to our assumptions about the evolution of specialized, and medicalized, hospitals for the insane although these assumptions are based on the experiences of countries larger, richer, and medically more sophisticated than the Danish kingdom was then.

But Denmark has a charm for the medical historian. Government was centralized, and the monarch absolute, to a degree that struck even contemporary observers as faintly comic.[2] With the exception of the journalist Riegels, all the Danish physicians, jurists, and architects mentioned here held a position in the slow-moving crown bureaucracy. It is not therefore hard to plot the course of Danish official thinking about lunatics between 1790 and 1820. At any point in this period, fewer than a score of persons were involved in anything more ambitious than meeting the lunatic's need for shelter, food, and linen. There were not many Danish doctors, no mad-doctors, and no books about lunatics aside from legal commentaries and a few Latin dissertations whose texts, judging from the titles, were either charmingly cranky or safely imprecise.[3] Without distracting atmospherics generated by political upheaval, medical in-fighting, or a flourishing private sector in the form of madhouses, the voices of this score can be heard with a clarity impossible in more complex societies. Themes emerging during a reading of the Danish documents, we realize, had been sounded elsewhere too; doubtless with more elegance but rarely with such intelligibility.

As it happened, Christian VII (1749–1808), grandson of George II of England and by God's grace King of Denmark and Norway, the Wends and the Goths, Duke of Schleswig, Holstein, Stormarn, Dithmarschen, and Oldenburg, was mad.[4] Contemporaries who found it hard to reconcile lunacy with the king's status as the incarnation of an empire which had once been a force to reckon with, reported that his passions were ungoverned and his extravagances embarrassing enough to demand constant supervision after the late 1760s.[5]

It is tempting to suggest that the gulf that existed between the concepts of 'regency' and 'lunacy' might have been bridged, as it was in the Britain of Christian's brother-in-law George III, by an articulate and confident corps of mad-doctors if such had then existed in Denmark. However, the available sources are inconclusive, and vague about chronology; and it is not clear how much, and when, members of the court circle let alone the general public knew about the king's condition and were willing to label it 'madness'.[6]

In the 1770s and 1780s Danish physicians had no right to claim any particular expertise in handling lunatics. Nor were they inclined to look abroad for help. Danish architects, however, resigned to the idea that their country's buildings offered no models worth emulating, all aspired to study abroad. The architects who sat on the St Hans Hospital Rebuilding Commission may have encouraged their fellow commissioners, the doctors, to widen their horizons. It is significant that long before the first bibliography of foreign psychiatric works appeared, in 1821,[7] long before foreign experts were cited in the protocols and journal articles, the St Hans commissioners ordered architectural drawings and copies of institutional regulations from Britain, Austria, Spain, Germany, and Russia. Every educated Dane could have read the German Romantic theorists, and Pinel's *Traité*, for example, soon appeared in German translation; but it was buildings that were needed in Denmark and the duchies. Architects and doctors, all in the civil service, worked together; and the first codification of the tenets of clinical psychiatry was so closely bound up with the planning and construction of the new St Hans and the Schleswig Asylum that the historian runs little danger of overemphasizing theory at the expense of planning and practice.

Architects and doctors

Ideas and associations aroused by words like 'peasant' and 'peacefulness', 'vegetation' and 'variety' impinged on Danish thinking about cemeteries, painting, schools, and farms at the turn of the eighteenth century. 'Picturesque' theory coincided with the development of the new building type, the insane asylum, too.

Period terms ('baroque', 'neo-classical', 'Romantic') customarily applied by students of the fine arts have also been used by medical historians, of course;[8] but this essay constitutes no attempt to define a picturesque period in Danish psychiatry. The picturesque is anyway not an era, but a suitable subject, like a picture, particularly a landscape; a way of doing things, like a maker of pictures who must prefer singularity, irregularity, and haze to the academic ideal, symmetry, or hard outlines. Architects placed buildings among artificial wildernesses and waterfalls, terrains carefully shaped to look natural. The sensitive spectator was to be reminded of a painted landscape. Brand-new buildings sported ready-made aggregates of classical porticoes and medieval towers, suggesting that their fabrics represented the cumulative result of accretions over the ages, that they had grown in a way exactly analogous to the landscapes around them. This kind of architecture is 'picturesque'.

Some of the strands which came together to form the picturesque can also be found in the psychiatric literature of the period; architects and doctors had, after all, been brought up to the same vulgarized psychology and historiography. Two themes can be mentioned.

The first is the belief that emotional responses could be manipulated through the presentation of calculated visual stimuli. For architects, this truism granted special urgency to their insistence that buildings be given 'character'.

> The art of characterizing, that is to say, rendering tangible with material forms those intellectual qualities and moral ideas which can be expressed in edifices; or to make explicit, by the agreement and suitability of all the constituent parts of a building, its nature, its propriety, its use and its purpose: that art, I say, is perhaps the most delicate and difficult of all the secrets of architecture both to understand and to develop.[9]

Every structure has its own nature, use, and purpose: taken to its limits, the criterion of character, isolating every building from every other building, would make typology impossible. In this we detect the picturesque insistence upon variety and a multiplicity of appearances at the expense of academic ideality;[10] there are echoes in medical theory.[11]

Thus 'character' became a multi-purpose tool in the hands of architectural theorists, especially the French; but it is fair to define it summarily as the medium through which a building announces its purpose in its external form. In other words, it was taken as self-evident, by 1800, that a theatre should not look like an arsenal; and a hospital for paupers could no longer look like a palace. It was a maxim, indeed, that misplaced character was not only ludicrous, but immoral and dangerous. At the simplest level, an over-elaborate façade on a pauper hospital financed by public charity (as opposed to private or royal philanthropy) could well discourage further donations;[12] or an insane asylum which looked like a prison would reinforce public prejudice and unfairly distress inmates and friends.[13] At the most elevated level, 'art without eloquence is like love without virility' as the architect Ledoux magnificently phrased his credo that the designers of such expressive façades should and would be a potent force in the creation of a new world order.[14] Plans which segregated and channelled were of course important, but the proper presentation of architectural character on the front of the building could instil even the casual passer-by with the desired civic virtues.

Sometimes the emotions to be aroused by a façade were negative ones: the sight of a prison was supposed to terrify and unsettle.[15] Similarly, moral-therapeutic attempts to counteract inappropriate and excessive emotion, or even insane delusions, with the stimulation of counter-emotions sometimes had to depend on the inculcation of fear. In 1821 Thaarup wrote approvingly of the 'good-natured and humanitarian conduct' and 'calm and sober firmness' which St Hans's physician Seidelin mustered in the face of his trying and extravagantly emotional charges; and, without irony, that the 'love and fear' he aroused obviated the necessity for more coercive methods such as the circulating swing used at the Berlin Charité.[16] German institutional practice was inevitably well known in Denmark but Danes congratulated themselves on avoiding the excesses associated with, for example, J.C. Reil's *Rhapsodieen über die Anwendung der psychischen Curmethode* of 1803, which we can assume Seidelin had read.[17] With the elaborate devices and visions Reil advised the doctor-artist to use and to stage, to arouse emotions just as specific and selective as the delusions they were intended to counter, psychiatric theory becomes most precisely analogous to architectural character theory.[18]

The second theme apparent in the writings of both architects and doctors around 1800 is the idealization of a primitive, prelapsarian classicism which had not yet lost its respect for nature and its workings and so achieved a timeless rationalism. For architects, this rationalism was supremely manifested in the post-and-lintel system presented by the Doric, Ionic, and Corinthian orders of classical antiquity.

The self-discipline and quietude to be instilled by moral therapy was occasionally explicitly identified as 'classical' by the therapists themselves. Pinel, for example, suggested that the 'precepts of enlightened morality' offered by Plato, Seneca, Tacitus, and Cicero were more effective prophylactics than any number of nostrums.[19] Some looked to the classical Golden Age for the origins of moral therapy itself: the inclusion of an entry called 'Agriculture' in the *Dictionnaire des sciences médicales* seems surprising, until we read in it that doctors of antiquity recommended frequent walks in gardens laid out with many varieties of plants for those suffering from nervous disorders.[20]

More generally, medical practice in the Golden Age was supposed to have avoided fruitless theorizing in favour of 'diligent observance of plain matters of fact'. So wrote Francis Clifton in his *State of Physick* (1732) about the Aesculapian dynasty's 700 years of medical practice.

> The study of the *Ancients* has given way, in a great measure, to the philosophy of the *moderns*: and, tho' we have *Theories* in abundance, and treatises without number; yet, to our great misfortune, we can find but little in 'em to be depended upon.[21]

The last word should be given to Joshua Reynolds, who summed up antiquity, nature, and custom in the third of his 'Discourses'. Representing academic idealism at its most vigorous and convincing, Reynolds reminded the artist that his task was to transcend 'peculiarities, and details of every kind'. Too often, however, a painter acquired the 'second nature' of artificial custom if he had not 'chastised his mind, and regulated the instability of his affections, by the eternal invariable idea of nature.... It is from a careful study of [the ancients'] works that you will be enabled to attain the real simplicity of nature.'[22] Like Pinel, Reynolds took it for granted that his readers would make the connection between moral and emotional life; that they would understand the importance of the distinction between nature interpreted customarily and nature observed, as the ancients had.[23]

The architects and doctors who met to discuss the rebuilding of St Hans Hospital, and who corresponded about the construction of the Schleswig Asylum, thus shared the same myths: all thought it self-evident, for example, that lunatic asylums should have a few trees planted around them. My conclusion is not as bathetic as it seems, however. It will emerge in the story of the construction of the two hospitals that even the common landscaped ground of the picturesque could not preserve the accord between the two professions in Denmark or elsewhere; that the theory of psychiatry and the theory of architecture had begun to diverge irrevocably by 1820.

Lunacy in eighteenth-century Denmark

'Danish Law', a late-seventeenth-century compilation of earlier legal codes, specified that anyone could bind and bring a 'furious' lunatic before the authorities. The lunatic's family was then obliged to appear and 'receive' him or her. This had been the law since the Middle Ages; in 1683 it was specified that if the family could not afford to keep the lunatic, then secure custody was a public responsibility.[24]

There were very few places for lunatics in eighteenth-century Denmark and there was no possibility that any but the most violent could be taken. In a nordic country of timber-framed buildings, trustworthiness with fire and candles was an important criterion of sanity for the poor; many disappointed applicants faced a future of providing the sole support for their families when an hour's absence could mean a return to a burnt-out house. In 1732 the workman Peder Sørensen wrote to the king to ask

> if mercy could not be extended to me and to my sick son Frederich Christian so he could go either to Frederiksborg or Elsinore Hospital. He has had his sickness for fourteen years and no remedies or advice could help, so his weakness grows worse and worse and because he can avoid neither fire nor water when the sickness comes on him, I am afraid that harm shall come to him some day and I, a poor man, shall die of sorrow.

The county's lieutenant-governor and the Bishop of Zealand together advised the civil service that Peder Sørensen's son

> is doubtless furious . . . in that case he cannot be taken into any hospital for not only would that be in violation of the hospital's charter but would also occasion great inconvenience to the other almsfolk there. Certainly there are a couple of cells [*daarekister*] at Elsinore Hospital . . . but we do not know if the applicant would want his son in one of these, even if a place were free.[25]

The *daarekiste* (plural *daarekister*, literally 'mad box') to which they referred was a wooden box typically about 3 metres (9.8 feet) square (see Figure 1.1). A small hole admitted some light and air and the box held a plank bed and a latrine. It was built of heavy planks; in Jutland dialect, to confine a lunatic was reportedly to 'plank' him.[26] The *daarekiste* was concurrently therapeutic medium and restraint; and itself a building type of some antiquity,[27] unvarying construction, and universal application. Providing shelter, and apertures for the ingestion of food and the effluence of human waste, it was the institution in miniature,[28] or a projection of the lunatic's own body. Quiet lunatics at St Hans stayed in 'rooms', 'apartments', or 'chambers'. But when the fury took them they were moved to the *daarekiste*, a word with no domestic connotations at all.[29]

Ordinances of 1709 and later specified that all the larger hospitals should set aside a couple of cells for the insane,[30] but *daarekister* could be found attached to a variety of other building types well into the nineteenth century in Denmark. From the inmate's point of view it made no difference if the *daarekiste* stood apart in the grounds or yard, or was installed in

Figure 1.1 Johannes Wiedewelt; 'So Paars with a certain dignity entered the daarekiste'; illustration to Ludwig Holberg's *Peder Paars* (c. 1770). Copenhagen, Library of the Royal Academy of Art

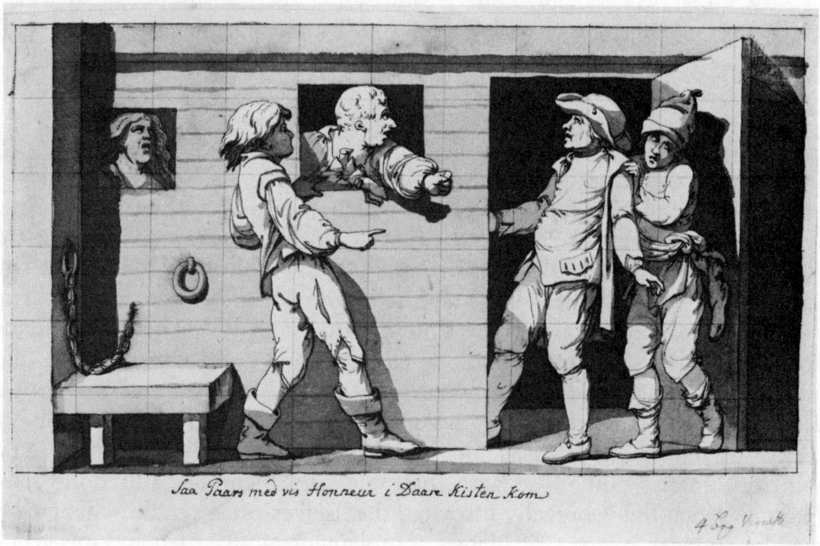

the cellars or some peripheral wing of a hospital, gaol,[31] poorhouse, town hall, or private home.[32]

The physician Ole Jørgen Rawert visited seventeen hospitals, that is, most of the civil hospitals then in Denmark; and his little travel diary, published in 1821, makes lively reading. The arrangement of sixteen *daarekister* at Odense Hospital, he wrote, burlesquing the then-flourishing genre of psychiatric travel literature, 'was not unlike the way in which I have seen pigsties organized in Germany'.[33] About the nine 'holes' for lunatics in the courtyard at Elsinore Hospital, he ruminated:

> lunatics are supposed to be able to stand greater cold than healthy people but in Denmark, generally speaking, we go a little too far in testing just how much cold they can stand: here they get just as little warmth in the winter as at most places.[34]

The presence of a stove in the castle gatehouse, shared with miscreants, at Frederiksborg; or a corridor at Rakskov Hospital so that one room need not be used as access to another: these were enough to ensure commendation.[35] Even at the new county hospital at Næstved, founded in 1817, the three *daarekister* were installed between the mortuary and the operating room; the inhabitants of the latter facilities were presumably insensible of the cries emerging from the planked rooms.[36]

The same year, Thaarup reported that the Zealand *daarekister* were gradually being demolished as the communes began to send their insane to St Hans at Bistrupsgaard;[37] but it would be decades before their complete extinction, particularly in Jutland where the asylum at Aarhus was not opened until 1852. Against this background, the institutions at Bistrupsgaard and Schleswig look rather better.

St Hans Hospital

Denmark's largest concentration of lunatics was to be found in St Hans Hospital, the old plague hospital to which the insane, then in a former leper hospital, were first moved in 1619. In the eighteenth century the hospital, by then officially known as 'St Hans' although commonly still called the 'Pesthus',[38] held not only the insane but the oldest, weakest, and wretchedest of the Copenhagen Poor Board's almsfolk: they, the 'incurables', were the crippled, blind, cancerous, apoplectic, consumptive, and simply bedridden who had nowhere else to go. In 1701 and 1703 royal ordinances had specified that the *spectaculeuse*, beggars maimed or 'so badly scarred in the face that one must be disgusted to see them' should join the lunatics and those with 'horrible' and incurable afflictions at St Hans.[39] When the venereally diseased, themselves often terribly disfigured, were introduced in 1772, St Hans's complement of unsettled and unsettling inmates was complete.[40] Its patients were precisely those excluded from Frederiks Hospital, one of the first in Europe explicitly devoted to clinical instruction and the treatment of curable illnesses, which opened for 300 of Copenhagen's poor in 1757; and from the Poor Board's own General Hospital.

Between 1619 and 1769, a century and a half precisely, St Hans was moved four times, always to more or less decrepit buildings outside the city walls. It was twice moved, in 1651 and 1769, to the site of the former royal farm, or Ladegaard. The civil and military authorities responsible for the infirm and insane in Denmark never had a very wide selection of sites available should circumstances force them to move their charges. Remote, undesirable, and cheap plots and buildings had often already served a comparable function for another department. In this way the Ladegaard, for example, successively hosted over the course of more than a century the Pesthus; the complex which served as the army's almshouse, madhouse, and prison; the Pesthus again, by then known as St Hans Hospital; a workhouse; and finally a penitentiary.[41]

By the end of the eighteenth century, however, the institutions which had been shifted in and out of crumbling buildings on the edge of the city began to find permanent homes which became indissolubly identified with the institutions themselves. As Samuel Johnson had put it in 1758, public charity was a process which first identified a distinct group of unfortunates, and then built 'peculiar houses for their reception and relief'.[42]

Psychiatric reform in Copenhagen had to begin with the perception of lunatics as a distinct category in the confusing welter of misery that St Hans's inmates presented to the observer; and then the amelioration of their ghastly conditions of confinement. This involved the separation of different kinds of inmates because the proximity of a furious lunatic, or a syphilitic with running sores threatened the well-being of a convalescent just as much as damp walls did.

In the last two decades of the eighteenth century, the Poor Board was subjected to steady critical pressure in the form of a series of journal articles by Niels Ditlev Riegels (1755–1802) whose part in the coup of 1784 had led to his dismissal from court service with a handsome pension giving him the leisure to pursue his interest in medical history and social problems. Although he was radical and suspect to many of his contemporaries, Riegels's articles calling attention to the dreadful conditions in St Hans did prompt a stream of donations and legacies upon whose disbursement he kept a careful watch during the 1790s. His posthumous rehabilitation was complete when his most disputatious suggestions were accepted as commonplaces; and indeed Riegels had a sharply focused eye and a prophetic pen. It was inevitably he who pointed out, in 1788, that St Hans's poverty meant that the 'mad, half-mad and alcoholic' had to share a day-room there. He paid graceful tribute to the serious courtesy prevalent in this odd company huddled around a single stove, but regretted the impediment presented to cure, or even comfort: 'Those who have *raptus* cannot be taken care of, or eased, and the drunks infect them all.'[43]

Architecture, scrutinized by the reformer's critical eye, now had to do more than shelter. Muddle and overlap between buildings and functions seemed incongruous and prompted complaint: at the end of the century it seemed worth noting for the first time that the building beside the town hall in Nykøbing (Falster) held the apartments for the town hall's caretaker, the pump house, the town gaol, a 'dungeon', a *daarekiste*, and the municipal and county courts.[44] This arrangement had doubtless worked perfectly adequately for years, but the new rule was one house, one function; and function was the criterion which still defined a building type.

The codification of building types was therefore important work, and architects emphasized the importance of 'character' in formulating these typologies. In this way they assumed control over the planning of the new institutions; character was, after all, their own arcanum.[45] Earlier hospitals, for example, had been built without effective interference from the medical brotherhood. The architect of the model Frederiks Hospital, Niels Eigtved, managed to avoid consulting with any doctors until 1754, a good two years after his drawings had been approved. By then the hospital's outer walls were built, but the medical establishment was still uncertain about the kinds of patients the new hospital was intended to admit. A hurriedly produced report followed the architect's meeting with leading physicians; the latter suggested, for example, that the proposed combination of laundry and slaughterhouse in a single room was not wholly desirable. To be fair, their demand that vaulted cellars be installed beneath four wings which had already been built was ludicrous. If the architect did not know much about clinical practice, the doctors understood less about how buildings went up. Eigtved died soon after, and his successor simply ignored the doctors.[46]

It did not take long for physicians to strike back. In 1771, John Aikin made the architect assume responsibility for the ignoble economies of charitable committees when he wrote that there were two incompatible personalities involved in the planning of a hospital: the architect who attempted to pack the space with as many beds as possible, and the physician who would rather have decent ventilation.[47] J.R. Tenon complained, in 1788, that even when hospitals were purpose-built, it was by architects with an eye to aesthetic effect, not practical arrangements or proper hygiene.[48] I will return to this debate again; it is mentioned here to point up the degree of consensus Danish architects and physicians achieved by the end of the century.

After 1769, St Hans was housed in buildings originally erected for the army's almshouse and detention centre, at the Ladegaard. The site was low and damp; and although quite new, the buildings were in very poor condition because they had been built on the cheap. It was claimed in the 1780s that St Hans's inmates were effectively exposed to the elements. A scabies epidemic and a sharp increase in the incidence of venereal disease was, by 1787, putting enormous pressure on the Poor Board's hospital bed-space and the board wanted to move and enlarge St Hans. The hospital was, however, popularly considered to be a collection of maniacs, syphilitics, and lepers, and attempts to move it in from the periphery met with insurmountable opposition in the last two decades of the century. Protesting householders near one proposed site were supported by the Collegium medicum, which noted that the presence of the insane could inconvenience local residents. The collegium concluded, furthermore, that three smaller hospitals, one for each of the main classes of inmate at St Hans, would be preferable to the unwieldy agglomeration then under one roof.[49]

One of the collegium's members was the physician Christian Elovius Mangor (1739–1801) who is credited with having been the first to suggest separating the different classes at St Hans. A few years later, in November 1794, Mangor was given a seat on the new commission created to investigate the rebuilding of the hospital. Its other members included the architect, Professor C.F. Harsdorff (1735–99), a former police chief and deputy mayor, a professor of obstetrics, and a surgeon. They were charged with deciding, first, if the funds available could best be applied to an enlargement of the old structure or the diversion of facilities to one or more different sites; and second, how the accommodation for the lunatics could be improved 'so their care is made easier and their cure, if possible, promoted'.[50]

Two years before, the architect Andreas Kirkerup had prepared plans and elevations illustrating his proposed enlargement and reconstruction of the buildings at Ladegaard.[51] With its careful provision of separated facilities for the venereally diseased, incurable, and insane; and, for the latter, 'honette' chambers for paying patients, *daarekister* for the 'extremely insane and furious', and observation cells for convalescents, Kirkerup's was a sensible plan which would have represented a distinct improvement (see Figure 1.2). It was, however, decided at the commission's first meeting in early 1795 that there was no sense in rebuilding at the unhealthy Ladegaard site. In any case, new ideas appeared in the reports and memoranda the commissioners began to submit. Most importantly, although St Hans had to remain, formally, a single institution for legal reasons, it was thought that the different classes of inmate had to be housed in separate buildings. Furthermore, the hospital must begin to attract a fee-paying clientele in the private sector and that meant lunatics; middle-class venereal patients were scarcely likely to prefer public hospital care to treatment at home, and the 'incurables' were paupers by definition. St Hans had long suffered a shortage of suitable accommodation for fee-paying lunatics and it was recognized that the market had scarcely been tapped.[52] Related to this question was the desideratum that the *daarekister* and their inhabitants had to be as far as possible from the other mad inmates, particularly the convalescent; but not so far as to handicap the fast transferrals from observation cells to *daarekister* which were sometimes necessary.

This last formula is repeated again and again in the commission's papers, which are permeated with their horror of the lunatic's screams. The *daarekister* were sturdy, but not sound-proof and the insane 'in their quiet periods should not hear too much lamentation from their furious fellows through which their own paroxysms might be aroused'. Madness was quite literally contagious and doubtless attendants feared the infection too.

It was with subtle irony, therefore, that Riegels called himself the voice of the silently suffering of St Hans. It was not the fault of the citizens of Copenhagen, he wrote, that the desperate need of the city's charitable foundations had not been met, for

> How could anyone dream that the mad, repulsive, abandoned, who cannot speak for themselves, nor send up their shrieks to the ear of the people, that their conditions are not better? Yes! that they are even being punished because they are repulsive.[53]

Riegels had experienced the unendurable din of St Hans's *daarekister* for himself, but he knew the difference between noise and communication.

In 1798, the architect C.F. Harsdorff presented his fellow-commissioners with architectural drawings showing three buildings, one for each class of inmate, angled around a roughly pentagonal court.[54] The pavilion for the insane had a complex plan which gave the paying patients a wing to themselves; the *daarekister* were placed at the end of another long wing which doubled back on itself, in dog-leg fashion, to distance the furious as much as possible from the paying patients and the rest of the hospital. On Harsdorff's plan the clinical state (and, to some extent, the social status) of each patient is mapped by his or her distance from the central courtyard.

Figure 1.2 Andreas Kirkerup; proposed reconstruction of St Hans Hospital (1792) showing an elevation of the church and sections of (left) cells for paying patients and (right) cells for the 'extremely furious'.

Copenhagen, Municipal Archives

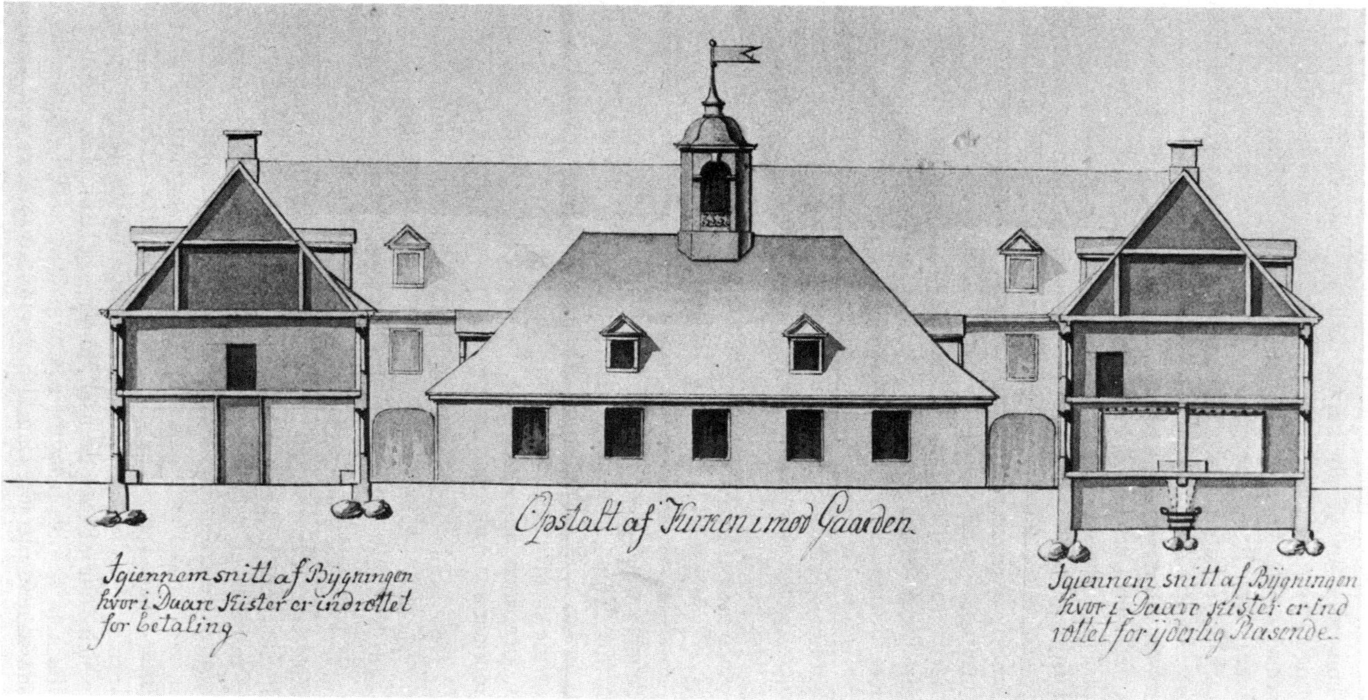

In terms of the evolution of the asylum 'type', Harsdorff's plan represents an advance on Kirkerup's, not only because it physically isolated the lunatics but because Harsdorff used the building plan as an instrument with which to mute the distressingly infectious roars and screams from the *daarekister*.

Harsdorff died the following year, in 1799. Other commissioners died or retired and in March 1802 three new members, including the deputy mayor and physician Jens Bang (1737–1808) and the builder, Major Philip Lange (1756–1805) were appointed to bring the commission up to strength. The revitalized commission rejected Harsdorff's plan, in part because in it 'too many were grouped around common passageways, where one could provoke another and a single screamer disturb all the rest'; and, more fundamentally, because they had decided to throw all their efforts and most of their resources into the planning of new accommodation for lunatics alone. They made it quite clear in their submission to the king in June 1802 that this decision was not only made because the lunatics were suffering but also

> because a family responsible for, and troubled with, someone mentally ill, would not hesitate to seek apartments for him in a well-appointed hospital for the insane, where all pains are taken and care directed towards a cure if possible.

At the new St Hans, the fees of the rich were to subsidize the care of the poor.[55]

Major Lange had prepared a sketch for a new building, and his colleagues asked him to work this up for presentation to the king. They decided at the same meeting to ask the Foreign Office to obtain reliable and detailed drawings of the 'circular' building for the mad in Vienna and St Luke's Hospital in London. Building plans and descriptions of institutions in Toledo, Lübeck, and St Petersburg were also received eventually, but these were of lesser interest. And, whatever Lange's first idea looked like (the sketch does not survive) his finished design was a replica of the 'Narrenturm' in Vienna, built in 1784 to accommodate dangerous lunatics at Joseph II's Vienna General Hospital.[56] While Vienna's example of a separate department for lunatics at a general hospital was influential, Lange's imitation of the Narrenturm's hollow cylindrical form was unique (see Figure 1.3). It was a surprising choice of prototype: the Narrenturm had been notorious since the day it opened and this may be the reason Lange's project was quietly dropped and new drawings accepted from Jens Bang in July 1804.[57]

Bang's professional qualifications are unique in the history of hospital design. During his medical training he had also attended architectural classes at the Academy of Art, where he took a major prize in 1765 and subsequently lectured on architecture, perspective, and anatomy. He later prospered as a physician and surgeon, in itself a combination of trades by

Figure 1.3 Philip Lange; first floor plan and elevation of a lunatic asylum (St Hans Hospital) (1802).
Copenhagen, National Museum

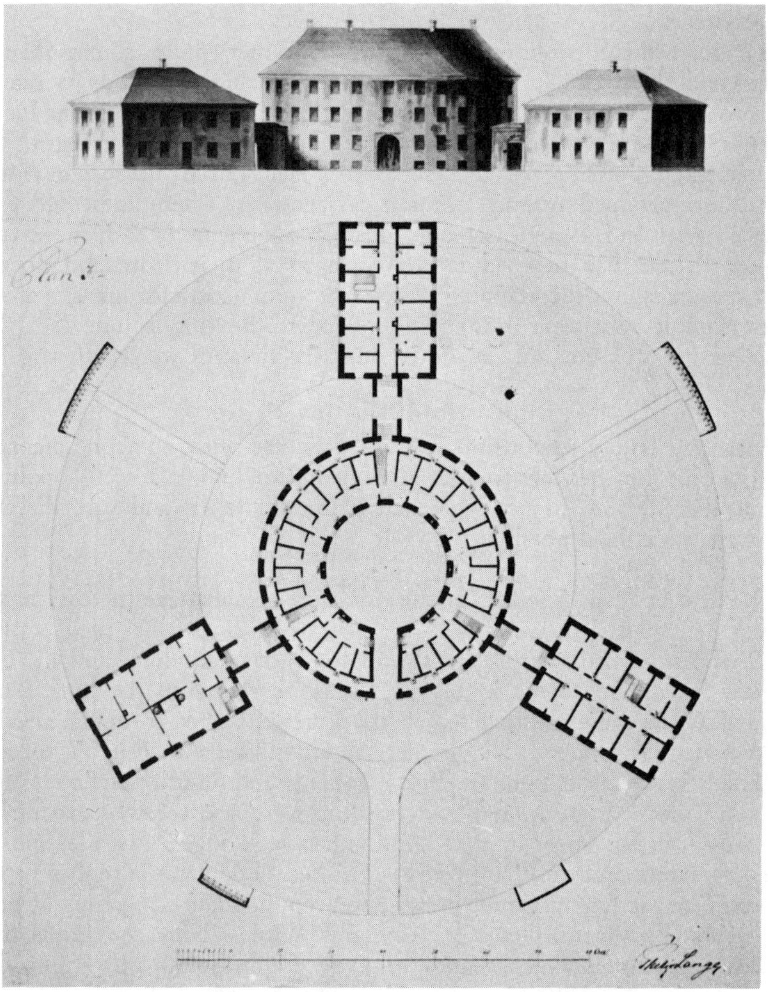

no means taken for granted. Obituarists would emphasize that he was peculiarly fitted to design a hospital.[58]

His drawings for a new asylum were submitted in the autumn of 1804. In outline, it would have formed a clover-leaf enclosing a central square court and, flanking it, three more courts with semicircular ends (see Figure 1.4). The two smaller courts at the sides were bounded by semicircular latrine blocks, and that at the top by a curved cell-wing with *daarekister*. The latter feature may have been inspired by the example of the Vienna

Figure 1.4 Jens Bang; detail, ground floor plan of a lunatic asylum (St Hans Hospital) (1804).
Copenhagen, Library of the Royal Academy of Art

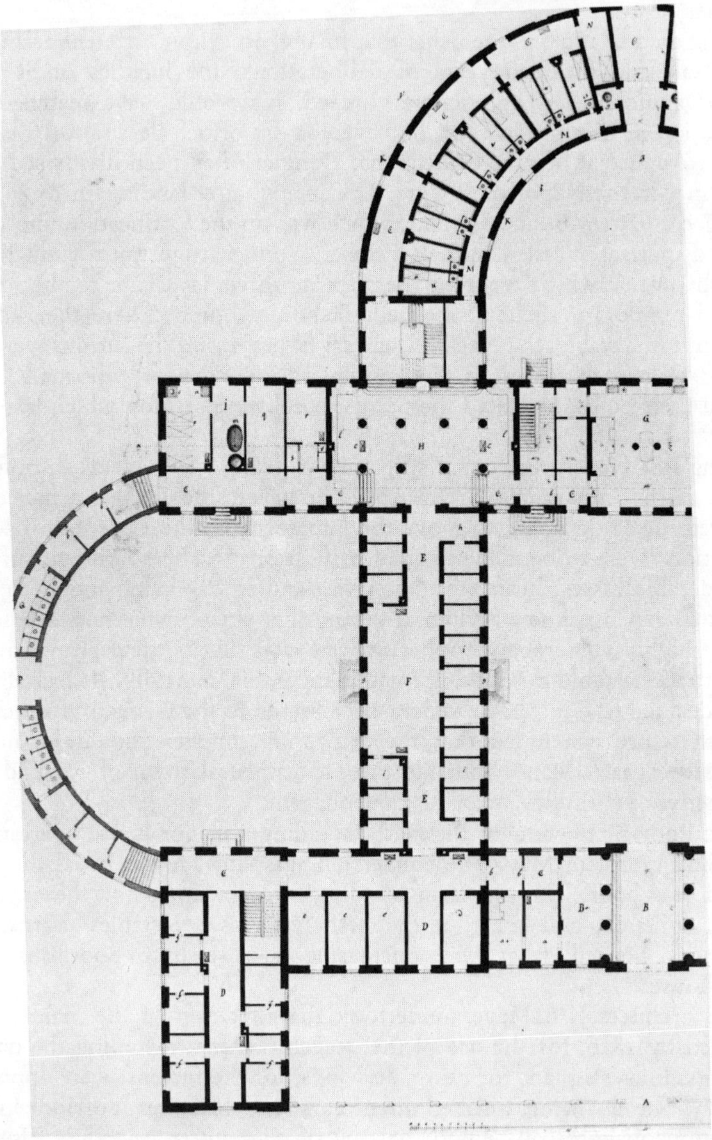

Narrenturm, although the connecting corridor at Vienna ran on the inner curve and that in Bang's wing was on the outer, or longer, side of the curve. The difference is important because Bang thought that in this way it would become 'more difficult for those under confinement to see one another'.[59]

Bang died in 1808, in the belief that finally, after four different architects' proposals and fourteen years of deliberations, the lunatics of St Hans would come to a proper home. Indeed, his would have matched any institution in Europe. In 1807, however, as the British fleet sat off Elsinore after 2 August, it became evident that Denmark had been ill-advised in its allegiance in the Napoleonic Wars. The enemy, after landing on 16 August, installed a battery beside St Hans, which was on the fortification line. After some dispute about the length of a ceasefire on 26 August, it was finally the British cavalry which escorted the patients three days later to the first of several temporary shelters, in Frederiksborg Church. There the venereal were put in a stable, the placid insane sat in pews, and the furious were laid bound by the altar even as the hospital's former pastor, who had finally joined their ranks, mounted the pulpit to deliver a sermon which lasted all night.[60]

Bang's St Hans project was still viable in early 1808, when an obituary called it his 'monument'.[61] In April, however, the Danish Chancellery ordered the Poor Board to move the inmates from the Ladegaard because alterations were to be made to the fortifications.[62] The board had suffered considerable losses during the hostilities and it was in no mood to construct an expensive new asylum at yet another site on what now seemed to be the highly vulnerable periphery of the city; and particularly when that construction would do nothing for the 'incurable' almsfolk. (It had already been decided to transfer the venereally diseased to the General Hospital.) It was therefore concluded that the remaining inmates should be moved to Bistrupsgaard Manor, outside the old cathedral town of Roskilde, 30 kilometres (18½ miles) west of Copenhagen.

The Poor Board bought the land, including a manor house overlooking Roskilde Fjord, in May. The conversion was slow, for as usual the Poor Board was poor. The old farm buildings were adapted for the crippled, blind, epileptic, and some of the 'lethargic' insane: stables, barns, and cowsheds housed what was, increasingly, a separate poorhouse and workhouse.[63]

The architect J.A. Meyer undertook the alteration of the main house, finished by 1810, for the use of the peaceful insane, including the paying patients. Meyer's plans for new side wings, for the furious, were approved in 1813. The east wing, finished three years later, had a rear corridor for the collection of night-soil behind the row of *daarekister*, and the cells were warmed by an oven in the corridor: such rudimentary arrangements prompted one observer to boast, perhaps accurately, that it was the equal of anything then in Europe.[64]

Riegels had been the first to suggest that all St Hans's patients could benefit from rural surroundings. In 1797, eleven years before the farm was purchased, he proposed the hospital's removal to an estate where the 'respectable sick of all classes' could be accommodated in the manor house. The next step would be the construction of small

> country houses like miniature towns around the manor house; one envisaged here the drunkards' town, the lunatics', the venereals', the melancholics'; and every house would have its own garden which every inmate, unseen and unrecognized, could tend as he liked . . . it would ideally be in the tending of these gardens that the very best medicine would be found.[65]

Riegels painted a vivid picture of an idyll far away from the noise of the city, where 'in the bosom of country life' St Hans's sickly inmates would emulate the pure and innocent customs of the locals, and fall into the natural rhythms of sound sleeping and healthy eating. The 'respectable' inmate of the manor house would be transformed from a 'supplicating Copenhagen citizen' into a 'gainful, healthy country man'.[66] The Hogarthian vignette of urban life, with its madness, venereal disease, and alcoholism, would be replaced by a picturesque landscape.

The benefits of country life were self-evident in the eighteenth century; who would dispute the advantages it presented to the care of the insane? Even this had classical sanction: the encyclopaedia article 'Agriculture', mentioned above, assured the reader that the doctors of antiquity recommended country walks for those suffering from nervous disorders because they knew that the varied aromas and 'vegetal emanations' soothed the senses and presented delightful views 'without offering the picture of physical and moral misery' associated with animal existence.[67] Pinel suggested in 1801 that patients be situated in 'locations most appropriate to counteract their delusions' and proposed that melancholics in particular should be placed in agreeably planted surroundings.[68] The four plans submitted for the rebuilding of St Hans Hospital, which in so many ways subsume the evolution of pesthouse to psychiatric hospital, had increasingly emphasized the gardens: Kirkerup had suggested that 'shady trees' be planted; Bang let it be understood that the 'garden, where the inmates can be assigned work according to their strength and desire' was a key feature of his design.

The official report published about the move to Bistrupsgaard explained that the insane and the incurably ill could only benefit:

> The former disturb and are disturbed in the city . . . the confined air can impede their cure. With respect to the latter, it is not advisable to accumulate more unemployable people in the city than is absolutely necessary.[69]

Indeed, there were still hopes at this early stage to be able to move all Copenhagen's orphans, beggars, and unemployed immigrants out to Bistrupsgaard, where they would form a 'poor colony' which in its productivity and self-sufficiency would, one assumes, compare favourably with Denmark's real colonies. These plans came to nothing; in the meantime, it was noted that work could be found for some of the epileptic and cancerous in the country. The cultivation of medicinal plants was mentioned along with time-honoured activities like spinning.[70]

The idealization of rural life for the insane was reinforced by the belief that the patient's removal from family and neighbourhood could speed his or her recovery,[71] and by the earnest wish of family and friends that the business of cure, or at least confinement, be conducted as discreetly as possible. In the jargon of asylum prospectuses of the day, lunatics with 'friends' signified lunatics with money behind them; and privacy was a commodity offered most cheaply and easily by an institution with plenty of land. In concluding his proposal that St Hans be moved to the country, Riegels hinted at the possibility of a significant increase in income, 'if it is converted to a pleasant, anonymous and decorous place for rich and distinguished venereal-, mad-, alcoholic- and decrepit people ... the foundation must only keep its patients anonymous, each in clean and roomy quarters; and for this half-timbered houses are proposed ... with individual gardens'.[72] Between the bathing, fresh air, agreeable walks and drives in the grounds, and home-grown produce, it would be a sorry drunk or syphilitic who did not have a good time. Robert Reid similarly described the proposed Edinburgh Asylum where persons 'whose friends object to their associating with the patients, may be accommodated' in small houses scattered around the estate.[73]

Esquirol pretended to despise the asylum class system, which he saw as the peculiarly English vice, but his vision of the ideal institution was, in 1818, not too different from Riegels's or Reid's. In advocating purpose-built insane asylums in his essay 'Des établissements aliénés', he pointed out that the higgledy-piggledy, architecturally additive buildings then the norm could not separate patients according to the character of the malady.[74] Thus objecting to hospitals which had grown up in a quasi-organic fashion and which were therefore, strictly speaking, picturesque, Esquirol did advocate the sort of ready-made picturesque which architects of his day were practising. Although he argued that mental hospitals should be built new, with the symmetrical arrangement of the necessary subdividisons, this regularity did not extend to the appearance of the separate pavilions he advocated for each category. Uniformity was a 'vice' in designing the pavilions; Esquirol emphasized that with its pavilions, courtyards, and little roads, the asylum should have the atmosphere of a country village.[75]

The seclusion of the insane was always justified from their, and not their relatives', point of view. Crowded urban asylums which had admitted casual visitors were already notorious. Visitors 'only wanted to satisfy their curiosity, and thought to see wild animals in human beings' wrote Gøricke.[76] There was an alternative vision of the pre-history of psychiatry, of course; and innumerable evocations of a past in which incurable and incomprehensible insanity was shut away for ever in some 'remote prison or obscure dungeon'[77] read oddly when juxtaposed with contemporary exhortations to remove lunatics to decent remoteness and obscurity in the countryside.

The patient's right to peace and privacy from 'curious observers' was one reason advanced for St Hans's move away from the city and, later, for the elaborate vetting and constant supervision to which all callers at St Hans and the Schleswig Asylum had to submit. The institution 'should be so quiet . . . that all classes should almost feel themselves at home'.[78] Home, however, might not have been so quiet: at Bistrupsgaard, visitors were not allowed to engage in any unnecessary conversation with the 'unfortunate inhabitants', and they were never allowed to ask them their names.

Immediately after the publication of the report[79] about the move to Bistrupsgaard, the jurist and educator J.H. Bärens, editor of the journal *Penia*, which was devoted to all issues affecting the poor, published extracts from the report with a commentary revealing him to have been not entirely in accord with its authors. Bärens agreed that St Hans had to be moved out of the city, but objected to a site quite so distant, pointing out that 'it is not seldom the surest way to improvement for [the insane] who do have good periods, to see relatives and friends' and it was rather too bad if the latter could not visit except with the sacrifice of time and money which they could ill afford.[80] His colleagues did not try to answer Bärens's controversial therapeutic point, and confined themselves to remarking that almsfolk supported with public funds had no grounds for complaint wherever they were put.[81]

The Poor Board's report had outlined the medical advantages to be derived from concentrating the insane in one location.[82] For Bärens, however, the insane could give lessons to us all: 'a lunatic hospital is ultimately a school for the teacher, the public physician and the philosopher in general'.[83] Riegels had anticipated him here, too:

> You mighty and rich, visit [St Hans] assiduously and believe me, here is to be found greater wisdom than in the orations and promotions of the academies, for here reason reveals itself in its full brilliance. Its absence teaches us about the evil cancers which we must daily struggle against.

The 'cancers' are the emotions which, unchecked, could push us into madness.[84] This is no romantic vision of the mad as saner than the rest of us; even as he advocated rural and picturesque surroundings, Riegels reminded his readers that self-discipline must be of neo-Spartan toughness.

At Bistrupsgaard, according to the apologists for the move, the insane would enjoy beautiful surroundings, healthy victuals, and pure water for bathing and drinking. Satisfying and productive labour would be easy to arrange,[85] and the construction of accommodation would be cheaper.[86] The almsfolk could have houses 'like most of the prosperous peasant families have' with clay walls and thatched roofs. Since a disastrous fire in 1795, building regulations had prohibited these in the capital, and the price of construction materials and labour had increased enormously in Copenhagen. The Poor Board claimed that the shortage of cheap housing had caused its rolls to swell, but now these artificial problems created by urban conditions could be left behind.[87] The 'cottage' style was then becoming a fashionable alternative in England, as vernacular building achieved legitimacy with the help of the picturesque current,[88] but at Bistrupsgaard there would be no choice.

The vast majority of St Hans's inmates were from the lower classes. At the end of the eighteenth century, many had emigrated to the capital in search of work, and were living there when they became mad: further proof of the threat urban life posed to mental stability. What the advocates of the picturesque did not point out, however, was that so many other lunatics were brought in straight from the country that St Hans's admission figures peaked in July and August when there was time to spare from farm work.[89] Indeed, the hospital represented one of the few legitimate escapes from the countryside. Until 1800, Danish male peasants between the ages of four and forty were compelled to live on and work the land assigned to them. Ostensibly a measure to ensure a supply of men for the army, *stavnsbaand*, or compulsory residence on the domain, in fact protected landowners from the age-old ambition of the peasant to better himself or herself on better land, in the city, or abroad.[90] Advocates of female *stavnsbaand* argued that peasant women fell into alcoholism, and worse, in the city.[91]

Riegels's eloquence on the subject of the simple and pure habits of the country-dwellers signals his place in the avant-garde of Danish social thinking in the late 1780s: most of the earlier literati were under no illusions. The peasant was slovenly, superstitious, suspicious, obstinate, and drank too much.[92] In 1788, however, it was announced that *stavnsbaand* would be abolished. This act, perhaps the least of the agricultural reforms then in motion, nevertheless caught the imagination of artists and writers who, almost overnight, created an iconographic genre quite new to the kingdom: life on the land, and those who lived it. The peasant woman, who in the city had been a troublesome Pandora, was now Ceres.[93] All the rhetoric about St Hans's move to Bistrupsgaard, even the fabric of Bistrupsgaard itself, with its manor house, cowsheds, and stables, can be seen as part of this artistic development.

At Bistrupsgaard St Hans's insane got their own physician in Johan Henrik Seidelin (1786–1855), a new kind of medical specialist who kept track of developments abroad. According to Esquirol's encyclopaedia article of 1818, the King of Denmark had ordered the construction of an insane asylum after the English bombed St Hans. This was not quite true but Esquirol did not have a high opinion of the English anyway. 'Dr Weidelin [*sic*] will send me the plans which I will publish in my book' (he did not).[94] Unfortunately Seidelin's expertise took the unhappy form of an increasing enthusiasm for Reil's 'psychic curative methods', including beatings, induced hunger and thirst, and the strapped chair. He was finally dismissed in 1831.[95]

In 1818, however, the Poor Board could still report with pride that St Hans's move to a 'convenient, larger and lighter' site where the insane could exercise and work in the open air had not only improved their health and strength, and cheered their appearance, but had also significantly altered the very character of their madness. The doctors did not have to resort so often to restraints or punishments, for 'the raging scream and the uproarious noise by which the insane in the old hospital always expressed their condition' was now only periodic; and the paroxysms themselves were shorter and milder.[96] The insane were no longer repulsive, to be counted among the *spectaculeuse*. The screams and cries about which the Rebuilding Commission had written so often were finally muffled, as rural peace replaced urban turmoil.

The Schleswig Asylum

If in Copenhagen the insane suffered through simple poverty and neglect, their plight in the prisons of the royal duchies of Schleswig and Holstein was the very stuff of reformist rhetoric. Here the narrative has an obvious protagonist in the person of Carl Ferdinand Suadicani (1753–1824) who by the turn of the century not only held important civil posts but was physician-in-ordinary to both the Duke of Augustenburg and his brother-in-law Frederik, the Crown Prince, son of Christian VII. Suadicani first protested against conditions in the prisons in 1783.[97] An idea to build an asylum near the medical school at Kiel, made in 1805, had to be dropped during the Napoleonic Wars; but when Suadicani proposed in 1816 that the lunatics be moved out of the last of the prison-madhouses and a mental hospital be erected in his home town of Schleswig, a royal ordinance to these ends appeared the following year.[98]

Plans were drawn up by a local contractor. They were, predictably, found wanting by C.F. Hansen (1756–1845), Denmark's Chief Inspector of Buildings, who controlled all public construction in the kingdom. Letters and conversations between him and his old friend Suadicani followed; the Schleswig Asylum, built to Hansen's plans, opened in the autumn of 1820.

Suadicani was appointed one of the asylum's directors. He did not live much longer; obituarists would delicately refer to the melancholia clouding his later years.[99] He had seen too many meteors ascending and disappearing again in the heaven of theory, he was reported to have said, to do anything but follow the only certain course at the sick-bed: that of nature.[100] A reformer of the style already shaping myth in his own lifetime, Suadicani belonged to a generation of physicians nostalgic for Greece as it was when doctors sought, not Byzantine theory, but natural truth. In recommending the asylum's foundation, he contrasted the murky horror of the 'death sentence' which confinement in the old prison-madhouses had meant, with the imminent dawn when the insane would enter the healing light of the sun.[101]

At Hansen's asylum four wings, each lined with arcades, surrounded a square courtyard for the quieter lunatics, who in wet weather could take exercise in the loggias behind the arcades.[102] (See Figure 1.5.) At the top of the asylum, facing north, was a semicircular court called the 'raging court' (*Tobhof*) terminated by a curved *daarekister* wing for the most violent inmates. Hansen had sat on committees together with Jens Bang before the latter's death a decade earlier[103] and the Schleswig Asylum's curved wing was undoubtedly borrowed from Bang's St Hans plan. It was the Schleswig Asylum, and not the motley collection of buildings at Bistrupsgaard, which represented the real fulfilment of the St Hans commissioners' endeavours.

In 1817 Hansen wrote in connection with the Schleswig project that 'the beauty of a new public building, of whatever type, lies in the fact that one can, in regarding the exterior, at once roughly imagine the function of the interior'. In the case of a lunatic asylum, he continued, the most important considerations were of course healthy and convenient accommodation, and security, but then he returned to architectural character: 'of course such a building requires *no architectural* splendour [but rather] . . . a truly convenient arrangement . . . linked with a simple, regular exterior'.[104] Hansen was still preoccupied by the character theory he had learned at the Danish Art Academy forty years earlier. For him, the 'beauty' of a public building depended on the legibility of its character: how, then, did he intend the façades of the Schleswig Asylum to be read?

Hansen practised a stringent neo-classicism and none of his buildings has much ornament, but the asylum is particularly severe. Its decorative features are wholy architectonic: the entrance to the curved wing, for example, is flanked by columns of exaggerated, primitivistic squatness. Most of the ornament is supplied by 'rustication', the term applied to masonry (or, as here, imitation masonry) in which the joints between the stones are emphasized, or the stones worked to exaggerate their texture, giving an impression of rustic simplicity.[105] The columns at the main entrance were banded by rough, heavy rings as if they had been abandoned before completion; inside the square court, the entrances to the large day-rooms Hansen planned in each of the side wings were laterally rusticated (see Figure 1.6). Aside from these gestures the asylum was, as Hansen promised it would be, plain and orderly in the extreme. The roof has a steeper pitch than those on his other buildings, and the asylum's proportions are reminiscent of the local, rural vernacular. It is tempting to see the building as a manifestation of Reil's suggestion that an asylum look like a dairy farm.[106] But in Hansen's day the arcades, these kinds of columns, and the use of rustication would have conjured up primitive classicism and its associated moral qualities.

Frugality, providence, industriousness, and self-containment were virtues long associated with early antiquity, and they had just been attributed to the Danish peasant. The cure of the Schleswig lunatics was to be effected through the continuous busy-work that was one cornerstone of the 'psychic cure'; emotional reticence, or thrift, would follow. Hansen's rus-

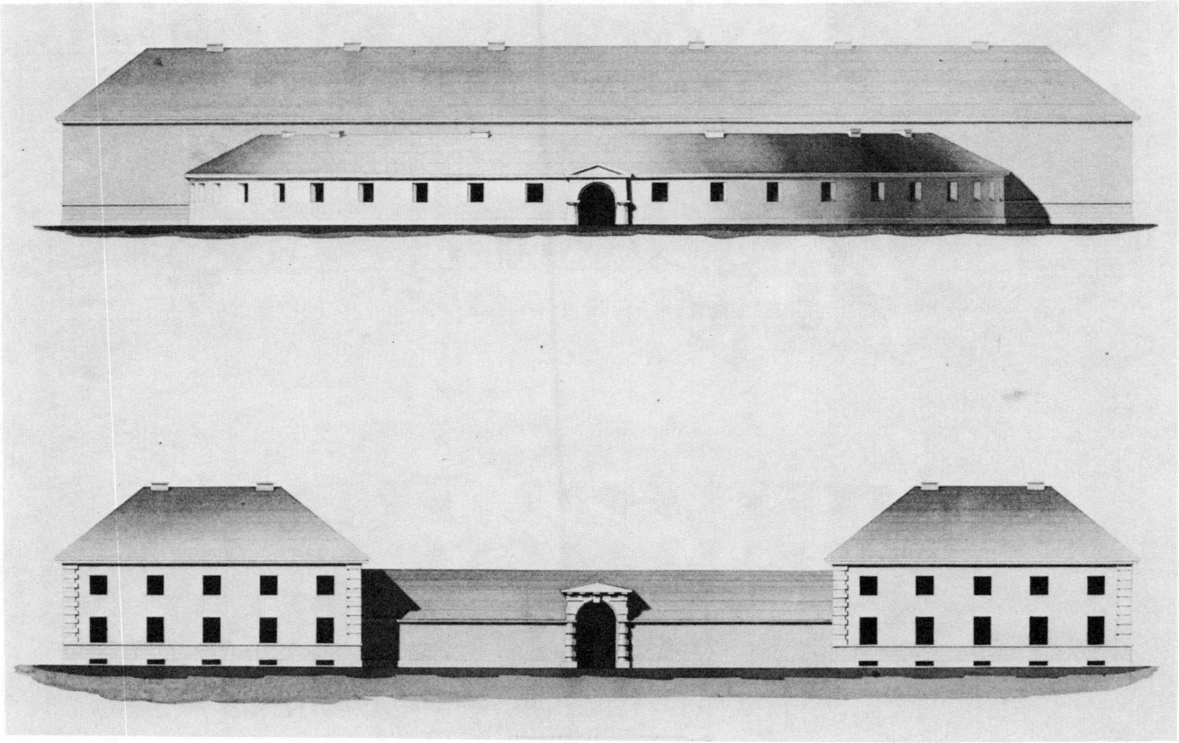

Figure 1.5 C.F. Hansen; elevations of the Schleswig Asylum (1817), showing (top) the curved wing with daarekister and (bottom) the main entrance.
Copenhagen, Library of the Royal Academy of Art

Figure 1.6 C.F. Hansen; elevations and sections of the Schleswig Asylum (1817). Copenhagen, Library of the Royal Academy of Art

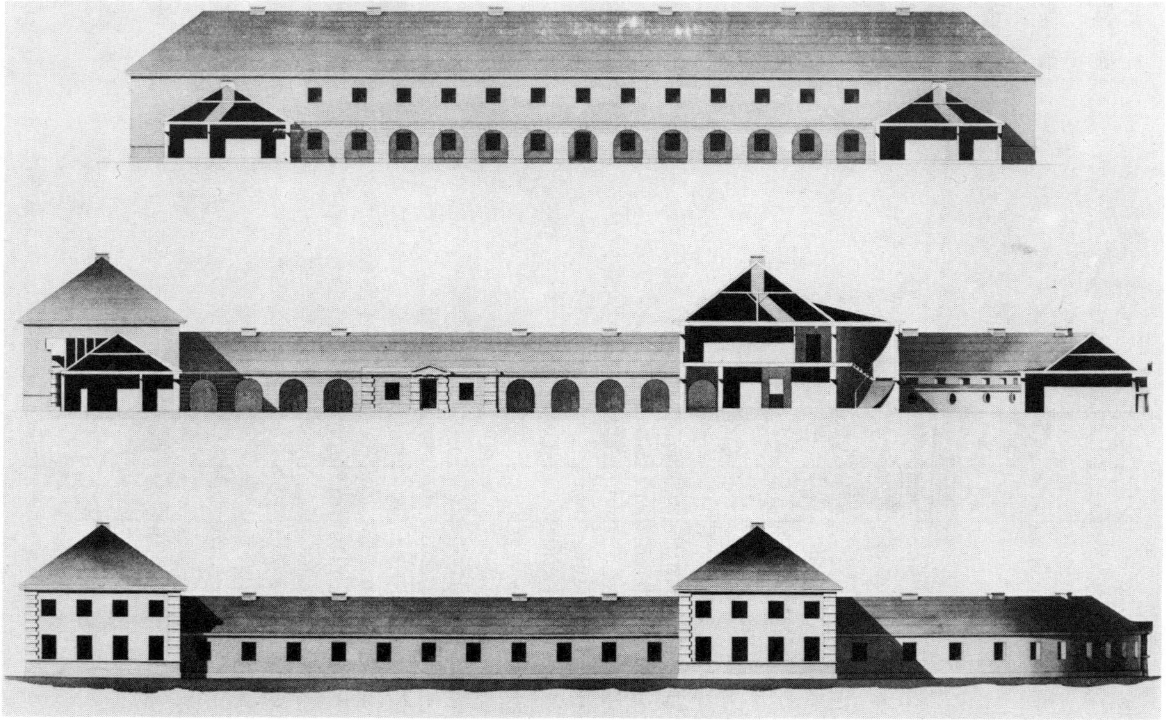

tication was to signify, and even promote, an uncomplicated, uncommunicative, hard-working life, sustained by clean linen and good food, through which the mad and the maddening were to be restored to reason and, above all, quiet.

At Schleswig, patients were expected to occupy themselves constructively according to their capabilities and social standing. Peter Willers Jessen (1793–1875), the first medical director, placed great emphasis on the therapeutic qualities of 'work and activity and order'. 'Educated' inmates were permitted to look at picture books; the rest were to help in the gardens.[107] Jessen wrote in 1828 that the 'perfection, diversification, and expansion of the means to occupy the patients constructively is only possible through the linkage of the asylum with an agricultural operation' but his request that the asylum be allowed to buy more land was refused that year.[108]

Patients of all classes could benefit from the soothing variety provided by a picturesque setting. A visitor described it in 1827 as

> on an elevation near St Jürgen's water-mill north of [Schleswig's] Old Town.... The building is situated gracefully and offers charming views on the one side to the mill and on the other, beyond a valley divided by a brook, to the city.[109]

The layout of the gardens 'in the English [i.e. picturesque] style' had just been completed then. Patients of the 'educated' class could enjoy a plantation of trees, a lawn, a 'hermitage', and a bowls alley. The poor and quiet insane had their own flower beds. Potentially violent inmates could take fresh air in courts north of the building where they were enclosed, picturesquely enough one supposes, by a barrier of thorns.

Building campaigns which have made Hansen's asylum unrecognizable today began as early as 1821 when Jessen proposed a number of alterations, most importantly the partial walling-up of the arcades around the square courtyard to ensure 'the complete separation of the sexes'. Hansen must have regretted the loss of his loggias, but he had to agree.[110] Jessen had no hand in the planning of the hospital; and circumstantial evidence suggests that he would have preferred panoptical surveillance to picturesque elegance. In 1828 he published a review essay which referred approvingly to the asylums at Glasgow and Limerick which had adopted, as he wrote, the 'radiating' or 'windmill' plans of the best new English prisons. Indeed, he continued, it was only logical to adapt such plans to asylums, based as they were on the principles of 'health, security, surveillance and correction'.[111] One wonders what Suadicani, who had devoted most of his career to getting lunatics out of prisons, would have thought of his protégé's enthusiasm for the penal type.

There was a wide fee-scale for private patients at Schleswig. The fees charged to local authorities for the care of their pauper lunatics were also considered high; the medical journalist J.C.W. Wendt hinted that if the building had not been so expensive, the institution could have afforded to care for as many 'desperate unfortunates' as St Hans. 'Although the institution is on the grand scale, and architecturally impressive, I think just as highly of the simple rural Bistrups [gaard] . . . where the new buildings are less imposing, but convenient.'[112] 'What need is there for palaces or magnificent buildings', he asked, 'when one had convenient arrangements at a site as beautiful and salubrious as St Hans's?'[113]

Not even Hansen's enormous personal authority was proof against the old suspicion of architects and their extravagance. Ironically enough, picturesque thinking gave it an added edge as critics, applauding the new tendency to surround asylums with therapeutic gardens,[114] decided that the grounds, no matter how extensive, could have embraced just one more vista if the building had not been so expensive. In 1818, the splenetic J.G. Spurzheim claimed that

> a building which costs a hundred thousand pounds is of less use than another might be which would cost half the sum, if the other half was expended in the purchase of fields surrounding it.[115]

Jessen must have ruminated on the same lines when he was refused permission to buy more land.

The idea that the architect, unleashed, would gleefully dissipate public funds on columns and cornices anyway inappropriate to a pauper hospital thus continued to symptomatize a prevailing uncertainty about where control over the new building type should reside, a tension between doctors and architects. Two years before the Schleswig Asylum opened, Esquirol wrote that the 'plan of a mental asylum is not at all a trivial thing to be left up to architects alone' even as Spurzheim exploded:

> Who shall make the plan? Who shall decide on its adoption? The architect, who is fond of his art, and likes to display architectural beauties . . . ? Or medical men, who have paid particular attention to insanity?[116]

The medical men soon won control over, and even the credit for, the planning of the new institutions. Jessen's successor at Schleswig, Julius Rüppel, published a book about the hospital in 1872 in which he described the main building as 'after the specifications [*nach Angabe*] of Esquirol' and a neighbouring block (which Hansen also designed) as 'after the specifications of Prof. Dr Jessen'.[117] Hansen's name is nowhere mentioned.

The notion that Esquirol was somehow involved in the planning of the Schleswig Asylum, or had even designed it, is an old and tenacious one.[118] If it were true, the asylum would be the earliest example of Esquirol's involvement in any new hospital construction, as Rüppel did not fail to point out.[119] But there is no evidence to support the thesis, and the question is raised here only to illustrate the thoroughness with which Hansen's name was eradicated from the record. Jessen, who in any case would have preferred a radiating plan, was a German nationalist;[120] and Rüppel's book appeared when the asylum was at last sitting in bitterly won

German territory,[121] but one suspects that a German architect's name would have been forgotten too.

Conclusion

In Denmark, the refinement of the tenets of clinical psychiatry was inevitably mediated by the St Hans Rebuilding Commission and its commissioners, doctors and architects who were all salaried state officials and who could, therefore, be introduced to the deliberations easily and economically. The two professional groups collaborated in harmony. Much of the commissioners' time was spent in talk of damp-coursing and night-soil and it was with relief, and in a spirit of high seriousness, that they turned to a vision of trees, brooks, and fjords. They wanted to believe that the beauty of Bistrupsgaard's setting would compensate for the inadequacies of its buildings, that it would transform the irritable urban lunatic into a serene countryman or -woman, that new iconographic construction.

Country folk had always crowded St Hans in Copenhagen; in the duchies, it was they who had to pay for the expensive new asylum, for the building fund had been raised by a plough tax.[122] Planned by two elderly friends, the Romantic physician Suadicani and the neo-classical architect Hansen, the Schleswig Asylum provides a rare example of a hospital for lunatics designed as an instrument for the techniques of moral therapy, whose façades, drawing on both the picturesque and the classical ideals, were themselves instrumental with their legible architectural character. The result was a beautiful building but it was already too old-fashioned for its youthful medical director, for whom plan was infinitely more important than façade. Even an architectural supremo like Hansen could not prevent Jessen's alterations to the building fabric in 1821.

Physicians like Jessen began to assume control over the shape of buildings, which had become indistinguishable from the hospitals they housed. By that time, function was inseparable from type in architectural theory too. This convergence, which architects had thought would inevitably lead to their control over social operations like the housing, and therefore the care, of lunatics, actually signalled the reverse. The hospital-building type was the hospital itself and it was therefore medical men, not architects, who took over its planning in the Danish kingdom and in the western world. Asylums would continue to find picturesque settings, but these were no longer assumed to have the enormous potency with which Danish architects and doctors together credited the gardens between 1790 and 1820.

Notes

1 K. Doerner (1981) *Madmen and the Bourgeoisie*, Oxford: Blackwell, p. 221.
2 Thomas Malthus's diary entry of 30 May 1799: 'It seems to be agreed that the

King of Denmark, tho' by law the most despotic monarch of Europe, has the least power of exercising that despotism.' Malthus referred not to the king's mental condition, but to the inefficiency and corruption of his officials. P. James (ed.) (1966) *The Travel Diaries of Thomas Robert Malthus*, Cambridge: Cambridge University Press, p. 39.

3 According to A.H. Rasmussen, in 1777 there were thirty-four practising physicians in Denmark (excluding Norway and the duchies), of whom twenty-one were in the capital: 'Laegedom', in A. Steensberg (1971) *Dagligliv i Danmark i det syttende og attende Århundrede*, Copenhagen: Busch, vol. 2, p. 207. On books published about insanity in eighteenth-century Denmark: F. Thaarup (1821) 'Om St Hans Hospital og Claudi Rossets Stiftelse paa Bidstrupsgaard', *Penia*: 54; H. Helweg (1915) *Sindssygevaesenets Udvikling i Danmark*, Copenhagen: Lund, pp. 36–9 and B. Zalewski (1984) 'Det hårde kors af vanvittighed. St Hans hospital i det 18. århundrede', *Historiske Meddelelser om København*: 33.

4 V. Christiansen (1906) *Christian VIIs Sindssygdom*, Copenhagen: Gyldendal, Christiansen's monograph formed part of a genre of retrospective diagnoses stimulated by Kraepelin's identification of *dementia praecox*. It is, however, a useful summary of the available sources of information about Christian's behaviour. Excellent English sources about aspects of the period are W.F. Reddaway (1912) 'Struensee and the fall of Bernstorff', *English Historical Review* 27: 274–86; and W.F. Reddaway (1916) 'King Christian VII', *English Historical Review* 31: 59–84.

5 The private correspondence of highly able statesmen, in regular contact with Christian, reveals that even as they acknowledged their allegiance to a 'roi imbécile' they told themselves and each other, at first, that his extravagances were merely the fruits of a self-indulgent character. Christiansen, *Christian VIIs Sindssygdom*, p. 70.

6 According to the memoirs of Christian's former tutor, the Swiss E.S.F. Reverdil, popular rumours were circulating as early as 1771 that the king was held in seclusion, perhaps drugged, by one of various court factions which then spread the rumour of his 'imbecility' to protect itself; however, he wrote long after the event. E.S.F. Reverdil (1858) *Struensée et la Cour de Copenhague 1760–1772*, Paris: Roger, pp. 246–7.

7 (1821) 'De vigtigste Skrivter over Afsindighed, og Vanvittighed', *Penia*: 48–54. Wendt's short bibliography is presented as a supplement to that in *Penia*: J.C.W. Wendt (1827) *Meddelelser om Anstalter for afsindige i Tyskland og Danmark*, Copenhagen: Jacobsen, p. 63n. N.D. Riegels is, as usual, the exception: his article of 1798 refers to 'Citizen Pinel's' work at the Bicêtre, and he often cites the admirable English spirit of public charity and their institutions for the insane. (1788) 'Pesthuset some det er, og hvorledes det kunde blive', *Kjøbenhavns Skilderi* 2: 285; (1798) *Noget ganske Nyt om pesthuset*, Copenhagen: Holm, p. 8.

8 We associate attempts at medical periodization, and in particular the concept of 'Romantic medicine', with German scholars of earlier generations: G. Rosen (1951) 'Romantic medicine: a problem in historical periodization', *Bull. Hist. Med.* 25: 149–50; and W. Leibbrand (1937) *Romantische Medizin*, Hamburg: Goverts, p. 174, comment. Both mention, for example, Sigerist's characterization of Harvey as a 'baroque' scientist. The recent official history of Copenhagen University's medical school calls the period between 1788 and

1842 the 'romantic interlude': V. Møller-Christiansen (1979) in J.C. Melchior (ed.), *Københavns Universitet 1479–1979*, vol. 7, *Det laegevidenskabelige Fakultet*, Copenhagen: Gad. Such attempts can indeed be traced back to the German Romantics themselves, some of whom wrote remarkably programmatic medical histories: Leibbrand, *Romantische Medizin*, p. 174.

9 A.C. Quatremère de Quincy (1788) *Encyclopédie methodique d'architecture*, Paris: Panckouke, vol. 1, p. 501, s.v. 'Caractère'.

10 A. Vidler (Spring 1977) 'The idea of type', *Oppositions* 8: 103; C. Rowe (January 1974) 'Character and composition', *Oppositions* 2: 48.

11 Foucault's remarks about how 'classificatory medicine' gave way to 'perspective distribution' are suggestive when taken in conjunction with contemporary developments in architectural theory: Michel Foucault (1976) *The Birth of the Clinic*, London: Tavistock, pp. 4–7, 89, 119, 176–7.

12 A. Forty (1980) comments: 'The modern hospital in England and France', in A.D. King (ed.), *Buildings and Society*, London: Routledge & Kegan Paul, pp. 69, 72. See also C. Stevenson (1986) 'The design of prisons and mental hospitals in the neo-classical period; with special reference to the work of C.F. Hansen', University of London PhD thesis, pp. 66–70 on character theory as it pertained to the proper appearance of hospitals.

13 A. Digby quotes John Bevan, the architect of the York Retreat, who 'commented at an early stage of planning that "if the outside appears heavy and prison-like it has a considerable effect upon the imagination"'. A. Digby (1985) 'Moral treatment at the Retreat, 1796–1846', in W. Bynum, R. Porter, and M. Shepherd (eds), *The Anatomy of Madness*, London: Tavistock, vol. II, p. 54.

14 C.N. Ledoux (1804) *L'Architecture considérée sous le rapport de l'art, des moeurs et de la législation*, Paris: Nobele, vol. 2, p. 61.

15 On prison façades see Stevenson, 'The design of prisons and mental hospitals', pp. 75–80.

16 Thaarup, 'Om St Hans', 76.

17 Helweg, *Sindssygevaesenets Udvikling*, p. 39, suggests that at least one Danish book of the period (O.D. Lütken's *De afflictionibus spirtualibus*, published 1821) drew heavily on Reil. The *Rhapsodieen* is, however, not mentioned in the psychiatric bibliography ('De vigtigste') published that year.

18 Doerner, *Madmen and the Bourgeoisie*, pp. 198–206 on Reil.

19 Pinel (An IX [1801]) *Traité philosophique sur l'alienation mentale*, Paris: p. 36. See K. Grange (1961) 'Pinel and eighteenth-century psychiatry', *Bull. Hist. Med.* 35: 443–51 for a very useful analysis of Pinel's conception of 'moral' therapy as specifically directed towards the regulation of excessive and inappropriate emotion; cf. Digby, 'Moral treatment at the Retreat', p. 53 for references to similar thinking in operation at the Retreat.

20 Entry by Tollard (1812): *Dictionnaire des sciences médicales*, Paris: Panckoucke, vol. 1, p. 201.

21 F. Clifton (1732) *The State of Physick Ancient and Modern*, London: Bowyer, pp. 3, 7, 124.

22 J. Reynolds (1778) *Discourses on Art*, London, pp. 76, 84, 88.

23 Grange, 'Pinel and eighteenth-century psychiatry', 443. Pinel's 'hypothetical' morality ('axioms related to the pursuit of virtue') can be compared with Reynolds's 'second nature' of artificial custom.

24 Zalewski, 'Det hårde kors', 29.

25 H.F. Rørdam (1897–9) 'Sindssyges Vilkaar i aeldre Tid', *Kirkehistoriske Samlinger*, 4th series, 5: 406–7. The author quotes other comparable petitions in the bishopric's archive.

26 J.S. Dalsager (1941) *Helsingør almindelige Hospitals Historie*, Elsinore: Steffensen, p. 103.

27 M. Jochumsen (1981) *Sindssyges vilkår i aeldre tid*, Copenhagen: Dansk Plejerforening, p. 44 and Rørdam, 'Sindssyges Vilkaar', 402–3: the word is used in records dating from the fifteenth century.

28 Bethlem Hospital was, for example, described as a *'daarekiste'* in the mid-eighteenth century: *Ordbog over det danske Sprog*, s.v. 'Daarekiste'.

29 Doerner, *Madmen and the Bourgeoisie*, p. 166 on the *Dollkasten* in the German states 'whose policy aspired towards autarky against all alien influences... This spatialization reached its extreme in an appliance that was designed to keep the dangerous expansion of the insane to a minimum and eradicate it: the *Dollkasten* – the mad-box – movable boxes or cases designed to restrain the mobility of their rebellious contents for as long as deemed necessary.' I have found no evidence for mobile *daarekister* in Denmark.

30 Repetitions of this ordinance, which eventually covered Norway too, were necessitated by the hospitals' unwillingness to take lunatics. Helweg, *Sindssygevaesenets Udvikling*, p. 57n, lists them; Zalewski, 'Det hårde kors', 30–1 comments.

31 *Daarekister*, in a pinch also used for felons, were found in gaols well into the nineteenth century: see Helweg, *Sindssygevaesenets Udvikling*, pp. 62, 64–5.

32 On *daarekister* in private homes see Rasmussen, 'Laegedom', p. 269: families could receive parish or Poor Board funds to construct private *daarekister* and after the death of the original occupant these were often rented out. In 1840 J.R. Hübertz, taking the first census of the insane in Denmark, calculated that for the 2,398 lunatics and idiots there were around 500 hospital places: the rest must be with their families or in private *daarekister* of which he found 133, some horrible and none cheap. Helwag, *Sindssygevaesenets Udvikling*, pp. 66–8.

33 O.J. Rawert (1821) 'Er Danmark tilstraekkeligen forsynet med Sygehuse og er disse, som de bør vaere', *Penia*: 36.

34 ibid., 41.

35 ibid., 41, 42.

36 A plan is given in Guldberg (1841) 'Udsigt over Virksomeden af Praestø Amts Sygehus', *Bibliothek for Laeger*, NS, 5: 18. Rawert, 'Er Danmark', 34, 45. The operating room, surely noisy itself at times, in turn separated the *daarekister* from the sick-rooms, which leaves one wondering which sounds were being insulated from whom.

37 Thaarup, 'Om St Hans', 113.

38 Zalewski, 'Det hårde kors', 23–4: the origin of the name 'St Hans' is obscure. In 1651 a decree accompanying the hospital's first move to the Ladegaard, specified that 'a' St Hans Hospital should be provided there for the 'insane, plague-ridden and others with contagious diseases': it seems to have been used as a kind of generic term. See V. Christiansen (1913) 'Københavns Hospitalsforhold i aeldre Tid', in K.M. Nielsen and E.A. Tscherning (eds) *Københavns Kommunehospital 1863–1913*, Copenhagen: Københavns Kommune, pp. 12–13 on the earlier history of the hospital.

39 O. Nielsen (1877–92) *Københavns Historie og Beskrivelse*, 6 vols, Copenhagen: Gad, vol. 3 (1881), p. 343; vol. 5 (1889), p. 250; vol. 6 (1892), pp. 47–9.

40 By that time some of the disfigured *spectaculeuse* could be accommodated in a special small hospital in Hillerød: see N. Gustafsson (1958) *Det gamle Hillerød Hospital*, Hillerød: Pallesen.

41 K. Carøe (1919–20) 'Hospitalsnød i København i Slutningen af det 18. Aarhundrede', *Historiske Meddelelser om København*, 1st series, 7: 449–50; F. Olsen (1934–5) 'Ladegaarden udenfor Nørreport i Kjøbenhavn og dens Kirke', *Historiske Meddelelser om København*, 3rd series, 1: 129–34; Zalewski, 'Det hårde kors', 23.

42 (6 May 1758) 'Charities and hospitals', *The Idler* 4: 20.

43 Riegels, 'Pesthuset som det er', 248. Cf. J.N. Wilse (1790–8) *Reise-Iagttagelse i nogle af de nordiske Lande* 5 vols, Copenhagen: Poulsen, vol. 3 (1792), p. 161: of the 320 inmates at St Hans Hospital 'are some venereal, some furious or weak-witted, and some drunks; each of these three [groups] needs a separate and suitable arrangement and subsequently a cure'. E.K. Sass (1986) *Lykkens Tempel: Et maleri af Nicolai Abildgaard*, Copenhagen: Ejler, p. 116, quotes a diary entry from 1802: 'The notorious writer Riegels is dead. He had wit, [was] the only one to put himself out for madness; and fought for the good, most people think, out of a spiteful heart.'

44 V. Holm (1922) 'En ny Daarekiste', *Lolland-Falsters historiske Samfunds Aarbog* 10: 78.

45 A. Vidler (March 1977) 'Architecture, management and morals', *Lotus International* 14: 4–7, on the architect's efforts to consolidate his position as the 'central agent of progress' and the 'peculiarly ethical slant' of the 'unambiguous expression of character, the constituent ingredient of an architecture that actively participated in the formation of society'.

46 H. Lund (1969) 'Frederiks Hospital og Frederiks Stad', *Kunstindustimuseets Virksomhed*, Copenhagen; with references to the numerous histories of Frederiks Hospital.

47 John Aikin (1771) *Thoughts on Hospitals*, London: Johnson, p. 13.

48 J.R. Tenon (Spring 1975) *Mémoires sur les hôpitaux de Paris*, quoted in L. Greenbaum, 'Measure of civilization: the hospital thought of Jacques Tenon on the eve of the French Revolution', *Bull. Hist. Med.* 49: 47. A. Scull's introduction to his anthology (1981) *Madhouses, Mad-doctors and Madmen*, London: Athlone, discusses the doctors' usurpation of the care of lunatics in eighteenth-century England (p. 7). Scull suggests that the asylum building itself became a weapon in this struggle as psychiatric legitimacy then 'rested heavily on the public's (especially the wealthy public's) response to the asylum'. The debate I describe, although scarcely a sustained dialectic, can be interpreted as one offshoot of this struggle.

49 Carøe, 'Hospitalsnød i København', 456–7, 466–7. The Collegium medicum was the health directorate: physicians, surgeons, and apothecaries had seats on it.

50 On Mangor see Bärens's obituary (1806) in *Penia*: 38–9; and Carøe, 'Hospitalsnød i København', 465. I have traced the history of the St Hans Rebuilding Commission's deliberations in detail in an illustrated article in the Yearbook of the Danish Society for Architectural History: (1986) 'Plans for reaccommodating lunatics at St Hans Hospital, 1791–1808', *Architectura* 8: 82–112, where references to the documents in the Copenhagen Municipal Archives are given; and shall do no more than recapitulate here.

51 Stevenson, 'Plans for reaccommodating lunatics', 85–8.

52 Accommodation for paying patients seems to have been available at St Hans

since its earliest days: see Carøe, 'Hospitalsnød i København', 468; Zalewski, 'Det hårde kors', 49 describes the shortage of 'honette' chambers there in the 1780s.

53 (1789) 'Taksigelse', *Kiøbenhavns Skilderie* 3: 117.

54 Stevenson, 'Plans for reaccommodating lunatics', 92–3.

55 ibid., 95. For other examples of this kind of proposed bookkeeping see Doerner, *Madmen and the Bourgeoisie*, p. 71 (Liverpool Asylum); A. Bailey (1971) 'An account of the founding of the first Gloucestershire County Asylum', *Transactions of the Bristol and Gloucester Archaeological Society* 90: 178–9 (Gloucester Asylum) and (1807) *Address to the Public respecting the Establishment of a Lunatic Asylum at Edinburgh*, Edinburgh: Ballantyne, (Edinburgh Asylum).

56 Stevenson, 'Plans for reaccommodating lunatics', 96–9.

57 On the General Hospital see E. Lesky (1967) 'Das Wiener Allgemeine Krankenhaus', *Clio Medica* 2. Contemporary criticisms of the Narrenturm are cited in Stevenson, 'Plans for reaccommodating lunatics', 99; to these can be added T. Bateman (1806) 'Some account of the General Hospital and Medical School at Vienna' and (1807) 'Further account of the Medical School at Vienna', *Edinburgh Medical and Surgical Journal* 2: 491–6; and 3: 122–5.

58 On Bang see J.H. Bärens (ed.) (1806) *Penia*: 192; (1808) *Penia*: 98–9; V. Klingberg (1810) 'Bangs Necrologie', *Bibliothek for Laeger* 2; and H. Weitemeyer (1907–8) 'Graverboligen på Assistenskirkegård og Jens Bang', *Historiske Meddelelser om København*, 1st series, 1: 65–93.

59 Stevenson, 'Plans for reaccommodating lunatics', 105.

60 V. Christiansen (1907–8) 'København under Belejringen 1807', *Historiske Meddelelser om København*, 1st series, 1:123. The losses to the hospital's inventory are listed in J.H. Bärens (ed.) (1807) *Penia*: 283–7 and (1808) *Penia*: 72, 133.

61 Bärens (ed.) (1808) *Penia*: 19.

62 [O. Malling] (1808) *Beretning om St Hans Hospitals og Claudi Rossets Stiftelses Forflytning til Bidstrupsgaard*, Copenhagen: Schulz, pp. 8–9.

63 Summary in Helweg, *Sindssygevaesenets Udvikling*, pp. 49–51.

64 Rawert, 'Er Danmark', 42.

65 N.D. Riegels (1797) 'Pesthusets Skiebne fra 1788 til 1796', *Fornuftens og Menneskehedens Rettigheders Archiv* 9: 242.

66 'Pesthusets Skiebne', 239, 241.

67 *Dictionnaire des sciences médicales*, vol. 1, p. 201.

68 Pinel, *Traité*, p. 179. According to Goldin, melancholics were placed close to the trees at the new Salpêtrière loges of the late 1780s: J.D. Thompson and G. Goldin (1975) *The Hospital*, New Haven & London: Yale University Press, p. 56.

69 [Malling], *Beretning*, pp. 13–14.

70 (1808) 'Beretning om St Hans Hospitals og Claudi Rossets Stiftelses Forflytning til Bidstrupsgaard', *Penia* 3: 250. This article is a summary review of the published *Beretning*, with Bärens's commentary.

71 W.L. Parry-Jones (1972) *The Trade in Lunacy*, London: Routledge & Kegan Paul, p. 233: 'through the period under consideration, an important feature of the treatment of insanity was, in fact, the strong belief in the therapeutic value of severing the patient's association with his home and the prevention of early or indiscriminate visiting by relatives and acquaintances'.

72 Riegels, 'Pesthusets Skiebne', 249–50.
73 R. Reid and others (1809) *Observations on the structure of hospitals for the treatment of Lunatics*, Edinburgh: Ballantyne, p. 77.
74 According to Esquirol printed without change in his (1838) *Des malades mentales considérées sous les rapports medical, hygiénique, et médico-legal*, 3 vols, Paris: Ballière, vol. 2, p. 421 (cf. p. 398).
75 Esquirol, *Des malades mentales*, vol. 2, pp. 414, 423–6.
76 A. Gøricke (1831) 'Det i Odense oprettede Hospital for Afsindige', *Bibliotek for Laeger* 14: 81.
77 ibid.
78 Andrew Halliday (1827) *A General View of the Present State of Lunatics, and Lunatic Asylums, in Great Britain*, London: Underwood, p. 2.
79 On St Hans's restrictions see Thaarup, 'Om St Hans', 108–12; on Schleswig's, Wendt, *Meddelelser om Anstalter*, p. 14.
79 [Malling], *Beretning*.
80 (1808) 'St Hans Hospital forflyttes til Bidstrupsgaard's', *Penia* 3: 228–9.
81 'Beretning' [in *Penia*], 267–8.
82 ibid., 246; 'St Hans Hospital', 228.
83 ibid.
84 Riegels, 'Pesthuset som det er', 232.
85 'St Hans Hospital', 215.
86 'Beretning' [in *Penia*], 248.
87 [Malling], *Beretning*, pp. 15, 16.
88 Rowe, 'Character and composition', p. 49.
89 Zalewski 'Det hårde kors', 26, 44.
90 J. Christiansen (1983) *Rural Denmark 1750–1980*, Copenhagen: Central Cooperative Committee, p. 18.
91 K. Kryger (1986) *Frihedsstøtten*, Copenhagen: Landbohistorisk Selskab, p. 13.
92 F.S. Skrubbeltrang (1978) *Det danske Landbosamfund*, Copenhagen: Den danske historiske Forening, p. 261.
93 Kryger, *Frihedsstøtten*, pp. 16–23.
94 J.E.D. Esquirol (1818) 'Maisons d'aliénés', *Dictionnaire des sciences médicales* Paris: Panckoucke, vol. 30, p. 59.
95 Helweg, *Sindssygevaesenets Udvikling*, p. 54. The Poor Board's report of 1818 (quoted below), while generally approving of the 'psychic curative methods', noted that their application in Denmark stopped short of the 'rotary machine' used at the Berlin Charité, although it was used at Schleswig (cf. Thaarup, 'Om St Hans', 76).
96 Thaarup, 'Om St Hans', 74.
97 H. Laehr (1893) *Gedenktage der Psychiatrie und ihrer Hülfsdiscipline in allen Ländern*, 4th edn, Berlin: p. 286; M. Barth (1958) 'Der Geschichte der Psychiatrie in Schleswig-Holstein', Kiel University diss. med. p. 4; D. Jetter (1966) *Geschichte des Hospitals: Westdeutschland von den Anfänge bis 1850*, Wiesbaden: Steiner, p. 205.
98 D.V. Lafrenz (1982) 'Das Irrenhaus bei Schleswig', in G. Wietek (ed.), *C.F. Hansen 1756–1845 und seine Bauten in Schleswig-Holstein*, Neumünster: Wachholz, p. 25; J. Rüppel (1872) *Summarischer Bericht über die Irrenanstalt bei Schleswig*, Hamburg: Haendcke & Lehmkuhl, p. 1; Barth, 'Die Geschichte der Psychiatrie', p. 5. According to T. Grodum, Kiel had been proposed again so medical students could study the insane; but Schleswig was chosen at

Suadicani's suggestion: (1982) 'Sindssygehuset i Slesvig', *Dansk medicinhistorisk Årbog*, 124.

99 G.P. Petersen (ed.) (1827) *Schleswig Holstein Lauenburgische Provinzialberichte* 16: 563–4.

100 (1824) 'Carl Ferdinand Suadicani', *Staatsbürgerliches Magazin* 4: 140.

101 The *Bericht* of 11 May 1816, quoted in Barth, 'Die Geschichte der Psychiatrie', p. 5.

102 More detailed information on the Schleswig Asylum will be found in the last chapter of my dissertation: 'Design of prisons and mental hospitals', pp. 237–73.

103 C.M. Smidt (1978) 'C.F. Hansen og hans indflydelse på arkitekturen i Danmark *c.* 1800–30', Copenhagen University dissertation, pp. 44, 57, 99.

104 Quoted Lafrenz, 'Das Irrenhaus', p. 26.

105 The definition is taken from H. Osborne (ed.) (1970) *The Oxford Companion to Art*, Oxford: Clarendon Press, s.v. 'Rustication'.

106 Lafrenz, 'Das Irrenhaus', p. 27.

107 Wendt, *Meddelelser om Anstalter*, p. 15.

108 Quoted in Rüppel, *Summarischer Bericht*, p. 48; see Helweg, *Sindssygevaesenets Udvikling* p. 73 on Jessen's attempts to buy land.

109 J. von Schröder (1827) *Geschichte und Beschreibung der Stadt Schleswig*, Schleswig: p. 236.

110 Lafrenz, 'Das Irrenhaus', p. 27 has summarized the alterations conducted under Jessen and his successors.

111 [P.W] 'J' [essen] (1828) in *Magazin der ausländischen Literatur der gesammten Heilkunde ... zu Hamburg* 16: a review of F. Holst (1828) *Beretning, Betaenkning og Indstilling fra en til at undersøge de Sindssvages Kaar i Norge*, Christiania [Oslo]: Lehmann. Holst's book comprised a report about plans for a new insane asylum in Christiania (by then no longer part of the Danish kingdom): his own plan consisted of a hub with four attached radiating wings along the lines of the Glasgow Asylum. See Stevenson, 'Design of prisons and mental hospitals', pp. 258–9.

112 Wendt, *Meddelelser om Anstalter*, pp. 20–1.

113 ibid., 68.

114 For example, William Stark's Dundee Asylum, designed in 1812, like Schleswig opened in 1818. T. Markus interprets it as the culmination of Stark's steadily more 'picturesque' thinking: (1983) *Order in Space and Society: Architectural Form and its Context in the Scottish Enlightenment*, Edinburgh: Mainstream, p. 20.

115 J.G. Spurzheim (1817) *Observations on the Deranged Manifestations of the Mind, or Insanity*, London: Baldwin, Craddock & Joy, p. 217.

116 Esquirol, *Des malades mentales*, vol. 2, p. 421 (part of the essay first printed in 1818); Spurzheim, *Observations on the Deranged Manifestations*, pp. 214–15, 217.

117 Rüppel, *Summarischer Bericht*, pp. 5, 7.

118 The earliest published reference is probably that in J.R. Hübertz (1844) 'Bemaerkninger om Daarevaesenet, anstillede paa en Rejse i Danmark og Tyskland i Aarene 1841–2', *Bibliotek for Laeger*, 2nd series, 10:77, who was actually more critical than any of his successors. He credited Esquirol with the design of the main block, but continued that he 'seems to have had it in mind, that the institution would serve only one of the sexes', which goes part-way

towards reconciling the discrepancies between the building plan and what we know of Esquirol's thinking about architecture as it had progressed by 1818, the year the building was started. Hübertz's source of information was Rüppel. On the whole question see Stevenson, 'Design of prisons and mental hospitals', pp. 253–6.

119 Rüppel, *Summarischer Bericht*, p. 2.

120 Doerner, *Madmen and the Bourgeoisie*, p. 223.

121 Rüppel, medical director at the asylum from 1845 to 1879, neatly survived the entire Schleswig-Holstein Question. Grodum ('Sindssygehuset i Slesvig', pp. 137, 139–40) suggests that Rüppel was merely anxious to gloss over all Danish involvement in the foundation of the asylum.

122 Helweg, *Sindssygevaesenets Udvikling*, p. 72.

CHAPTER TWO

Asylums in alien places: the treatment of the European insane in British India

Waltraud Ernst

I

In the opening section of Frank Richards's *Old Soldier Sahib* – one of few working-class autobiographies – the author muses about his youth in the 1890s as a miner in South Wales, when he had been enthralled by a former soldier's 'wonderful yarns of India', a place which was described to him as being 'a land of milk and honey'.[1] The subsequent account of soldiers' duties and adventures in the colony at the beginning of the twentieth century, however, reveals that they lived in somewhat of a fool's paradise. The idealized vision of a poor man's bonanza in the east had been nurtured for over a century not only by wily recruiting officers but also by men like Richards.[2] For members of the higher classes, too, the prospect of taking a share of the Orient's bounty had a strong appeal. In their case the period when *really* big and quick fortunes could be made was seen to have been the few decades between the battle of Plassey (1757), which opened the way for British control of Bengal, and the time of the reforms introduced by Lord Cornwallis in his capacity as Governor-General (1786–93), which cleared the way for the administration of British India on 'Western' principles.

As it happens, this is also the period when the first lunatic hospitals were established for the reception of those members of the European communities in Bengal, Madras, and Bombay whose minds were seen to have become 'afflicted with derangement'. It is not the intention to suggest that the rise of the fabulously and perhaps maddeningly rich nabob and the emergence of the European lunatic asylum in India may be related in more than a contingent way.[3] Whilst the hopeful nabob was concerned with quick acquisition of riches, it was rather the loss of, or anxiety about, them which was frequently linked with the necessity to provide for the reception of suddenly unfortunate members of the higher middle classes as well as for military servants for whom the vision of a 'land of milk and honey' had turned sour. The emergence and development of India's European lunatic asylums may thus merely be seen to reflect one of the less illustrious and less presentable aspects of European colonial life and personal ambition in the east, which – as a Bombay asylum superintendent put it in 1852 – was grounded in 'disappointed love, blighted hope, and crushed ambition'.[4] Here we will, however, be less concerned with the social and personal implications of 'weakness, folly, dissipation, and crime', said to have been characteristic of European asylum inmates,[5] but rather with the socio-political context within which asylums for the European mentally ill emerged towards the end of the eighteenth century, and with the diverse administrative developments these institutions underwent in the three presidencies of Bengal, Madras, and Bombay up to 1858.

Originally designed for the reception of as few as five to fifteen Europeans, and established with the express aim of 'affording security against the perpetration of those acts of violence which had been so frequently committed by unrestrained lunatics',[6] by the 1850s each of the three asylums confined as many as 100–150 patients of various racial backgrounds and of both 'violent' and 'tractable' dispositions.[7] Along with the increase in asylum population went a changing perception of what was regarded to be proper quality of provision. The asylum reformer Sir A. Halliday, for example, referring to asylum reports of 1819, praised the East India Company's asylums in India in that they 'surpass many of the European establishments that have long been considered as the most perfect of their kind'.[8] Only a few decades later, in the 1850s, Dr J. Macpherson, superintendent of the Calcutta Lunatic Asylum, was quoted lamenting that 'we are doubtless below par in our treatment of the insane'.[9] Halliday and Macpherson's diverse assessments are certainly of a kind to point up a change in emphasis concerning the management of institutions and inmates rather than merely a deterioration of provision. However, such diverse if not incompatible evaluations at different periods are not confined to expert judgements on Indian institutions alone. In the colonial motherland itself, the criterion of what was seen to constitute adequate institutional regimes shifted once the early-nineteenth-century asylum reformers' preoccupation with institutional management, moral therapy, and non-restraint in small-scale asylums gave way to concern about the cure-efficiency in what Scull has described as the 'mammoth asylums' for the lunatic poor, established towards the middle of the nineteenth century.[10] What is striking, however, in both Halliday's and Macpherson's evaluations is their unquestioned point of reference, namely the standard of asylum provision in the British Isles rather than any reference to Indian social-medical systems. It may well be argued that the comparison of institutions in the colony with those in the metropolis itself is only to be expected, as it merely goes to exemplify the nature of a colonial situation. Nineteenth-century colonizers not only assumed the general superiority of their ideas and institutions *vis-à-vis* the allegedly less 'enlightened' and less 'humane' indigenous 'customs', but also conceived it as their duty to spread European civilization. Moreover, we are here dealing primarily with the treatment of members of the colonial rulers' own community, namely Europeans. Taking British psychiatric developments as the yardstick against which to measure institutions in India therefore seems to be a plausible concomitant to colonial expansion, if not a necessary constituent of the civilizing mission – not to speak of the British authorities' responsibility for providing a rejuvenating institutional back-up for those servants in the colony whose vision of India may have become one of 'the land of regrets'.[11] The crucial point here is that institutionalized European psychiatry became a seemingly necessary companion of the European colonial community in India at a time when the nature of British presence in the east changed considerably – however much this process may have been assisted by developments in British medical sciences.

The East India Company's organizational development between the early eighteenth and the early nineteenth centuries was both reflected in and sustained by a corresponding reorganization of the European community itself. It had been the male adventurers and merchants who came to India for commerce at the beginning; it was the soldiers and administrators who after Plassey accompanied them to annex and govern; and finally it was European women who increasingly were to round off the hitherto more or less exclusively male community during the last century of British presence in India. Emily Eden, accompanying her brother, Governor-General Auckland, on his tour of the Upper Provinces (1837–9), grasps one aspect of these changes when pondering the entertainment at a hill-station of North India:

> Twenty years ago no European had ever been here, and there we were, with the band playing the 'Puritani' and 'Masaniello', and eating salmon from Scotland, and sardines from the Mediterranean, and observing that St. Cloup's potage à la Julienne was perhaps better than his other soups, and that some of the ladies' sleeves were too tight according to the overland fashions for March, &c.; and all this in face of those high hills, some of which have remained untrodden since the creation, and we, 105 Europeans, being surrounded by at least 3,000 mountaineers, who, wrapped up in their hill blankets, looked on at what we call our polite amusements, and bowed to the ground if a European came near them.[12]

The underlying trend of the social changes occurring among Europeans in India – one important aspect of which was captured by Emily Eden's episode – was towards the transplantation to India of the grander style of the English way of life by members of the middle classes, the social diversification and stratification of the European community, and a gradual withdrawal from Indian life that steadily grew into racial discrimination. In terms of population figures the change had been similarly distinct. The British community which had amounted to no more than about 2,000 members in the 1750s, had increased to about 100,000 a century later. A large proportion – about half of the latter figure – belonged to the lower classes of British society, with military servants accounting for about two-thirds of the total number.[13]

It is within this context of the changing face of British colonialism at the turn of the eighteenth century, and the changes in the social stratification of the European community in British India going along with it, that the emergence and development of the 'European Insane Hospital' has to be set. The institutional history of European asylums in British India did not merely *duplicate* the institutional and medical paradigms extant in the British Isles at the time. Although regulations for asylums in India were based on English select committees' and the metropolitan commissioners in lunacy's recommendations, they were implemented in various different ways, dependent both on the presidential governments' diverse policy emphases and on the professional preferences as well as the personal commitment of asylum superintendents. Whilst drawing on British medical ideas and practices, lunacy provision in British India experienced a certain 'colonial twist' which led to the emergence of three different ways of disposing of mentally ill Europeans. To these we now turn.

II

The first lunatic hospital for Europeans in Bengal was established some time prior to 1787.[14] It was privately owned and provided for but few patients in a presidency with not more than 2,000–3,000 'inhabitants of respectability'.[15] No standard admission policy was as yet laid down. Only in 1787, when Assistant Surgeon W. Dick offered his medical services and the lease of his private lunatic asylum to the Government of Bengal, would anything like a more organized and regulated system of institutional provision emerge. The practice of 'boarding out' public patients became the norm. Dick would charge the government a fixed sum per patient, and in addition draw house rent, surgeon's salary, and pay for the four European invalids employed as attendants as well as an allowance for each patient's personal *cooly* or servant. Most asylum inmates appear to have fallen into the category of 'public patients', thus being paid for by the military, naval, or civil authorities. In imitation of military pay regulations civilians were ranked accordingly; gentlemen were afforded the equivalent of a lieutenant's pay, whilst lower-class patients were provided for like private soldiers.[16]

This arrangement was to a certain extent comparable to the system in England, where parish officials disposed of the insane within their administrative boundaries by making them over to the care of private madhouse owners for a stipulated rate. The system in Bengal was, however, structurally less straightforward in so far as the private contractor was at the same time a government employee. It was this union of asylum proprietor, medical superintendent, and government servant in a single person which was open to corruption due to the potential of personal gain at the company's expense. A further major difference between systems in Bengal and England was that in the east the authorities paid the expenses for both first- and second-class patients and not merely for people who in England would have been designated 'paupers'.

On Surgeon Dick's return to England, in 1802, it was decided to establish what sounds like an institution more favourable to the public treasury, namely a 'Government Asylum'. In the event these proved to be empty words, as an arrangement similar to the one under Dick was retained. The housing and the provision of victuals and clothing were entrusted to an appointed assistant surgeon, who was also responsible for the patients' medical treatment at fixed rates.[17] Significantly, objections against this 'innovation' were raised by the company's authorities in London rather than by the local government in Bengal. In line with the findings of the select committee on the better regulation of madhouses in England (1815/16) the notion that the medical officer in charge of the asylum might be 'allowed to derive [any] benefit, directly, or indirectly from his situation beyond the salary ... allowed to him', was found objectionable and by order of the court of directors of the East India Company had to be discontinued.[18] Consequently the commissariat was ordered to provide the institution's supplies, and the government's control was strengthened by obliging both the medical board and the chief magistrate of Calcutta to examine monthly the asylum and to draw up a report on its management and on the state of every single patient. It was also ordered that case books ought to be kept.[19]

Despite the court of directors' apparently progressive stance and the seemingly large extent of public control over the place's internal management laid down in the regulations, petty corruption still prevailed virtually unhampered by the local authorities. Some three decades later the local authorities in Bengal admitted that the system during the first two decades of the nineteenth century was 'on a scale of liberty to all connected with the institution which those accustomed to the more exact and healthier administration of the public resources of the present day [1847] can scarcely contemplate without astonishment'.[20]

At the time, however, the government's attention could conveniently be directed away from the accounts and towards a less intricate, but more pressing, matter: the asylum building had by 1815 become 'utterly inadequate' and new premises had to be looked for.[21] The news about the government's plan to do away with the derelict building travelled fast among Bengal's 5,000 or so Europeans: an informed assistant surgeon promptly suggested a plan which promised to save the government's expenses and, incidentally, to ensure a regular income to himself and his business partner. In future mentally ill people of European origin were to be sent to England and a 'House of Reception' was to be kept on a small scale only to take care of patients in transit.[22] The plan was adopted on account of its (relative) cost-efficiency and from 1821 onwards the government's public patients as well as some private patients were prior to embarkation sent to an asylum, later known as 'Beardsmore's Bedlam'.

Mr I. Beardsmore, former soldier and subsequently a keeper in the early 'Government Asylum', reserved thirteen rooms for public patients and drew a rate which was much lower than the one charged hitherto, but still well above the average rate in England.[23] The contract with Beardsmore and later with his wife was to outlive several demands for the asylum's abolition. Only in 1856 was it revoked in consequence of the reorganization of the Indian Medical Service by the then governor-general, Lord Dalhousie, and his promotion of state intervention in public welfare.

During the nearly four decades of its existence Beardsmore's asylum created the dilemma common to many contracted-out service institutions in the public sector: the tension between the government's attempts to guarantee effective control of provisions and to pursue at the same time a policy of non-interference. This situation was aggravated not only by the diverse views on state intervention held by successive governor-generals, but also by the various authorities and interests involved. Beardsmore, the private entrepreneur, was faced with authorities more often in conflict than in agreement with each other; the medical board, the governor-general and his council, as well as, less visible to him, the court of directors and the parliamentary board of control in London.

The medical board as the officially acknowledged body of medical experts, was vested with the immediate control and responsibility for the presidency's medical affairs and institutions. Thus it had the potentially important duty of overseeing the lunatic asylum's efficient management and of preventing any abuse of its inmates. Formally its task could be compared to that of the board of metropolitan commissioners in lunacy in England. However, the medical board as a regulatory controlling agency with potential powers of inspection did not work entirely satisfactorily.[24] In many instances the board showed a propensity either to interfere heavy-handedly in professional medical matters, or to fail to 'exercise the powers vested in them . . . sufficiently at the onset', and thus to engender a 'lax system, which then they were unable to improve'.[25] The government itself did not seem to enforce orders effectively, to pursue a consistent public health policy, or to be sure to what extent it wanted to endow the medical board with discretionary authority.[26] The inability to define the board's authority and enforce efficient control and supervision without interfering with professional medical judgement was equally characteristic of the medical officers, the Bengal government, and the court of directors. The situation of undefined authority and responsibility is evidenced by several disputes between the board and the asylum proprietor.

One area continually pregnant with controversy was the classification of patients. Whilst certification was to be undertaken prior to admission into the asylum – by a medical committee in the case of military servants, by the marine surgeon in the case of naval employees, and by two medical officers whenever civilians were involved – it was the subsequent process of classing patients according to 'previous station and circumstance' which led to tugs-of-war between asylum proprietor and medical board.[27] The charges allowed to the madhouse owner depended on a patient's class category, and as the profit margin was higher in the case of first-class inmates, Beardsmore's interest tended to be served better with the greater part of the asylum population being designated as 'first-class'. The three members of the medical board were, however, less inclined to make use of the twice as expensive first-class category, and frequently downgraded patients – to the repeated irritation of the asylum proprietor. An ambition to do justice to the government's accounts cannot have been the sole motive for such cost-effective measures, as the board members were on other occasions not at all disinclined to engage in arrangements from which they themselves or colleagues rather than the public treasury would profit. Long-standing personal animosities – nurtured in the philistine hot-house of pretentious Calcutta society – and professional arrogance on the part of medical board members against the soldier-turned-madhouse-owner – who, they sneered, 'pretended to no medical knowledge' and consequently should be their subordinate – partly accounted for the bitterness and fierceness exhibited in the repeated disputes.[28]

These controversies are also of a kind to point up the importance that was attributed to an ever-increasing extent to questions of social class and racial background. By the early nineteenth century the European community in Bengal had developed into a hierarchically structured society – a 'middle-class aristocracy'[29] – which was obsessed with preserving social precedence amongst its own kind and fiercely defended its assumed exclusiveness *vis-à-vis* people of other races. Whilst military and naval hierarchy as well as the company's civil staff were conveniently structured, the ranking of civilians unconnected with any of the company's services constituted some problems. Among the latter it was mainly people of mixed race whose social position was less easily defined as they might have been fathered by a person of some standing though undoubtedly be considered inferior due to their Indian blood.[30]

Despite squabbles over classification of lunatics – which would in most cases only be settled after government arbitration – segregation within the asylum was strictly based on patients' gender, social class, and race, whilst medical considerations concerning the nature of the disease were of subordinate importance. For most of the first half of the nineteenth century emphasis was placed on the adequate transfer of the main characteristics of European society's social stratification and segregation into the lunatic asylum. The inmates remained what they had been in society outside – members of a certain gender, race, and class, with the corresponding status to which consideration and comfort was seen to be due.

The racial composition of the asylum population changed considerably over time. Take the example of G. Swinton, a military officer, who was admitted to Beardsmore's asylum in July 1825. Although born in India, and the son of a European father and an Indian mother, he was on account of his officer status provided for as a first-class patient. He consequently was entitled occasionally to take his food at the asylum proprietor's family table – provided his behaviour was orderly and he was willing to participate in polite conversation. Together with the only other first-class inmate he would be allocated his own separate apartment, which was furnished with hanging lamps and had washing facilities and other utensils in a partitioned corner. Although he would have to share toilet facilities with second-class inmates he was unlikely to have to socialize with any of the thirteen ward-patients who then lived in less comfortable buildings in small cells, spartanly equipped with wooden bedsteads. Some thirty-five years later, in 1859, Swinton still happened to be an in-patient. About 1,200 patients had by then passed through the asylum and the average asylum population had increased considerably, to about seventy patients, eight of whom were then designated as first-class inmates. People of Swinton's mixed race would now largely outnumber those of pure European origin – as the latter were within each year sent back to England. At the age of seventy-six and suffering from 'dementia' Swinton would enjoy the superior comforts still afforded to patients of the 'better classes'.[31]

A less lucky Eurasian who had been admitted only two years after him, in 1827, would in contrast have experienced a much more thorough change in provision. Mrs Nelson, born in India, and without independent financial means, was provided for as a second-class patient. She had formerly, in the 1820s, 1830s, and even 1840s enjoyed a 'degree of ease and luxury, that [she] never could have expected to procure for [herself] in health', and which, it was reported, may even have been 'irksome' to her 'from its novelty'.[32] Such generous consideration bestowed on second-class patients owed much to the asylum proprietor's endeavour to keep rates up in order to maintain a reasonable profit and to keep attracting private patients who might be deterred from making use of the institution in case it had the reputation of a downmarket, low-class establishment. The situation was to change drastically, however, once a government investigation asserted in 1850–1 that the cost for the upkeep of poor lunatics in Bengal showed the 'extravagance' with which the Beardsmores conducted their institution.[33] In consequence second-class inmates like Mrs Nelson were from 1856 onwards to be put on a low dietary regime, and provided for on a standard more akin to that prevalent in army hospitals.

The take-over by government in 1856 of the former private madhouse certainly did more to economize than to improve second-class patients' condition. The 'Government Lunatic Asylum' was, however, from the date of its foundation in 1856 onwards, to become the model for future asylums in Madras, Bombay, Delhi, Rangoon, Colombo, Lahore, and Karachi. Up to that date asylum provision for Europeans in the two subordinate sister-presidencies – Madras and Bombay – differed in certain respects.

III

Just like the institution in Bengal, the Madras Lunatic Asylum evolved from a profitable private enterprise to a low-budget public institution towards the middle of the nineteenth century. It was established in 1793, by Assistant Surgeon Valentine Conolly, who was to set in train both a lucrative business and a procedure for the disposal of insane persons, which was regarded as most humane and judicious by the authorities.[34] Between five and fifteen patients – of mainly European parentage and all walks of life – were received into the institution during the first few years.[35] The accounts praising Conolly's achievements are divided between mention of personal profit on the one hand and public benevolence on the other.[36] On his return to England he had accumulated great wealth and was acknowledged as one of those formerly less well-off Englishmen who returned from India as wealthy nabobs.[37] He settled down in London, comfortably seeing his five sons through education in prestigious colleges and thus preparing them for promising careers – as military officers and members of the civil service in India. Before embarkation Conolly had sold the asylum buildings for three times the premises' estimated value to another medical practitioner who expected the asylum to be a good enough income source to enable him to imitate his predecessor's rise to fortune.[38] When in 1815 the asylum changed hands once more at a highly inflated price, the government finally objected to the sale and transfer of the lease it had entered into with Conolly on the grounds that 'the principle of selling not merely the building, but the charge of the patients contained in it' was unacceptable.[39] The then-owner, Surgeon J. Dalton, consequently had on his return to England's green and pleasant land contracted an agent to run the property, and had no involvement whatsoever with the institution's day-to-day affairs.[40]

Whilst in Bengal the union of function of resident proprietor and superintendent in the person of Beardsmore, and the Bengal government's failure to clarify management and control structures had caused continuous disputes between madhouse owner, medical officers, and government, the Madras authorities, in contrast, took steps towards administrative systematization as early as 1808. Despite transient petty rows amongst medical practitioners as to what constituted a reasonable level of profit for the madhouse owner, the comparatively stringent contractual conditions imposed upon the proprietors by the government worked relatively effectively.[41] The early abolition of rates and introduction of one-off allowances in 1809, the definite vesting of authority for admission and classification in the medical board, and the curtailing of property speculation in regard to the asylum buildings and the government's lease, contributed towards the institution's more or less tranquil development during the following five decades.

As in Bengal, Eurasian and Indian asylum inmates were to remain in India, whilst mentally ill Europeans were once a year routinely embarked for Europe.[42] On arrival in England those patients who had neither recovered nor died during the long voyage around the Cape would usually be admitted into 'Pembroke House', Hackney. This private lunatic asylum had become the main receptacle for the company's insane servants ever since the institution's owner, a Dr G. Rees, had in 1818 offered to provide especially for mentally ill persons returning from India. Rees was styled 'physician to insane persons returning from India, under the patronage of the Honorable East-India Company' and claimed to have 'restored to health and reason' three-fourths of his patients. Although Pembroke House was not the only institution in Britain to receive patients who were transferred from the three Indian asylums in the east, it nevertheless provided for the majority of formerly institutionalized returned expatriates. By 1892 about 500 lunatics who had a claim on being maintained by the company had passed through the asylum in England.[43]

Despite the periodic repatriation of Europeans (from 1821 onwards), the asylum building in Madras soon became overcrowded. Asylum returns show a slow but constant increase in the asylum population for the period from about 1800 to 1850.[44] During the first two decades of the century the number of Europeans was to rise to about twenty. In consequence of the deportation policy the number of Europeans fell again to an average of about ten patients, whilst in contrast the number of Eurasian and Indian patients increased drastically between the 1810s and 1850s (fourfold and sevenfold respectively). By the 1850s first-class patients were outnumbered more than ten times by second-class inmates of mainly Eurasian and Indian description. This circumstance caused the authorities to make concentrated efforts to avoid having high-class Europeans admitted into a public institution frequented by lower-class patients, as the asylum, it was argued, was 'unsuited' for persons of officer's rank.[45] Institutional alternatives such as convalescent homes and sanatoriums were, however, lacking in the town and immediate vicinity of Madras.[46] This calamity was resolved to a certain extent by the Madras government's attempts, less pronounced than Bengal's, at the centralization of asylum provisions. Up-country European lunatics were at times confined in local gaols, garrison hospitals, or asylums without ever being admitted to the specialized central institution in Madras[47] – a practice which had caused much correspondence in Bengal due to the authorities' insistence on a centralized policy of confinement and on strict and discriminating principles of institutional segregation.

There prevailed a further and most striking difference between practices in Madras and those in the superior presidency. The Madras asylum provided for the reception of both Europeans *and* Indians.[48] Whilst there existed separate wards for the different races, the propriety of confining Indian and European lunatics in the same compound was not apparently questioned. In Bengal, in contrast, any suggestion of racial intermingling was outrightly and vehemently rejected. In 1820, for example, the authorities in London proposed that the specialized institution for European lunatics in Bengal should be closed down, as due to routine repatriation of the mentally ill it was no longer needed as a permanent establishment. The medical board was alarmed and went to great pains to explain that such procedure was utterly inconceivable from the point of view of the local European community. The crucial point was that the court of directors had ordered that Europeans awaiting passage be temporarily kept in the 'Lunatic Asylum for Natives', near Calcutta.[49] To accommodate European lunatics for however short a period in an establishment meant for Indians was, the medical board argued, neither practical nor expedient. The board further held that 'even were not the propriety of mixing Europeans labouring under mental derangement with natives in the same unfortunate condition, in itself very questionable', the institution for Indians was not adequately fitted to cater for the 'comfort of the European'.[50] The nature of the argument appealed to the court of directors, and the Bengal government was finally permitted to retain institutional segregation. The economy of keeping two distinctly separated systems of mental health care in Bengal – one for Indians and another for Europeans and Eurasians of all but the lowest classes – had been questioned once more, in the 1840s. Again an innovation was suggested by a person based in England, rather than by a long-standing member of the European Bengal community. This outsider suggested the establishment of a single, large-scale, cost-effective 'panopticon' for the mentally ill of all races and descriptions.[51] This proposal, too, was rejected by the government in India on the grounds that it aimed at imitating, unmodified, the English system, and thus neglected the local European community's aversion to the mixing of Indians and Europeans.[52]

In stark contrast to such a determined stance against racial integration, a somewhat more permissive – albeit not indifferent – attitude was manifest in Madras, at least at the beginning of the century. Despite occasional objections to confining higher-class Europeans in a public asylum, no fundamental doubts as to the propriety of receiving Indians into the European asylum were raised. Towards the middle of the nineteenth century, however, in Madras, too, the principle of maintaining social distance between Europeans and Indians came more to the fore. It was, however, exclusively members of the upper classes whose exemption from admission into the asylum was discussed. The authorities' hesitation in sending upper-class Europeans to the multiracial asylum was partly also occasioned by the derelict and 'highly dangerous' state of the buildings.[53] They were by the 1840s long past their best – mainly because the late, benevolent Conolly had made use of construction material of an inferior quality.[54] When the erection of a new and larger asylum was at long last decided (in 1851),[55] well-off Madras citizens who owned homes in the planned asylum's neighbourhood petitioned against the project. The main argument ran that the institution would create a nuisance – even 'great injury' – as well as declining property prices in the vicinity.[56] Whilst the maintenance of social distance between the races was apparently not insisted on as doggedly as in Bengal (as long as inter-racial contact could be restricted to within the confines of the madhouse), the prospect of a large-scale asylum for deranged people of all walks of life bordering too closely on Europeans' private compounds, seemed to disturb the local residents' peace of mind. Class prejudice, racial sentiments, and the need to keep a psychological as well as spatial distance from the mad asserted themselves here. As had been argued by one medical board member some decades earlier, to bring a gentleman – whether of sane or of temporarily weak mind – into close proximity with 'maniacs of all countries and of the lowest ranks of life', would be inappropriate.[57] In an attempt to prevent any adverse effects on the amenities and peace of mind of local residents, the government delayed the long overdue reconstruction still further. It was not until long after the revolt of 1857 that work would finally begin in 1867[58] and construction be completed some years later (in 1871). Until then the asylum personnel and inmates had to put up with overcrowded and structurally dangerous premises, and would have to make alternative arrangements for the boarding-out of inmates for whom adequate provision was seen to be available within other institutions.[59]

IV

Whilst Madras developed from what had been called an 'enlightened presidency' during the late eighteenth century to somewhat of a social and commercial 'backwater' in the course of the nineteenth century,[60] the town and presidency of Bombay seem to have undergone the reverse process. The acquisition of new territories around the turn of the eighteenth century and the victory over the Marathas (1818) who had been feared – by the British and other Indian rulers alike – as aspirants to supremacy over India, were the start of a steady expansion. The opening of the overland mail route (1837) as well as the putting in at Bombay (1854) of Suez-bound P & O steamers, which had earlier taken the East Indiamen's Cape route, were to contribute further to a bustling town and port life. Bombay's development from a small plot of land – ceded to the English crown by the Portuguese in the seventeenth century as a wedding present – to the literal 'gateway to India' was most dramatic during the first half of the nineteenth century. During this period of expansion lunacy policy, too, was to undergo similarly marked changes. Despite some local specificities the history of the Bombay Asylum points up in a particularly distinct way certain trends and themes characteristic of the company's stance towards its mentally ill.

The first question any of the governments in the three presidencies had to tackle was whether insane Europeans ought to be institutionalized or to be simply left to their fate. Due to the peculiarity of temporary expatriates' lives in an alien country, neither family nor parochial relief could be relied upon, so that confinement within company establishments appeared to be the most adequate response on such – initially – rare occasions as when one of the few European civilians or military servants became mentally ill. The alternative of leaving distressed Europeans to wander about in European towns or Indian states was felt to be undesirable not least because of the anticipated embarrassment this might cause to the British self-image and Indians' respect of the white man's assumed superior character. Institutional provision for lunatics in Bombay is reported to date back as far as 1670, when some rooms in the hospital were set aside.[61] Once institutionalization had become a routine measure, the next problem with which the local government was faced was one of finance and space. How could an ever-increasing number of lunatics in rapidly expanding towns and provincial stations be accommodated at the least expense to the treasury? Should *any* deranged person – whether violent or merely harmlessly 'idiotic' – be secluded from European society for the sake of public peace and order and sentiments of racial prestige? If admission was restricted to certain groups – as it was during much of the nineteenth century – what was to be the criterion for deciding on a person's eligibility for confinement? Was it to be their racial background, social standing, relation to the company's services, or rather the social intrusiveness of their affliction, or perhaps the individual's pain and suffering? The importance attributed to these various aspects changed not only with the financial circumstances but with the people involved in the decision-making process. The question was also always highly controversial.

The Bombay government in the early decades favoured the confinement of any European, Eurasian, or even Indian lunatic who was sent to the asylum by either the military or civil authorities.[62] In 1820 the governor-in-council rejected the Bengal notion of establishing separate 'Native Lunatic Asylums' – a decision based as much on the recognition that the demand for asylum provision in Bombay was not yet urgent, as on the less stringently pursued policy of racial segregation and a preference for largish central institutions.[63] A couple of decades later, however, this decision was to be revised on account of the overcrowding of asylum wards.[64] Bombay's European and Indian population had increased steadily and so had the number of Indian and Eurasian lunatics who had been admitted alongside Europeans. Furthermore, in the absence of adequate facilities in newly 'settled' areas, patients from the outstations were also sent to the metropolis.[65] In consequence of such unexpected developments, the magistrate and officers of police were ordered to refrain in future from sending 'harmless' lunatics to the asylum.[66] It appears that this order was in practice applied to Indians and Eurasians and not to Europeans who were still admitted regardless of their symptomatic behaviour. Again, the decision to impose selective admission restriction did not remain undisputed. The police authorities were against it on account of the expected disruption of public peace and order from non-violent though irritating 'idiots' roaming the city's streets.[67] Officials such as Governor Falkland opposed it on humanitarian grounds. He considered institutional confinement as a measure of social relief for the 'friendless lunatic',[68] and it constituted in his opinion an obligation on any civilized government to provide 'for the reception and treatment on the most approved system of the unfortunate victims of a calamity the heaviest which can well befall a rational and responsible being and the most entitling him to sympathy and assistance from his fellow men'.[69] Similar arguments had been employed in Bengal and there, too, had been rejected on predominantly financial grounds.

The disputes about admission restriction are significant as they expose some basic features of early-nineteenth-century lunacy policy. First, they reveal the wide spectrum of official ideas about the extent to which government ought to make institutional provision for the European as well as for the Indian mentally ill. This is strongly intertwined with the various points of view in regard to the nature of colonial state administration in general and the company's responsibility for the social welfare of its subject people in particular. This broader question of what the nature of the colonial state ought to be was as yet unresolved and was a matter of controversy for people from a wide variety of ideological viewpoints, such as the evangelical, romanticist, utilitarian, and liberal approaches. Secondly, the continued disputes indicate the precedence finally accorded to peace and order, racial considerations, and the prevention of violent behaviour against person and property, rather than to treatment-orientated considerations such as whether a mentally ill person could be cured or at least their condition alleviated by early treatment. Governor Falkland pointed out in 1849 what he considered to be the regrettable consequence of such a pragmatic setting of priorities, expressing his indignation that a mentally disturbed person should be debarred from 'all professional aid merely because he may be quite inoffensive'.[70] Thirdly, not only government officials but medical officers, too, were divided on the question of who was to be regarded as a fit subject for admission into the Bombay Lunatic Asylum. Taking recourse to different medical concepts and ideological premises they gave their support to schemes as diverse as that the asylum 'should not be occupied with idiots and harmless imbeciles',[71] or that early medical treatment ought to be provided 'at the first onset of the disease' and prior to a person committing some criminal offence,[72] or else that one large-scale institution should be established or rather that separate asylums ought to be provided for the feeble-minded, the homicidal and former military servants of different races.[73] Doctors' various recommendations do not, however, appear to have particularly impressed the authorities anyway – a fact which may not be blamed so much on the practitioners' diverse preferences as on the government's insistence that, when it came to the outlay of public money it could not merely consider what is '*desirable*, but what can be afforded'.[74] Furthermore, medical practitioners were only just beginning to establish themselves within professional associations and lobbies which would have allowed for participation and leverage in socio-medical, decision-making processes.[75]

The persuasive power of reference to the accountant books was evident during most decades and in all government departments. The decision on whether or not certain institutional measures were to be implemented was, however, finally not always arrived at on economic considerations alone. The Bombay authorities had, for example, been renowned for their support for cost-effective, and easily controllable, panopticon-style public institutions, such as gaols.[76] When in 1820 the medical board asked for government sanction of new and considerably enlarged provision for the insane because of the 'defective state of the present lunatic asylum' – a private house owned by a surgeon – their plan was accepted on grounds of anticipated savings of expenses and a perceived need to rectify a situation which had been reported as having effected the 'agonizing suffering of some of the patients'.[77] Moreover, the proposed scheme was in congruence with the then governor's predilection for large central public institutions.

By the 1840s and 1850s this institution – providing for about 100 patients – had not only become hopelessly overcrowded so that harmless as well as homicidal patients were denied admission,[78] but in several of the expanding presidency's cantonments and provincial stations extensive accommodation for the insane had been established (e.g. in Pune, Surat, Ahmadabad, Lahore, Karachi).[79] Further, cells adjoining general hospitals or gaols had been set aside for the mentally ill in smaller places.[80] The Bombay government considered a revision of existing practices. It aimed at recentralization of provision; the mushrooming of small-scale establishments in the provinces should be checked; and one single asylum in Bombay should provide for all of the presidency's insane as, it was pointed out by the medical board, 'more benefit at a moderate cost would be produced on a certain number of insanes by their being accommodated and treated in large, rather than in small asylums'.[81] In this instance, however, the argument of economies of scale was not considered decisive. Officials in the Punjab and Sind – renowned for their strict and despotic military-style rule – argued that Bombay could hardly be considered a 'central' location as it was about 700 miles away.[82] The rationale behind the plan for a routine transfer of patients to the capital was questioned by pointing out that it made as much sense as sending lunatics from London to St Petersburg. Not only would the transport cost be considerable but the culture shock experienced by those sent away from their motherland would be detrimental to cure and would in addition tend to antagonize relatives. Such sensible reasoning – despite government aversion to provincial parochialism – could not easily be refuted.

Consequently a Benthamite mammoth asylum was in the event to be built neither in the provinces nor in Bombay – despite existing prototypes of large-scale penitentiaries. It would in any case not have been necessary for Europeans, because they were sent back to England, regardless of whether they were of tranquil or of violent disposition. In regard to the Indian and Eurasian mentally ill, in contrast, the need for large asylum complexes may have become pressing – had the authorities in the 1840s not decided against proceeding with their earlier policy of encouraging police officers and magistrates to recommend for certification any Indian or Eurasian whom they considered to be a public nuisance on account of behaviour interpreted as stemming from mental derangement. What seems to have caused the backing-down from the former relatively indiscriminate institutionalization policy was the government's gradual realization of the magnitude of the 'native' lunacy problem which it had generated by its street-clearing policy. An immensely large – and with every new annexation a growing – number of Indians and Eurasians potentially became eligible for institutional confinement. Had such a tendency been allowed to continue beyond the 1840s, British India would have seen the 'great native confinement'. However, people such as stone-throwing fakirs and hashish-smoking or 'indecently' dressed and recalcitrant mendicants who had formerly often without much hesitation been put into the European madhouse, were henceforth more frequently left at large.[83] The company's problem with European and Indian lunatics was thus economically and pragmatically solved by sending to England the former and by redefining whenever prudent the criterion for institutionalization of the latter.

V

The way in which lunacy policy was implemented in the three presidencies differed, largely in accordance with the priorities set for the administration of public affairs by the local governments. However, there are also some points which appear to have characterized all of them to some degree. First, towards the middle of the nineteenth century and certainly by 1856 the Bengal government's earlier *laissez-faire* approach was being revoked in favour of centralized state control of asylum provision. Segregative confinement of asylum inmates of various racial backgrounds came to be laid down by statute and implemented either by inter-institutional (Bengal) or intra-institutional (Madras, Bombay) segregation. Similarly, the quality of services was to undergo standardization to an ever-increasing extent, thus curtailing the freedom of action – whether to the benefit or detriment of patients – formerly enjoyed by asylum superintendents. Secondly, a certain tension between Victorian reformers' endeavour to make governments accept their alleged obligation to provide for the 'friendless lunatic' of any race and the company's pursuit of a cost-effective administration asserts itself to an ever-increasing extent. Thirdly, in Madras and Bombay the question of *European* lunacy was less easily dealt with independently from measures envisaged for the Indian insane. Unlike in Bengal, Europeans temporarily shared premises with Indians, and any change in policy towards the latter was consequently bound to have repercussions for the former. Fourthly, the earlier belief in the practicability and desirability of institutionalizing not only European but also Eurasian and Indian lunatics slowly faded. By the 1840s local governments had become alerted to the ever-increasing overall cost of asylum provision. Furthermore, whilst earlier it may have been envisaged that a few asylums here and there would adequately provide for the lunatics of the land, such a belief was increasingly exposed as wishful thinking by mid-century. Consequently sporadic measures of admission restriction were endorsed whilst the deportation of Europeans was speeded up. Although the steadily rising number of asylum inmates seems to attest to the company's continued and increased subscription to institutionalization and to a policy of asylum extension, the local governments' efforts were in fact geared towards restricting the growth of the European and Indian asylum sector. Finally, the repatriation of asylum inmates came to be the decisive factor in containing European lunacy.[84] Although the company's stance towards the expatriate lunatic essentially derived from and was guided by contemporary ideas and practices extant in Britain, institutions for the European insane in British India certainly avoided one phenomenon characteristic of asylums in Europe: due to their inmates' regular transfer to England they would never develop into what had been dubbed 'museums for the collection of insanity'.[85]

It appears then that the European lunatic asylums in British India saw but a short period when they prospered and flourished as lucrative, expanding income sources for house proprietors as well as permanent institutions of a comparatively high standard. By the time of Queen Victoria's succession at the latest the institutions' purpose had changed considerably. The 'European Lunatic Asylums' had shrunk to small separate European wards in the three main asylums. These were then run as temporary receptacles for people in transit, and thus did not usually engender much concerted effort on the part of medical superintendents to pursue detailed diagnostic assessment and psychiatric treatment. Specialized medical and moral treatment would, it was generally envisaged, be administered at Pembroke House, back home in England, and would thus make any short-term attempts at cure prior to the passage to England superfluous. This attitude may partly account for the occasional indifference and carelessness exhibited by medical practitioners in preparing inmates' case reports and in supervising patients' transfer to Europe. For example, a patient was once, apparently unwittingly, entered in the books as a 'Joseph Haydn, a musician and a maniac', and, on another occasion, a Mr Schultze, a German missionary, had on the basis of medical case descriptions been mistaken for a lunatic by the port authorities, and duly been embarked for the long journey around the Cape of Good Hope.

That medical practitioners and provincial governments should expectantly turn their eyes to Europe was characteristic not only of the way in which the mentally ill were ultimately disposed of, but also of the practice of initially dealing with socially deviant or invalid Europeans on location in the east by discreetly locking them away while preparing for their deportation. Furthermore, the idea of service in India as a temporary vocation with a view to retirement in England had been prevalent from the late eighteenth century onwards. By the middle of the nineteenth century this concept had taken a firm hold amongst the various strata of the European community in India, making anything resembling a fresh rise of the European asylum in British India ever more unlikely. An asylum superintendent summarized in 1851 the dominant medical view when he stated that 'in no instance, after an attack of insanity should a man be permitted to remain in circumstances and relations which are obviously so likely to lead to a relapse'.[86] Fanny Parkes, in contrast, expressed the more sentimental/

reflective view of many Europeans in British India – not confined to those with a romantic disposition or a weak frame of mind:[87]

> Oh! Western shore! what would I not give for your breezes, to carry away this vile Indian languor and re-brace my nerves![88]

Had the Orient's allure made people long for the alien shore, it was the memory of more familiar and temperate lands that was evoked in times of dejection, hardship, or personal failure. Psychiatric institutions for Europeans in India may well have been called 'asylums'; however, they fell short of being perceived as such – as the ultimate places of refuge for the European expatriate in an alien country.

Notes

This chapter is based on my PhD thesis (see note 7). I want to express thanks to Prof. K. Ballhatchet (School of Oriental and African Studies, London) who read through several long-winded versions of my thesis and provided valuable advice and information. I am further indebted to Dr D. Arnold (University of Lancaster) for his critical interest and helpful remarks. Special thanks are due to M. Williams (Brunel University) for struggling through my verbose, teutonic syntax with a clear Anglo-Saxon mind and an editorial pencil; and for putting up with elaborate story-telling – against his own better (conceptual) judgement.

A fellowship by the Wellcome Trust has provided me with the material resources necessary for the pursuit of further research.

1 F. Richards (1936) *Old Soldier Sahib*, London: Faber, p. 14.

2 For a precursor to *Old Soldier Sahib* see J. Shipp (1829) *The Path of Glory. Being the Memoirs of the Extraordinary Military Career of John Shipp, written by himself*, London: Hurst (rev. edn ed. C.J. Stranks (1969), London: Chatto & Windus).

3 J.M. Holzman (1926) *The Nabobs in England: a study of the returned Anglo-Indian, 1760–1785*, New York: privately printed.

4 India Office Records, London (hereafter IOR): Asylum Report, 31–3–1852, in Medical Board to Government, 24–5–1853; Bombay Public Proceedings, 9–7–1853, 4537, 69.

5 Asylum Report, 31–3–1852 (note 4).

6 IOR: Madras Government's Despatch to the Court of Directors of the East India Company, Military Department (hereafter Madras Military Letter), 18–2–1794, 88.

7 W. Ernst (1986) 'Psychiatry and colonialism: the treatment of the European insane in British India, 1800–1858', University of London unpublished PhD thesis.

8 A. Halliday (1827) *A General View of the Present State of Lunatics, and Lunatic Asylums, in Great Britain and Ireland, and in some other Kingdoms*, London: Underwood, p. 68.

9 J. MacPherson (1856) 'Report on insanity among Europeans in Bengal, founded on the experience of the Calcutta Lunatic Asylum', review in *Calcutta Review* 26:594.

10 A.T. Scull (1982) *Museums of Madness: The Social Organization of Insanity in Nineteenth-Century England*, Harmondsworth: Penguin (1st edn (1979) London: Allen Lane).

11 What far-reaching Nemesis steered him
From his home by the cool of the sea?
When he left the fair country that reared him,
When he left her, His Mother, for thee,
That restless, disconsolate worker
Who strains now in vain at thy nets,
O sultry and sombre Noverca!
O Land of Regrets!
'The Land of Regrets', Sir Alfred Lyall, 1885.

12 E. Eden [1866] (1978) *Up the Country*, London: Curzon, p. 293. Emily Eden ends her reflection, stating 'I sometimes wonder they do not cut all our heads off, and say nothing more about it.' Her vision nearly became reality in 1857.

13 Figures estimated from S.C. Ghosh (1970) *The Social Condition of the British Community in Bengal, 1757–1800*, Leiden: Brill. (1863) *Royal Commission on the Sanitary State of the Army in India*, 2 vols, London: Eyre & Spottiswoode for HMSO. D. Arnold (1979) 'European orphans and vagrants in India in the nineteenth century', *Journal of Imperial and Commonwealth History* 7: 106–14.

14 D.G. Crawford (1914) *A History of the Indian Medical Service, 1600–1913*, London: Thacker, vol. 2, p. 415.

15 Ghosh, *The Social Condition of the British Community in Bengal*, p. 61.

16 IOR: Medical Board to Government, 4–2–1788; Bengal Military Proceedings, 13–2–1788. (Cf. Board's Collections, 1801, 127, 2343, n.p.). W. Dick was later to become the East India Company's Examining Physician in London (1809–18).

17 IOR: the Court of Directors of the East India Company's Despatch to the Government of Bengal, Military Department (hereafter Bengal Military Despatch), 8–4–1816, 3.

18 IOR: Bengal Military Despatch, 8–4–1817, 6.

19 IOR: Bengal Public Letter, 28–10–1817, 9, 28.

20 IOR: Medical Board to Government, 20–10–1847; Bengal Public Proceedings, 21–6–1848, 6, 10.

21 IOR: Bengal Government's Despatch to the Court of Directors of the East India Company, Public Department (hereafter Bengal Public Letter), 28–10–1817, 9, 28.

22 IOR: Minute by Governor-General, 6–11–1818; Bengal Public Proceedings, 27–11–1818, 6. Committee for reporting on the proposed measure of sending Insane Patients to Europe, 12–1–1819; Bengal Public Proceedings, 22–1–1819, 31.

23 ibid.

24 IOR: Medical Board to Government, 20–10–1847; Bengal Public Proceedings, 21–6–1848, 6, 13, 27.

25 IOR: Summary of Correspondence relative to the Calcutta Asylum for Insane Persons, Undersecretary to Government, 30–12–1847; Board's Collections, 1852, 2494, 141,296, 15.

26 IOR: Bengal Public Proceedings, 13–7–1836, 23. The 'Medical Code' of 1838 contained 'no orders on the subject of insane hospitals' in contrast to the Code of 1819. See Summary of Correspondence (note 25), 16.

27 IOR: Note on Bhowanipore Asylum, no date; Board's Collections, 1852, 2494, 141,296, 112 ff.

28 IOR: Medical Board to Government, 31–5–1836; Bengal Public Proceedings, 21–6–1848, 6 (Enclosure).

29 F.G. Hutchins (1967) *The Illusion of Permanence: British Imperialism in India*, Princeton: Princeton University Press.

30 K. Ballhatchet (1980) *Race, Sex and Class under the Raj: Imperial Attitudes and Policies and their Critics, 1793–1905*, London: Weidenfeld & Nicolson.

31 IOR: Asylum Report, 14–6–1856; Bengal Public Proceedings, 24–6–1856, 52, no para. Summary of Correspondence (note 25), 40. Annual Return of Patients treated in the Asylum for European Insanes at Bhowanipore during the year 1859, 1–1–1860; Bengal Medical Proceedings, 12–1–1860, 37.

32 IOR: Medical Board to Government, 10–3–1851; Bengal Public Proceedings, 24–6–1852, 6.

33 IOR: Accountant General to Government, 21–3–1850; Bengal Public Proceedings, 28–8–1850, 13, no para.

34 IOR: Madras Military Letter, 18–2–1794, 88. Madras Military Letter, 16–10–1794, 6. Madras Military Despatch, 6–5–1795, 72.

35 IOR: Medical Board to Government, 15–2–1808; Madras Military Proceedings, 4–3–1808, 153 ff, 2400 ff. Medical Board to Government, 9–2–1821; Madras Military Proceedings, 9–2–1821, 12. Military Board to Government, 28–8–1846; Madras Military Proceedings, 29–9–1846, 441. Medical Board to Government, 10–1–1852; Madras Military Proceedings, 23–1–1852, 10.

36 Crawford, *A History of the Indian Medical Service*, p. 415. Madras Military Letter, 18–2–1794, 88. Madras Military Despatch, 6–5–1795, 72.

37 S. Lee and L. Stephen (eds) (1887) *The Dictionary of National Biography*, London: Oxford University Press, vol. 12, p. 24.

38 IOR: Madras Military Letter, 17–2–1802, 182. Madras Military Letter, 19–1–1821, 22 f., 30. Madras Military Despatch, 20–8–1823, 40 f.

39 Surgeon J. Dalton had bought the asylum for Rs 91,000. The building itself had been valued by government at only Rs 39,756. In 1815 Dalton wished to sell it for the sum of Rs 91,000 to a Dr Macleod. IOR: Madras Military Despatch, 20–8–1823, 40 f.

40 Crawford, *A History of the Indian Medical Service* (note 14), p. 415. Madras Military Proceedings, 29–9–1846, 441. Like many other medical practitioners Dalton, too, was a prominent Madras citizen, well known not so much for professional achievements but for family connections. His wife was a Catherina Augusta Ritso, said to have been the daughter of George III by Hannah Lightfoot. Although this family connection seems somewhat far-fetched – given the ages of the parties involved – it obviously did much to excite the European community's imagination.

41 IOR: Resolution, 13–12–1808; Madras Military Proceedings, 13–12–1808, 11517.

42 IOR: Madras Military Despatch, 24–5–1820, 12 f.

43 See advertisement by Dr G. Rees (February 1819) in *The East India Register and Army List*, London: Allen. The procedure of sending 'Indian Insanes' to Pembroke House was 'not affected by the transfer from the Company to the Crown in 1858'. See IOR: Records of Pembroke House and Ealing Lunatic Asylum, 'Indian Insanes', Memorandum. In 1870 patients were transferred to the newly established Royal India Lunatic Asylum in Ealing, where they were

provided for until 1892, when the remaining seventy-six patients were either transferred to other psychiatric hospitals or were handed over to the care of their family or friends. See W. Ernst and D. Kantowsky (1983) 'Mad tales from the Raj: case studies from Pembroke House and Ealing Lunatic Asylum. 1818–1892', *Papers of the Eighth European Conference on Modern South Asian Studies*, Taellberg: Sweden. See for a shortened version, Ernst and Kantowsky (1985) 'Mad tales from the Raj', *Transaction/Society* 3: 31–8.

44 IOR: Asylum Report, 15–2–1808; Madras Military Proceedings, 4–3–1808, 153 ff., 2400 ff. Medical Board to Government, 9–2–1821; Madras Military Proceedings, 9–2–1821, 12. Military Board to Government, 28–8–1846; Madras Military Proceedings, 29–9–1846, 441. Medical Board to Government, 10–1–1852; Madras Military Proceedings, 23–1–1852, 10.

45 IOR: Chief Magistrate and Superintendent of Police to Military Board, 21–8–1852; Madras Judicial Letter, 30–10–1852, 2. Medical Board, Superintending Surgeon, Chief Magistrate, Medical Officer in Charge to Government, no date; Madras Judicial Letter, 30–10–1852, 3. Madras Judicial Letter, 12–11–1850, 1 f.

46 IOR: Chief Magistrate and Superintendent of Police to Military Board, 21–8–1852; Madras Judicial Letter, 30–10–1852, 2.

47 IOR: Madras Public Despatch, 26–5–1824, 46. Madras Judicial Despatch, 8–9–1824, 44. Madras Military Despatch, 24–8–1825, 69.

48 IOR: The Asylum Returns of 1808, for example, mention the names of seven Indian patients. Madras Military Proceedings, 4–3–1808, 153–183.

49 IOR: Bengal Public Despatch, 28–6–1820, 94.

50 IOR: Medical Board to Government, 5–2–1821; Bengal Public Proceedings, 20–2–1821, 32, no para. For a description of the development of lunatic asylums for 'natives' see W. Ernst, 'The establishment of "Native Lunatic Asylums" in early nineteenth-century British India', in G.J. Meulenbeld and D. Wujastyk (eds) (1987) *Studies on Indian Medical History*, Groningen: Egbert Forsten.

51 IOR: G.A. Berwick, M.D. to Government, 5–3–1847; Bengal Public Proceedings, 26–5–1847, 12.

52 IOR: Medical Board to Government, 20–10–1847; Bengal Public Proceedings, 21–6–1848, 6, 41.

53 IOR: Superintending Surgeon to Medical Board, 23–1–1846; Madras Military Proceedings, 10–2–1846, 705.

54 IOR: Asylum Superintendent to Superintending Surgeon, 15–7–1846, in: Medical Board to Government, 23–7–1846; Madras Military Proceedings, 28–7–1846, 118.

55 IOR: Madras Military Despatch, 31–3–1852, 3.

56 IOR: Madras Citizens to Government, 28–11–1851; Madras Military Proceedings, 16–12–1851, 3702.

57 IOR: Minute of Second Member of Medical Board, in: Medical Board to Government, 15–2–1808; Madras Military Proceedings, 4–3–1808, 153–183.

58 Crawford, *A History of the Indian Medical Service*, p. 416.

59 Patients diagnosed as 'idiots' were sent to the infirmary for Indians while patients suffering from 'criminal insanity' were transferred to the gaol. IOR: Madras Public Despatch, 26–5–1824, 46. Military Board to Government, 28–8–1846; Madras Military Proceedings, 29–9–1846, 441. Medical Board to Government, 17–3–1852; Madras Military Proceedings, 6–4–1852, 62.

60 P. Woodruff [1955] (1971) *The Men Who Ruled India*, London: Jonathan Cape,

vol. 1, pp. 64–9. P. Spear (1980) *The Nabobs. A study of the social life of the English in eighteenth-century India*, London and Dublin: Curzon (enlarged edn [1932] 1963), pp. 66–79.

61 Crawford. *A History of the Indian Medical Service*, p. 400.

62 IOR: Medical Board to Government, 19–6–1820; Bombay Military Proceedings, 28–6–1820, no number (p. 3380), 12.

63 IOR: Medical Board to Government, 19–6–1820 (notes 62), 15.

64 IOR: Medical Board to Government, 24–5–1853; Bombay Public Proceedings, 9–7–1853, 4536, 15. Minute, 7–6–1849; Bombay Public Proceedings, 11–7–1849, 3610. Asylum Report, 31–3–1849, in: Medical Board to Government, 18–5–1849; Bombay Public Proceedings, 11–7–1849, 3609, 10.

65 IOR: Bombay Public Letter, 16–4–1851, 11. Superintending Surgeon, Karachi, to Commissioner in Sind, 1–2–1850, in: Commissioner in Sind to Government, 16–2–1850; Bombay Public Proceedings, 13–4–1850, 1999.

66 IOR: Minute, 7–6–1849; Bombay Public Proceedings, 11–7–1849, 3610. Asylum Report, 31–3–1849, in: Medical Board to Government, 18–5–1849; Bombay Public Proceedings, 11–7–1849, 3609, 10. Medical Board to Government, 19–6–1820 (note 62), 15. Minute, 7–6–1849; Bombay Public Proceedings, 11–7–1849, 3610.

67 IOR: Minute, 26–7–1849; Bombay Public Proceedings, 8–8–1849, 2.

68 IOR: Further Minute (Governor Falkland), 2–11–1849; Bombay Public Proceedings, 14–11–1849, 6288, 9.

69 IOR: Minute (Governor Falkland), 7–9–1850; Bombay Public Proceedings, 9–10–1850, 7655.

70 IOR: Further Minute, 2–11–1849 (note 68), 9.

71 IOR: Asylum Report, 31–3–1849, in: Medical Board to Government, 18–5–1849; Bombay Public Proceedings, 11–7–1849, 3609, 10.

72 IOR: Asylum Report, 31–3–1849 (note 71), 11.

73 IOR: Minute 7–9–1850 (note 69), no para. Minute (Governor Falkland) 28–2–1851; Bombay Public Proceedings, 4–4–1851, 2279. Based on previous recommendation: Medical Board to Government, 18–5–1849; Bombay Public Proceedings. 11–7–1849, 3608, 4. Minute, 22–10–1849; Bombay Public Proceedings, 14–11–1846, 6285. Separate Minutes of 25–10–1849; Bombay Public Proceedings, 14–11–1849, 6286 and 6286.

74 IOR: Separate Minute, 7–12–1850; Bombay Public Proceedings, 4–4–1851, 2269, no para.

75 In 1790 British India's first Medical Society was founded in Bombay. Not much is known about its members' activities and it can be assumed that its professional leverage was not very great. This slowly changed with the establishment of the Medical and Physical Society of Bombay (1838), which became particularly renowned for its *Transactions*. In 1845 the Grant Medical College was opened. Finally, the Bombay branch of the British Medical Association was established in 1889. See Crawford, *A History of the Indian Medical Service*, pp. 454–5.

76 Especially during M. Elphinstone's time as governor. He was backed by J. Mill, examiner of the company's records, and described as 'a sincere trumpeter of Panopticon' (J. Bentham to Col. J. Young, 28–12–1827, *Works*, vol. X, p. 577). Cf. E. Stokes [1959] (1982) *The English Utilitarians and India*, Delhi: Oxford University Press, p. 325, note I. The panopticon idea was later also realized in the Punjab. See ibid., p. 247.

77 IOR: Medical Board to Government, 19–6–1820 (note 62), 10 and 12. Asylum

Superintendent to Medical Board, 30–10–1820; Bombay Military Proceedings, 8–11–1820, no number, no para (p. 5884). Medical Board to Government, 3–7–1820; Bombay Military Proceedings, 19–7–1820, no number (p. 3715). Medical Board to Government, 3–8–1820; Bombay Military Proceedings, 9–8–1820, no number (p. 4172).

78 IOR: Medical Board to Government, 24–8–1850; Bombay Public Proceedings, 9–10–1850, 7105, 1.

79 IOR: Medical Board to Government, 3–9–1853; Bombay Public Proceedings, 30–11–1853, 8549, 13 ff.

80 IOR: Medical Board to Government, 19–6–1820 (note 62), 4 f.

81 IOR: Medical Board to Government, 22–6–1852; Bombay Public Proceedings, 14–7–1852, 5471, 1.

82 IOR: Proposed Establishment of a Central Lunatic Asylum at Bombay; Board's Collection, 1855, 2596, 157,738. The provincial officials' view was obviously shared by the London authorities. See India Public Despatch, 6–6–1855, 7 f.

83 In 1849 Dr W. Arbuckle, the then asylum superintendent, observed that the institution had previously been misused as a receptacle for what he called 'alleged lunatics'. He provided statistical evidence for this assertion, pointing out that with stricter observance of administrative rules and regulations the number of persons improperly confined in the asylum had dropped. IOR: Asylum Report, 31–3–1849 (note 64), 5.

84 This is not to say that deportation had been a measure applied solely towards the mentally ill. Far from it – European invalids, vagabonds, rogues, wily crimps, 'bad characters' as well as criminals and shady punch-house owners had been sent back to England ever since the eighteenth century. Lunatics were thus just one among many social groups whose presence in the colony was deemed undesirable and feared to occasion detrimental effects to commercial and imperial ambitions. See for examples of cases of 'European crimes in Bengal, 1766–1800' Spear, *The Nabobs* pp. 192–4.

85 F. Scott (1879) in the *Fortnightly Review*. Cf. Scull, *Museums of Madness*, p. 186.

86 IOR: Records of Pembroke House and Ealing Lunatic Asylum, Medical Certificates, 1852, Case of H. Strauch.

87 See for an example of nostalgia and despair, that expressed by a luckless young blacksmith – by the name of John Luck – from Market Deeping in Lincolnshire who had enlisted as a gunner in the East India Company's artillery in 1839. He wrote to his mother from Kanpur in April 1841: 'My Dear Mother i often think of the Diference of the 3 last new years days one to be comfortable at home the next to be tost by the billows to and fro and on the deck not able to help my self . . . and this new years day to be on the burning plain encampt among the howling of wild beasts . . . all my wandring through this world of care all my greaf and God have given me my share i still have hopes when my long campains is passed ham to return and die at home at last.' On hearing that his mother had bought him out of the army he wrote in July 1842: 'i ham so ancious to se my dear native home agane . . . i know too well this country would soon kill me.' IOR: European Manuscripts, 'My Dear Mother . . . if for ever o a due, sell not my ole close!', Gunner John Luck's letters from India, 1839–44, letters 6, 11.

88 Cf. Woodruff, *The Men Who Ruled India*, p. 316.

CHAPTER THREE

'Morbid introspection', unsoundness of mind, and British psychological medicine, *c.*1830–*c.*1900

Michael J. Clark

The student can study mild forms of mental disorder in himself . . . he will find such introspection of great assistance in comprehending the more advanced disorders of others.
Maurice Craig (1905) *Psychological Medicine*, p. 49

Introduction

Sir Henry Holland, successively Physician-Extraordinary to William IV, Queen Victoria, and the Prince Consort, long-serving president of the Royal Institution, and perhaps the leading society physician of early-Victorian London, thought that he was the first modern 'psychological physician' seriously to have drawn attention to the dangers of habitual self-absorption, 'morbid introspection', and exaggerated self-consciousness to healthy mind and morals, in his essay 'On Dreaming, Insanity, Intoxication, etc.' (1839, 1852). 'Certain cases of madness', he warned,

> depend on a cause which can scarcely exist, even in slight degree, without producing some mental disturbance; viz. *the too frequent and earnest direction of the mind inwards upon itself.*[1]

Holland and his fellow Victorian physicians were, however, only the most recent and very partial heirs to an ancient, highly complex cultural tradition, stretching back through the Renaissance to antiquity, which stressed the grave danger to health, morals, and sanity from habits of intense introspection, 'day-dreaming', and reverie, especially when pursued in solitude and under the influence of sedentary habits.[2] And at least since the Scottish physician John Reid had included a chapter on the 'injuriousness of solitude in mental alienation' in his *Essays on Hypochondriacal and*

Other Nervous Affections (1816, 1821), the dangers of morbid introspection and habitual self-absorption had been one of the most insistently recurring themes in Victorian psychiatric literature.[3] During the latter part of the nineteenth century, however, this persistent medical concern with the dangers of introspection and self-absorption took on a new intensity and force. Thus according to Henry Maudsley, himself incurably subject to the condition,

> An excessive self-consciousness is the sorest of human afflictions.... Is it not veritably in the long run more painful than cancer, more paralysing than paralysis, more demoralising than despair?[4]

'By self-introspection and self-analysis', he warned,

> a *morbid egoism* is fostered ... a tender conscience of that kind, overrating its own importance, may easily pass into insanity, unless counterbalanced by the sobering influence of active outward preoccupations and interests.[5]

Throughout the works of Maudsley, Charles Mercier, Daniel Hack Tuke, Thomas Clouston, William Bevan Lewis, and many other late-nineteenth-century British authorities on 'psychological medicine', 'morbid introspection', almost invariably in conjunction with habitual self-absorption and unnatural egoism, forms one of the principal constitutive elements of their conception of 'unsound Mind'. In their view, introspection and self-absorption, persistent abstention from ordinary social intercourse, and neglect of active pursuits all tended to weaken the will, undermine the 'natural' moral affections, and encourage idleness, eccentricity, and the growth of perverse or immoral tendencies. Absorption in purely 'subjective' states of consciousness, they argued, upset the 'natural' mental balance by impairing the capacity to receive and react to external impressions, and by withdrawing or suspending the control habitually exercised by the will and judgement over the succession of thoughts and feelings. This dethronement of reason and will in turn favoured the development of 'dominant', 'imperative', or obsessional ideas or trains of thought, of morbid emotional states, and of mental automatism, and thus by degrees passed over into actual mental disorder.[6] Introspection was further associated, on the one hand, with exclusive attention to morbid ideas suggested by disordered internal sensations, and thus with hypochondriasis and hysteria; and, on the other hand, with selfish, anti-social behaviour and perverse moral tendencies, and thus with 'moral insanity' and 'moral imbecility'.[7] More specifically, morbid introspection and habitual self-absorption were believed to be the most constant symptomatic accompaniments of the 'chronic delusional insanity of pubescence' – the *dementia praecox* of Kraepelin – and were thus inextricably bound up with inflated egoism, emotional religiosity, and what Bevan Lewis called 'secret sins and sexual vices', in the peculiar mental condition regarded as characteristic of this 'adolescent psychosis'.[8]

In this essay I shall not attempt to trace the origins of the Victorian psychiatric literature of 'morbid introspection' in the classic 'Melancholia' tradition of the Renaissance and previous epochs, nor shall I attempt to follow the theme through all its various manifestations in the arts and literature of the Victorian period. Rather, I intend to concentrate on certain aspects and associations of the late-nineteenth-century medico-psychological literature of morbid introspection which serve to highlight several most important aspects of later-Victorian psychiatric theory and practice. Accordingly, I shall begin by stating more clearly what 'morbid introspection' meant, and what role it played in Victorian psychiatric theory, before going on to discuss some of its more important secondary associations, notably with imagination; with 'dominant', 'imperative', or obsessional ideas; with hypochondriasis and hysteria; and with 'moral insanity' and 'moral imbecility'. Finally, I shall examine some of the implications which these ideas and associations were to have for the *practice* of psychiatry, especially for the 'moral management' of the insane, the 'mental hygiene' of childhood and adolescence, and the psychological interpretation and treatment of insanity.

'Morbid introspection' and 'unsound mind'

For the Victorian 'psychological physician', the state of 'morbid introspection' – the habitual turning of the mind inwards upon itself to the virtual exclusion of external impressions, accompanied by the temporary or partial suspension of will and judgement – was perhaps the most characteristic symptom of 'unsound Mind', and the very antithesis of 'mental soundness'. In his view, 'mental soundness' consisted in the capacity to register 'objective' stimuli and form correct perceptions of external reality, to make correspondingly exact and intelligent judgements, and to adjust one's conduct accordingly; while the criteria for determining it were the degree to which the mental 'powers' which served to sustain this 'objective' mental orientation – namely, the power of the reason to form correct perceptions and make 'just comparisons' between impressions and ideas, and voluntary control over the instincts, imagination, and feelings – were retained. As the physiologist William Carpenter put it,

> in proportion as our Will acquires domination over our Automatic tendencies, the spontaneous succession of our Ideas and the play of our Emotions show the influence of its habitual control; while our Character and Conduct . . . come to be the expression of our best Intellectual energies, directed by the Motives which we *determinately elect* as our guiding principles.[9]

This ideal conception of 'sound Mind' may be contrasted with Robert Brudenell Carter's vivid account of the state of mental imbalance and moral degradation consequent upon the enslavement of the will to a single 'dominant' or 'imperative' idea.

> If the human will be . . . completely surrendered to the dominion of an idea, the unnatural ruler is apt to run riot with its captive, – leading it into the depths of bigotry, or through the mazes of fanaticism; and always liable to be exhausted by the very violence of its own manifestations. Then follow the phenomena of mental reaction. The idea first in possession is succeeded by another, commonly of a directly opposite character; and, after the occurrence of a few similar changes, the mind loses its individuality, and, like a mirror, does but passively reflect the appearances [and suggestions] of external objects.[10]

These were extreme cases, but Victorian medical psychologists were almost unanimous in maintaining that the difference between sanity and madness was only one of degree – that the one passed insensibly into the other through a whole range of intermediate conditions exhibiting various degrees of departure from the ideal of 'sound Mind'. As Carpenter put it:

> *Between the state of the well-balanced Mind*, in which the habit of Self-control has been thoroughly established, so that its whole activity is directed by the Moral Will of the Ego – *and that of the raving madman*, whose reasoning power is utterly gone, who is the sport of uncontrollable passions, and is lost to every feeling of [morality] . . . *vast as the interval may seem, there is an insensible gradation.*[11]

It was for this reason that Henry Maudsley declared:

> It is in . . . *excess* that madness lies – in the *exaggerated development of natural passions of human nature*, not in the appearance of new passions in it[12]

explaining that

> the various biasses of prejudice, passion, temper, interest and the like, which turn the mind from the straight path of truth . . . are just the causes which, when carried to excess, tend towards madness or [some] other mental aberration.[13]

Madness and other, milder forms of 'unsound Mind' consisted, then, not in the introduction of any unfamiliar alienating influences into the life of the individual, but simply in the exaggeration, immoderate indulgence, or one-sided development of the natural instincts and feelings – in what John Conolly described as

> [the] mere aggravation of little weaknesses, or . . . prolongation of transient varieties and moods of mind . . . [the] exaggeration of common passions and emotions . . . or [the] perpetuation of absurdities of thought or action . . . of irregularities of volition, or of mere sensation, which may occur in all minds, or be indulged in by all men.[14]

Of all the mental conditions likely to favour the development of eccentric habits, unbridled passions, 'dominant' ideas, and selfish, immoral tendencies, none was more likely to do so than the state of 'morbid introspection', especially when practised under the influence of solitary pursuits and sedentary habits. 'Nothing tends so much to increase [the strength of immoral tendencies]', warned Carpenter,

> as the continual direction of the mind towards the objects of its gratification, especially under the ... influence of sedentary habits; whilst nothing so effectually represses it, as the determinate exercise of the mental faculties upon other objects, and the expenditure of nervous energy in other channels.[15]

It was, therefore, of the utmost importance that all right-thinking people should conscientiously eschew introspection and self-absorption, and instead cultivate healthy, outgoing pursuits and interests, and the special duty of 'psychological physicians' was to diffuse and inculcate these doctrines and habits, if the dangers attendant upon mental imbalance were to be avoided, and health, morals, and sanity to be preserved.[16]

The state of habitual self-absorption or 'morbid introspection' was, therefore, primarily implicated in the development of a great variety of abnormal mental states, ranging from mere eccentricity to chronic insanity, but all included within the elastic formula of 'unsound Mind'. The association of morbid introspection, exaggerated self-consciousness, and 'unnatural egoism' with mental disorder was thus fundamental, even causal, rather than merely symptomatic or accidental. Except perhaps in extreme cases of idiocy or dementia, the one could scarcely exist without the other. This association gave physicians a vague yet congenial notion, even a criterion, of what constituted 'unsound Mind' (and, by contradistinction, of what qualities made for 'sound Mind'); and thus provided a kind of base-line or starting-point from which an elaborate conceptual superstructure was to be evolved. This essay will attempt to trace some of the principal lines of departure taken from this starting-point, around which so much of the theory and practice of later-Victorian 'psychological medicine' were organized.

The problem of the imagination

As we have seen, the condition of 'sound Mind', in which reason and will governed the succession of thought and feeling, was familiarly contrasted with that of 'unsound Mind', in which reason and will were at least temporarily in abeyance, and emotion, nourished by imagination, held unchecked sway. There was nothing intrinsically unhealthy or immoral in the 'judicious exercise' of the imagination, provided that it did not exceed the bounds of due proportion. 'It is not ... the imagination that is allied [with] madness', Conolly explained, 'but its excess, in minds unendowed with a proportionate share of the other faculties.'[17] Indeed, it was generally accepted that, as the Scottish physician and moralist John Abercrombie put it,

> The sound and proper exercise of [the Imagination] may be made to contribute to the cultivation of all that is virtuous and estimable in human character.[18]

Following the tradition of Scottish moral philosophy, Abercrombie maintained that it was chiefly through the imagination that the characteristic manifestations of 'sympathy' – the sentiments of charity, pity, loving-kindness, forgiveness, and unselfish generosity – were aroused, and the human mind elevated to the contemplation of the Sublime, and thence to that of the Deity;[19] while Robert Dunn and John Morell stressed the role of imagination in the highest creative achievements of intellect, not merely in the arts and literature, but in science and philosophy as well.[20] But although it was recognized that imagination and reason were creatively blended together in the highest products of civilization and culture, there remained a fundamental antithesis, or at least a tension, between the original, unmodified character of imagination, and those intellectual and moral qualities of right reason, sound judgement, and volitional control which, in Conolly's words, 'enabled [an individual] to judge . . . and to act well in all ordinary emergencies', and which alone could ensure 'health and soundness of mind'.[21] Thus, according to Abercrombie, the imagination, when properly exercised, 'under the strict control . . . of reason and . . . virtue', could ennoble the mind and strengthen the moral sense; but left to itself, 'it tends to withdraw the mind from the important pursuits of life, to weaken the habit of [voluntary] attention, and to impair the judgement'.[22] Imagination, he warned, could either originate or give a semblance of reality to nightmares, hallucinations, irrational fears, obsessional ideas, unnatural or immoral feelings, and irresistible impulses; while excessive indulgence in 'works of fiction' encouraged licentious excesses, and could bring about 'a disruption of the harmony which ought to exist between the moral [sentiments] and . . . conduct'.[23] Brudenell Carter and Carpenter emphasized further that habitual indulgence of the imagination for purposes of emotional gratification or relief tended to paralyse the will, alienate the 'natural' moral affections, and predispose the subject to hypochondriasis and hysteria.[24] In later decades, medico-psychological commentators were, if anything, even less willing to acknowledge the benefits which 'judicious exercise' of the imagination might confer, while being no less concerned to stress the dangers inherent in its excessive indulgence. 'The excessive cultivation of the imagination,' warned Hack Tuke, 'castle-building, and the absorption of the mind in works of fiction, are highly detrimental to the mind's health';[25] while Theophilus Hyslop echoed Abercrombie's warning of more than half a century earlier, when he wrote:

> The imagination is a function . . . which requires most careful watching. In . . . 'day-dreamers' you have an example of the result of [its] exces-

> sive indulgence.... Such an individual is generally purposeless. With too diffuse a consciousness [of the kind typical of 'day-dreaming' and reverie] there is apt to evolve an unhealthy conceit, especially in adolescents.[26]

In the works of Hack Tuke and Hyslop, and in the similar contemporary admonitions of Mercier and Clouston, warnings against excessive indulgence of the imagination have lost something of the more universal application which they had for earlier commentators, and become more particularly associated with the special problems of the mental hygiene of adolescence. We shall return to this development later.[27] Here, however, I shall emphasize a more general aspect of the problem of the imagination. The imagination, it was agreed, was an original and essential mental power, whose judicious exercise could greatly enhance its possessor's quality of life – and, indeed, that of the community as a whole. But whereas its *regulation* was undoubtedly necessary for the preservation of sound mind and healthy morals, its *positive cultivation and development*, unlike that of attention, volition, or the 'faculty of just comparison', was not, and was, moreover, likely to prove highly detrimental. Whereas a lively, yet well-regulated imagination might conceivably bring real distinction to even the most ordinary pursuits, it was not absolutely necessary in order to achieve even very high levels of competence in the ordinary business of life, while the dangers which might ensue from its attempted cultivation were so great, and the prospects of real creative achievement so slight, that it seemed hardly worth the risk involved. As Conolly put it:

> The ordinary circumstances of life ... do not require the possession of genius.... The most enviable condition of mind is that by which an individual is enabled to judge ... and to act well in all ordinary emergencies. This is health and soundness of mind; the result of the harmonious action of all the mental faculties. It is compatible with great and useful acquisitions; but ... does not invent or add.... It does not prompt its possessor to challenge the attention and admiration of the world; but its utility is constant.[28]

Failure to cultivate the imagination might mean some sacrifice of life's potential for enjoyment and achievement, but for all save the most exceptional of men, the plenteous rewards of deliberate cultivation of the reason and will would amply justify the effort and self-sacrifice involved, and more than compensate for whatever might have been lost in the way of a richer imaginative life.

The danger of 'dominant' ideas

Closely bound up with the question of regulating the power of the imagination was the problem of 'dominant', 'imperative', or obsessional ideas or trains of thought. Victorian alienists devoted much attention to the legal and philosophical difficulties raised by the controversial diagnosis of 'monomania', that is, insanity with respect to only one mental faculty, idea, or train of thought;[29] but the category of 'monomania' was only one of many morbid mental conditions in which 'dominant ideas' were causally implicated and more or less conspicuously developed. Whenever the mind was turned in upon itself for long periods, to the virtual exclusion of external impressions, there tended to arise sooner or later some idea, feeling, or train of thought with a special interest or attraction for it; and unless the idea were speedily checked and rationally compared with other impressions or ideas, it would soon engross the attention, gain a morbid ascendancy over the will and judgement, and come to dominate the entire mental life and conduct. As Holland warned,

> the long persistence of the mind in one idea or feeling, not duly broken in upon or blended with others, is a state always leading towards [mental] aberration.

One of the commonest indications of the onset of insanity, he believed, was 'the predominance of a single impression [in the mind]'.[30] The 'natural', healthy condition of the mind, Hyslop explained, was 'poly-ideational', a state in which a number of different impressions, feelings, and ideas, arising both from within and without, were competing for attention on roughly equal terms. But under the influence of 'hyperattention' – the intense and exclusive direction of the attention towards one particular idea, class of ideas, or train of thought – the mind tended to pass into 'mono-ideism', a morbid state in which 'dominant' or obsessional ideas rapidly succeeded each other at the prompting of internal or external suggestions unchecked by the will.[31] In Hyslop's view, all the principal forms of insanity could be distinguished by the different ratios in which attention was divided between 'objective' and 'subjective' stimuli. Thus in states of depression, there was 'a tendency to subjective hyperattention, with a corresponding ratio of inattention to objective stimuli', and in 'states of mental exaltation', there was 'subjective inattention and a corresponding variation in objective attention, or hyperattention'; while in 'states of mental enfeeblement', there was 'absence of the power of attention to events both within and without'.[32] The degree of 'hyperattention' possible without serious risk of mental disorder could, he admitted, vary widely between individuals. But the very 'laws' of mental and 'neural' habit which made possible the systematic cultivation of voluntary attention made it all the more difficult to rid the mind of dominant ideas, once they had acquired some special attraction for the attention; and the only safe policy was therefore systematically to vary both the objects of contemplation, and the direction of the attention towards internal and external impressions respectively. Among the characteristic pathological products of morbid 'hyperattention', Hyslop listed not only frequently recurring imperative ideas, but also fixed delusions of grandeur, of persecution, and of external influence or control by unseen agencies, and the phenomena of 'irresistible impulses'.[33]

In his *Principles of Mental Physiology*, William Carpenter placed even greater stress on the danger of allowing the attention to become engrossed by dominant ideas or suggestions. 'The continued concentration of Attention upon a certain idea,' he warned,

> gives it a *dominant* power, not only over the mind, but over the body; and the muscles become the involuntary instruments whereby it is carried into operation.[34]

Unless such dominant ideas or habitual trains of thought were speedily brought to the test of 'Common Sense', and shaken off by an effort of will, they would quickly tend to overpower the judgement, annul their victims' power of self-determination, and reduce them to mere conscious automata. 'If the Mind should lose for a time all power of Volitional self-direction', he explained,

> it cannot recall any fact ... that is beyond its immediate grasp; its attention being engrossed with the idea that ... [is] before it ... no incongruity prevents that idea from presenting itself with all the vividness of reality; – it cannot bring any notion with which it may be possessed to the test of 'Common Sense', but *must* accept it as a belief, if it be impressed on the consciousness with adequate force; it cannot shake off the yoke of any 'dominant idea', however tyrannical, but *must* execute its behests.[35]

'Dominant' or 'imperative' ideas, Carpenter emphasized, could come about either as the result of repeated acts of selective attention to some idea or feeling arising spontaneously within consciousness, or by way of some suggestion from without accepted by the will. The phenomena of dominant or imperative ideas were thus closely akin to those of hypnotism, somnambulism, 'electro-biology', and other artificially induced states characterized by partial or complete suspension of the will and judgement, the complete possession of the mind by one idea or suggestion, and the automatic performance of its dictates.[36] In every case the will was fundamentally implicated, whether through deliberate choice or tacit consent; and in every case, the eventual outcome was the phenomenon of 'mental reaction' – the loss, either partial or complete, of mental and moral autonomy, and the consequent degradation of the individual. Carpenter recognized that the phenomena of 'Expectant Attention' were natural and ubiquitous, and might easily be evoked in otherwise perfectly healthy persons.[37] And just as the phenomena of 'Expectant Attention' might to varying degrees be evoked in almost anyone, so also the original power of the will to resist temptations and overcome dominant ideas might vary considerably from person to person.[38] But he denied that there were any 'imperative' ideas, temptations, or suggestions which were absolutely beyond the power of individuals to resist, moderate, or offset. There were, indeed, people who had 'come at last so far as to have lost [their] power of self-control, as to be unable to resist ... temptation to what is known to be wrong'.[39] Such persons, however, although 'morally irresponsible for the particular act[s]' suggested by their dominant ideas, were nevertheless *'responsible for [their] irresponsibility'*, because they had 'wilfully abnegated [their] power of self-control, by habitually yielding to temptations which [they] know ... [they] ought to have resisted'.[40] Thus for Carpenter, belief in free will as the basis of moral responsibility remained unshaken by demonstrations of the ubiquity of the phenomena of mental automatism. The lessons to be drawn from the scientific study of these abnormal mental states were, first, the dangers of habitual self-indulgence and, second, the abiding responsibility of the individual for the continuous formation of his own 'Character' through the deliberate exercise of his capacity for moral choice.[41] Though few of Carpenter's contemporaries could match the systematic moral allusiveness of his rhetoric, this characteristic association of habitual self-indulgence with lack of will-power, 'dwarfed *morale*', mental automatism, and diminished responsibility may be traced throughout the Victorian medical literature of dominant ideas and morbid introspection.

'Morbid introspection', hysteria, and hypochondriasis

The association of morbid introspection and habitual self-absorption with hypochondriasis and hysteria is one of the oldest and most constant medico-psychological associations to have grown up around these themes since the Renaissance. In his *Essays on Hypochondriasis*, Reid had stressed this association, repeating Burton's famous injunction: *'Be not solitary; be not idle'*,[42] and this warning note was sounded throughout the Victorian literature of psychiatry and mental hygiene. Just as the exclusive direction of the attention towards some single idea, emotion, or train of thought tended progressively to increase its hold over the mind, and could eventually result in the complete subjugation of the reason and will, so, it was believed, the persistent 'morbid solicitation' of the attention towards some real or imagined bodily pain or ailment could eventually derange the vital functions, and even induce pathological changes in the organs themselves. Thus actual organic disease could succeed to hypochondriasis or hysteria through the excessive indulgence of morbid sensations and feelings, especially when combined with insufficient exercise and an unhealthy dietary regimen.[43] Brudenell Carter made this into one of the principal themes of his work on the pathology, prevention, and treatment of hysteria and allied nervous disorders. He went so far as to define 'introspection' as 'attention [given, whether voluntarily or involuntarily] to ... ideas suggested, directly or indirectly, by bodily sensations';[44] and argued that, since local bodily sensations were scarcely perceptible in conditions of physical and mental health, they must be regarded as pathological indications, and that sustained attention to them must therefore be hysterogenic, if not actually symptomatic of incipient hysteria.[45] Following Holland and Carpenter, Carter warned that persistent attention to real or imagined bodily pains or disorders would not only tend to increase their intensity and duration, but also make their spontaneous recurrence more likely, and even induce pathological changes in the circulation and nutrition of the parts affected, especially when accompanied by some strong emotion, a view reaffirmed by Hack Tuke in his work on the *Influence of the Mind Upon the Body* (1872).[46] Towards the end of the century Bevan Lewis was to incorporate the familiar identification of unconsciousness of bodily sensations with mental and physical well-being into a general Ego-psychology based on the evolutionary physiological psychologies of Spencer, Maudsley, and Hughlings Jackson, which sought to explain various morbid transformations of the Ego in physiodynamic terms. 'In healthy states of [physical and mental] activity', he argued,

> the ingoing [nervous] currents arouse ... none but the massive feeling of *pleasurable well-being* ... only when the bodily functions are deranged [do] we become ... conscious of the existence of our organs.

'So interblended, so inextricably interwoven is the web of sensuous feeling produced by [these] activities', he believed,

> that out of it arises the *central core* of the personality – the *ego*; around the latter there crowd ... impressions received from objective existences – the *physical* in contradistinction to the *physiological* environment.[47]

Bevan Lewis regarded painful awareness of morbid sensations arising from disordered bodily organs and functions as an almost universal feature of states of depression, responsible for many of the hallucinations and delusions which frequently accompanied them; while unconsciousness of such sensations was normally a sure indication of bodily and mental health.[48] He further associated these contrasting states of mind respectively with mainly 'subjective', or introverted, and mainly 'objective', or extraverted, mental outlooks, and thus came to identify healthy and unhealthy states of mind with '*object-*' and '*subject-*consciousness', to use Bevan Lewis's own terms.[49] 'The characteristic stamp of healthful mental operations', he believed, '[is] continuous and vivid realization of [the] distinction between the subject[ive] and the object[ive] world', which was only possible for minds in which states of 'object-' predominated over states of 'subject-consciousness'.[50]

It is well worth taking careful note of these important and characteristic associations and contrasts – between *extraversion*, *'objective'* states of consciousness, and *physical and mental health*, on the one hand; and *introversion*, *'subjective'* states of consciousness, and *ill-health*, on the other. To these may be added three further sets of associations and contrasts, strongly apparent elsewhere in Bevan Lewis's work, and repeatedly invoked by Maudsley, Mercier, Hack Tuke, Clouston, and other leading Victorian psychiatrists – namely, those between *healthy physical exercise*, in the form of 'manly sports and games', hard work, and other useful occupations, '*altruism*', and *sociability*, on the one hand; and *idleness, egoism* and 'selfish vice', and *unsociability*, on the other.[51] These associations and contrasts will recur frequently throughout the remainder of this essay.

To return, however, to the specific association of morbid introspection with hypochondriasis and hysteria – it is important to stress that this association involved more than a purely psychosomatic implication. Self-absorption and unnatural egoism were also principally implicated in the psychopathology of hysteria. 'The cardinal fact in the psychopathy of hysteria', wrote Horatio Bryan Donkin,

> is an exaggerated self-consciousness dependent on undue prominence of feelings uncontrolled by intellect ... the hysteric is pre-eminently an individualist, an unsocial unit, and fails in adaptation to organic surroundings.

Donkin's statement may serve as a useful introduction to the implication of unnatural egoism and self-absorption in the moral critique of hysteria.[52] According to Donkin, 'want of will-power', the 'mental correlative to hysterical paralysis', was the clearest and most constant accompaniment of the hysterical condition, while 'Indolence' was 'the foster-nurse of the hysterical temperament', since it 'gives every opportunity ... to beget the worst results of self-consciousness'.[53] Exclusive self-absorption, an unnatural, all-devouring egoism, selfishness, deceit, lack of will-power, loss of self-control, morbid suggestibility, and indifference to social and moral obligations were all seen as more or less constant accompaniments of the hysterical condition.[54] The characteristic mental and moral state of chronic hysterics was, according to Brudenell Carter, 'an union of selfishness and deceptivity'.[55] During the latter decades of the century, the mental and moral condition in hysteria increasingly came to be regarded as paradigmatic of the mental state in many other acute forms of mental disorder, and as the cultural stereotype of hysteria thus expanded so also its characteristic psychological and moral attributes became associated with a steadily wider and more diverse range of morbid mental conditions.[56] Principally through the aspects of moral depravity and anti-social behaviour, they became associated with 'moral insanity'; through those of defective volitional control and morbid suggestibility, with their wider implications of mental automatism, they became associated with cases of so-called 'impulsive insanity'; while through the aspects of exaggerated self-consciousness, want of will, moral depravity and anti-social behaviour, they became peculiarly closely associated with the 'insanity of pubescence' and the emergence of 'moral imbecility' in adolescents of strong 'neurotic' heredity.[57] More generally, unsociability, self-absorption, indifference to social and moral conventions, and selfish disregard for the needs of others, increasingly came to be seen as *generic* characteristics of the insane.[58] We shall return to several of these aspects later; here, however, I merely wish to note that whereas morbid introspection and unnatural egoism had begun as just two among a number of interrelated themes within medical psychology, having certain fairly specific clinical and pathological associations, during the course of the Victorian period their ramifications became so extensive that by the end of the century they had come to pervade much of the theory and practice of 'psychological medicine' and mental hygiene. In order to substantiate this claim, I shall now examine their influence on several important aspects of the practice of later-Victorian psychiatry, beginning with the institutional care and treatment of the insane.

'Asocialism' and insanity

The pervasive influence of the associations surrounding the concepts of morbid introspection and unnatural egoism is apparent in the conventional stereotypes of the insane found in late-nineteenth-century psychiatric literature, and in the implications for the theory and practice of 'moral treatment' which were drawn from them. Whereas earlier cultural stereotypes of the insane had tended variously to emphasize characteristics, such as unmeasured violence, animality, or childishness, which could not readily be associated with the condition of responsible adulthood,[59] later-nineteenth-century characterizations of the insane, in an ironic distortion of the original ideals of the pioneers of 'moral treatment', tended rather to emphasize those characteristics of the insane which most nearly resembled the behaviour of unsociable and/or morally degraded adults. Unsociability, bad manners, wilful disregard for polite usages and conventions, and indifference to social and moral obligations, were now regarded as the distinctive characteristics of the insane.[60] According to Clouston, 'asocialism', the egoistic withdrawal from ordinary social intercourse and obligations into introspective and solitary habits, was 'perhaps the most distinguishing feature' of the insane.[61] Maudsley, Mercier, Clouston, Bevan Lewis, Savage, Blandford, and Craig all stressed that the insane 'usually keep to themselves' – that whereas 'the healthy-minded man is gregarious: the insane [man] is solitary'.[62] Sudden tendencies to avoid company and seek solitude in persons of previously gregarious habits were frequently regarded as warnings of incipient mental disorder, especially when accompanied by depression and apparent physical exhaustion; while conversely, a return to more social habits was, according to Maurice Craig, 'one of the symptoms by which the physician knows when a patient with mental disorder has returned to health'.[63]

Psychiatrists' changing perceptions of the character of the insane were reflected in their conceptions of the underlying principles and purposes of 'moral treatment'. Thus according to William Octavius Sankey, it was '[a principal] object in the moral treatment [of insanity] to discourage solitary habits, and not to foster exclusive propensities';[64] while according to Bevan Lewis, the principal objects of 'moral treatment' in separate establishments for the insane were, first, to remove all mental and physical causes of excitement, exhaustion, and stress, and, second, 'to eliminate such noxious agencies as by self-indulgence, or by the influence of injudicious friends [and relations], have entered into the vicious circle of [the lunatic's] life', among which he included not only drink, sex, and drugs, but also 'solitary habits, and morbid introspection'.[65] Since the insane were principally characterized by their self-absorption and lack of any sense of social or moral obligations – since, indeed, there was a very real sense in which their morbid egoism actually *constituted* their diseased condition – the 'moral treatment' of the insane came increasingly to be seen as a process of more or less forcible extraversion intended to rouse the lunatic from his self-absorption and reawaken him to a proper sense of his social obligations. As George Fielding Blandford explained:

> By the moral control exercised personally by man over man, the patient's thoughts and feelings are to be directed from his morbid self-contemplation to that care and concern for others which is his normal state.[66]

Although lip-service continued to be paid to the moral therapists' original goal of individualized treatment, in fact the whole emphasis shifted away from individual treatment towards the forcible resocialization of the insane. Viewed in this light, the very impersonality of large asylums and their internal regimes no longer necessarily appeared as a grave disadvantage, as it had done to early advocates of 'moral treatment', but might prove advantageous, if not actually indispensable, for effective 'moral treatment'. Even the customary indifference of asylum attendants to patients' individual needs could now be regarded more favourably. As Blandford put it,

> when ... [a 'morbidly egoistic' person] is at home, he generally contrives to make himself the centre and focus of everyone's regard; and if away from home ... he may be able to do the same thing ... but place him in an asylum of fifty patients [Blandford was thinking of private patients, not 'pauper lunatics'], and he occupies at once merely the fiftieth part of the attention of those about him. He is given to understand that the establishment goes on just the same whether he is there or not, but that being there, he must conform to the rules, his going away depending to a considerable extent on his own efforts, and his observance of the precepts and advice which he receives.[67]

Thus even institutional processes of self-mortification could benefit the patient, when seen in their true medico-psychological relations. This ironic reversal of the traditional rationale and priorities of 'moral treatment' was, however, only one aspect of a much more general transformation in psychiatrists' attitudes towards the treatment of the insane which took place under the influence of evolutionary theory during the second half of the nineteenth century. I shall not discuss this point here, but will return to it in the concluding section of this essay.[68]

The 'nervous' child and the neurotic youth

Psychiatrists' concern with the intellectual and moral dangers of introspection is particularly apparent in later-Victorian medico-psychological discussions of the 'mental hygiene' of child-rearing, education, and adolescent socialization. According to Francis Warner, one of the pioneers of the medical examination of schoolchildren, and the leading late-nineteenth-century medical authority on the physiological aspects of education, 'introspection, as a brain-process [in young children]' was 'very exhausting, particularly when practised on retiring to rest in a half-dormant state'. It was, he said, '[a] mental habit [which] should [carefully] be looked for in children with brain exhaustion; it may result from exhaustion, or may produce it'.[69] Serious though this was, however, 'introspective tendencies' in children were chiefly alarming for their frequent association with 'the vice of selfishness', the development of a morbid, unnatural egoism, and precocious tendencies towards sexual vice and other forms of anti-social or immoral conduct. 'Alarm should be felt,' warned Hack Tuke, 'when the young seek solitude, and society is carefully shunned.'[70] 'Normal' children, it was believed, were 'naturally' sociable, and any tendency to avoid company or prefer contemplative to active pursuits was therefore to be regarded with grave misgivings. Thus Clouston wrote of children between the ages of 6 and 11 that 'This is naturally a very social age of life. The boy or girl who is not social is not healthy.'[71] 'If a child ever shows depression or mental pain,' he believed,

> some organ [most probably the brain] is disordered, [either] the child is being poisoned, by bad food or bad air, or some irritation is going on in its bodily processes.[72]

The entire late-Victorian medico-psychological literature on the physiological aspects of child-rearing, education, and socialization was founded on this unquestioned belief that young children were all cheerful extraverts, naturally gregarious and forever seeking to join with their peers in strenuous physical exercise, and that this constituted the sole and invariable course taken by healthy development. Thus the development of regular habits of sociability, involvement in group activities, participation in sports and games, and the copious expenditure generally of nervous and muscular energy, were all regarded as sure signs that physical, mental, and moral development were proceeding normally; while shyness, gloom, self-absorption, day-dreaming, and indolence were seen as alarming indications that the developmental process was going awry.[73] This ready assumption on the part of doctors that all tendencies towards introspection or solitary habits in childhood were symptomatic of some more or less grave departure from health, requiring prompt remedial and prophylactic treatment, is perhaps most clearly evinced by their growing perception of a special 'problem-class' of 'precocious' or 'nervous' children, of insane or 'neurotic' heredity,

> quick in mental action, [whose] spontaneous activity of the brain-centres is shown by the large amount of spontaneous movement which they exhibit; and on the intellectual side, [by] activity . . . often . . . up to the point of . . . exhaustion, in the amount of talk, in the questions asked, *or worse still, in habits of introspection . . . and excessive imagining*

as Warner described them.[74] Such children, it was believed, unless closely watched, and carefully monitored and regulated in their development, were peculiarly liable to suffer physical and mental breakdowns. In general, Warner recommended that 'precocious' children given to excessive introspection should be fed well and subjected to a vigorous hygienic regimen, to increase their 'impressionability',[75] and more specifically, that

> nervous, irritable children . . . are best cultured . . . by methods of manual training. . . . [They] require education in the faculty of receiving impressions capable of controlling them, rather than the implantation [!] of more thoughts – their spontaneity needs to be controlled to co-ordinate action, not stimulated to further activity.[76]

These views were echoed by Clouston in his *Hygiene of Mind* (1906). 'Undue nervousness and irritability in children', he warned, 'always indicate that the doctor is needed, and that the conditions of life should be changed.'[77] 'The child with a strongly nervous heredity or mental taint in ancestry,' he recommended, 'should be fed on milk, farinaceous diet and fruits. . . . It should be kept fat. Its faculty development should be repressed rather than stimulated.'[78] Like Warner, he recommended a predominantly physical and manual, rather than intellectual, culture for such children until a comparatively advanced age, combined with careful hygienic regulation and regular routine – these latter being invaluable stabilizing factors in children of 'nervous', volatile temperament.[79]

The special problems of the 'nervous' or 'precocious' child with strong neurotic heredity were often regarded as incipient or larval stages of the much more serious and intractable problems of 'adolescent neurosis', to which (so it was believed) they bore close hereditary and pathological relations. Hence psychiatrists were unanimous in proclaiming, with Bevan Lewis, that 'of all faults . . . introspection and subjectivity at this age should be avoided'.[80] 'At the period of adolescence,' Hyslop warned, '[the young male] . . . undergoes a mental evolution, with which . . . is developed an egotism that sometimes passes the border line of sanity.'[81] In adolescence no less than in childhood, introspective and solitary habits, and the occurrence of depression, signified some grave departure from normal, healthy development. 'Although [adolescent depression] may be slight, although the sufferers may be able to pull themselves together with an effort, yet it is unnatural', insisted Clouston, 'it is first cousin to actual disease'; and accordingly he prescribed purgatives, a vigorous tonic regime, mental rest, and a change of environment.[82]

However, medico-psychological attitudes towards morbid introspection in adolescence were peculiarly distinguished by the special emphasis placed on its association with 'secret sins and sexual vices' in the developmental neuroses characteristic of this epoch, and by the degree of moral revulsion and contempt which this association inspired. Sir George Savage was by no means untypical in his description of the shy, neurotic youth as

> alternately exalted and depressed, full of plans which never come to anything; he is self-asserting and conceited; then will-less, self-indulgent, and indolent. With the period of exaltation [in this 'manic-depressive' alternation] sexual desire becomes dominant, and may lead to immoral and degraded habits.[83]

We have already noted the familiar association between morbid introspection and 'immoral and degraded habits', 'secret sins', and 'solitary' or 'injurious vice', in the Victorian medico-psychological literature of adolescence.[84] But although these phenomena were indeed closely associated in the emerging late-Victorian clinical picture of 'adolescent insanity', there was a far more essential connection between them than mere clinical correlation. Much has been written during the past twenty-five years about the growing emphasis in nineteenth-century psychiatric theory on masturbation as both a 'cause' and a 'symptom' of insanity, culminating in the appearance in late-nineteenth-century clinical textbooks of a distinct nosological entity or 'variety' of 'masturbational insanity'.[85] Yet the almost invariable association of masturbation with morbid introspection and egoism in the clinical picture of 'masturbational insanity' has gone almost wholly unremarked. This association was, however, fundamental to the whole hypothesis implicating masturbation in both the physical and 'moral' causation of insanity. Indeed, it is impossible fully to understand later-Victorian psychiatry's apparent obsession with what Bevan Lewis called 'the vicious habit' without first examining this association and the reasoning which lay behind it.

Although the 'masturbatory hypothesis' was already more than a century old by the mid-nineteenth century, it enjoyed perhaps its widest currency and most authoritative status, and underwent its most elaborate development, during the latter decades of the century.[86] During this period, the themes of masturbation, morbid introspection, and unnatural egoism converged and became inseparably associated in the new medico-psychological perception of 'adolescent insanity'. Indeed, this association may be said to have played no small part in the actual constitution of a medical and social perception of adolescence which was to remain influential long into the twentieth century.[87] Perhaps the best and most detailed clinical-psychiatric descriptions of this new 'syndrome', with the differential diagnosis of 'simple' adolescent insanity from adolescent insanity 'complicated' by masturbation, are those given by Bevan Lewis in his *Textbook of Mental Diseases* (1889, 1899) and by Clouston in *The Neuroses of Development* (1891) and *The Hygiene of Mind* (1906).[88] According to Bevan Lewis and

Clouston, 'adolescent insanity' was a psychosis occuring shortly after the advent of puberty in both men and women of strongly 'neurotic' heredity, characterized by an irregular alternation of acute, maniacal with depressive or stuporose states. Generally, there was a preponderance of maniacal over depressive states, but this occurred less often, and to a much lesser degree, in adolescent males than in young women – the result, so Bevan Lewis believed, of the much greater prevalence of 'vicious habits' among men than women.[89] Typically, delusions of grandeur or superhuman powers in the maniacal phases alternated with delusions of persecution in the depressive phases, while both phases were frequently accompanied by aural and/or visual hallucinations, and not infrequently marked by suicidal impulses.[90] Morbid eroticism and moral perversities, hysterical or hypochondriacal complaints, furtive alcoholism, kleptomania and other manifestations of what Clouston called 'adolescent criminality' were other common accompaniments of the depressive phases.[91] 'All these [symptoms]', Clouston insisted,

> being liable to occur as adolescent psychoses in hereditarily neurotic families, should . . . be looked upon and treated from the medico-psychological rather than . . . the moral and disciplinary standpoints. Heredity and brain alone explain such divergencies from . . . normal social and mental types.[92]

This basic syndrome was significantly modified, however, when accompanied by habitual masturbation. According to Bevan Lewis, depressive, apathetic, and stuporose states, delusions of persecution, and auditory and visual hallucinations were all much more common in cases where masturbation was a complicating factor.[93] The 'morbid subjectivity' of the habitual masturbator typically revealed itself in overtly emotional religiosity, sudden, groundless apprehensions, frequent nightmares, extreme irritability and sudden, inexplicable changes of mood, long spells of listless apathy being punctuated by hysterical seizures, disagreeable behaviour towards close relations, and motiveless, impulsive conduct.[94] Whereas 'simple' adolescent insanity was not attended by any well-marked physical symptoms, the insane masturbator could usually be identified by his anaemic, debilitated appearance, languid circulation, weak extremities, slightly ataxic gait, and dilated pupils.[95] According to Bevan Lewis, 'egoistic sentiments' were prevalent in both ordinary adolescent insanity, and in cases complicated by masturbation, and were 'the fount from which issue extravagant schemes of action'.[96] But whereas in simple adolescent insanity, this egoism was 'ever tending outwards towards the realization of . . . phantom schemes', without any inordinate '*self-engrossment* [or] *abstraction*', in cases of 'masturbational' insanity the typical mental symptoms were

> a narrow repulsive egoism, flavoured by → pseudo-religious hypochondriasis, often with much shyness and reserve at first, but later on, obtrusive and unseemly [conduct].[97]

Finally, whereas in ordinary adolescent insanity the prognosis was comparatively favourable, in cases where masturbation was a complicating factor it was extremely poor, especially where there existed some strong 'hereditary predisposition' towards 'mental weakness' and/or 'moral imbecility'.[98] Such cases, Bevan Lewis and Clouston agreed, all too often ended either in chronic delusional insanity or in hopeless dementia, since persistent indulgence in 'the vicious habit' not only exacerbated all the characteristic symptoms of ordinary adolescent insanity, but caused permanent degeneration of the cerebral nerve-tissue.[99]

On first acquaintance, these accounts appear amply to warrant the charges of psychiatric stigmatization, persecution, and 'anxiety-manufacture' which have frequently been made against them.[100] But these judgements fail to grasp the importance of masturbation's association, on the one hand, with morbid introspection and unnatural egoism and, on the other, with the moral significance with which psychiatrists invested norms of mental and physical development. As we have seen, unnaturally intense introspection and morbid egoism were regarded as peculiarly constant accompaniments of mental disorder generally;[101] and although masturbation was sometimes regarded as an 'exciting cause' of insanity, and certainly as a complicating factor, still more was it regarded as an especially ominous *symptom* of mental and moral decay. Sexual perversions in general, and masturbation in particular, were regarded not just as moral enormities in themselves, but as peculiarly telling indications of an underlying and potentially far more serious mental and moral weakness characterized by failure of inhibition, unnatural egoism, and a deficient moral sense. As Bevan Lewis put it,

> the vice of masturbation ... [is] perhaps ... the best criterion of defective moral control ... [and] the symptom of a [grave] mental defect.[102]

From the evolutionary standpoint of psychiatrists like Bevan Lewis and Clouston, sexuality and mental action were both teleological processes intended by 'Nature' to serve certain specific purposes – namely, the reproduction of a progressively improved race, and the execution of responsible voluntary actions. Viewed in this light, masturbation and other 'unproductive' sexual deviations were perversions of Nature's goal in sexual reproduction *in the same way* that introspection was a perversion of her goal in mental action. Both vices sought to harness their parent 'functions' for purely selfish purposes, in flagrant disregard for Nature's utilitarian and altruistic purposes in instituting them, and for the moral ideal implicit in the normal development of the mental and bodily 'functions'.[103] The problems of morbid introspection, unnatural egoism, and sexual perversion in adolescents were thus inextricably bound up with psychiatrists' determination to emphasize the wider moral significance of physiological facts, when seen in the light of evolutionary theory. I shall conclude by examining the implications which these speculative-evolutionary views had for the theory and practice of later-Victorian psychiatry in more detail.

Introspection, egoism, and evolution

Much of the strength of medico-psychological hostility towards morbid introspection and unnatural egoism stemmed from their characteristic association with particular morbid states such as hypochondriasis, hysteria, and the 'insanity of pubescence'. But as the example of 'adolescent insanity' complicated by masturbation shows, this hostility went far deeper than any merely clinical association. For, when seen from the standpoint of evolutionary theory, morbid introspection and unnatural egoism appeared in a peculiarly negative light quite apart from any special pathological associations. With the addition of a dynamic, Spencerian evolutionary perspective, the hierarchical models of the structure and functions of the brain and nervous system developed by Thomas Laycock, William Carpenter, and John Hughlings Jackson seemed to take on great normative and teleological, as well as more purely psychological, significance.[104] From the standpoint of evolutionary physiological psychology, fully realized, responsible voluntary actions were, perhaps more than ever before, regarded as the proper ends of all healthy 'nervous' (and thus, by extension, 'psychical') functioning – as 'Nature's' chosen instruments for the furtherance of 'mental' and 'social evolution'. This placed a very high positive valuation, or moral premium, on responsible volitional action as the 'proper' end of all mental activity.[105] But this implied an equally strong negative appraisal of passive self-contemplation, which came to be regarded as at best a kind of imperfect realization, and at worst a wilful and corrupt distortion, of the final end of all healthy mental action. Morbid introspection and exaggerated self-consciousness thus came to be regarded as perverse deviations from the norm, evolutionarily regressive and even 'unnatural'. They marked the beginnings of mental and moral dissolution in the individual, and of degeneration in the race.

This consistently negative evaluation helps to explain some of the more particular associations of introspection and self-absorption with morbid mental and bodily states which we have already remarked upon. It also sheds light on the substantial rejection of psychologically oriented approaches to the interpretation and treatment of mental disorders by later-Victorian practitioners of 'psychological medicine'.[106] From the standpoint of speculative evolutionary social theory, every aspect of human thought, feeling, and conduct was invested with profound normative implications and teleological significance. The individual, it was assumed, must abstain from the gratification of his 'lower', more purely self-regarding instincts and feelings, and instead cultivate 'higher', more 'altruistic' sentiments, sacrificing his own interests to those of the 'social organism' or 'race' to which he belonged, while even the present happiness of society was to be sacrificed to that of future generations, in order to secure the progressive advancement of the 'race' in accordance with 'Nature's purpose' in 'social evolution'.[107] In the furtherance of this grand design, important instrumental roles were ascribed to the progressive supersession of 'subjective' by 'objective' states of consciousness, and of passive self-contemplation by purposeful volitional action, while psychiatrists increasingly came to see themselves as ministers and interpreters of these processes of 'mental evolution'. Their role was to be the trustees or guardians of society's mental and moral welfare, exhorting individuals to greater awareness and more responsible performance of their social functions by denouncing self-indulgence and self-absorption, and encouraging the formation of habits of self-denial, 'altruism', and voluntary regulation of thought, feeling, and conduct.[108] But these priorities seemed to militate very strongly against psychiatrists paying much attention to mere individuals or their problems and, in particular, against any kind of 'psychotherapy' which seemed to encourage morbid introspection, give individuals exaggerated notions of their own self-importance, and diminish their sense of social-evolutionary responsibility. As Maudsley put it,

> What such patients need to learn is, not ... indulgence but ... forgetfulness of their feelings, not ... observation but ... renunciation of self, not introspection but useful action.[109]

There was, he affirmed,

> but one true cure for suffering, and that is action ... a healthy mind, like a healthy body, should lose the consciousness of self in the energy of action.[110]

For the late-Victorian medical psychologist, the paradigm of healthy 'functional' action – psychological and social, as well as physiological – was the simple reflex act, in which consciousness had no essential part to play. As Maudsley put it,

> the plan of [the mind's] complex structure and function is the simple structure and function of a reflex act.... A disordered reflex act may be taken as the type of ... disorder of the most complex mental functions.[111]

Healthy psychological functioning was conceived of in Spencerian terms as the progressive 'organisation' of dynamic adaptations of 'inner, subjective' to 'outer, objective relations', in which consciousness was a progressively diminishing frictional quantity as the modes of adaptation became more perfectly organized as 'secondarily-automatic' or 'acquired reflex' actions.[112] In the 1850s, Morell and Dunn had seen the mind as 'struggling out of self' and 'beginning to throw itself into the objects around it, and to live in the world of outward realities', as it progressed from purely 'sensational' to 'perceptive' ('subject-' to 'object-') consciousness;[113] while in the 1870s and 1880s, Spencer, Jackson, Maudsley, Mercier, and Bevan Lewis saw 'mental evolution' as consisting in the progressive supersession of states of 'subjective' (or self-) consciousness by states of 'objective consciousness', which were themselves destined gradually to fade away as the modes of adaptation which they represented became more perfectly 'organized'.[114] It was for this reason that Maudsley came to envisage 'freedom', man's evolutionary goal, as a state of perfect instinctive and reflexive adaptation to his environment, in which self-consciousness had been completely superseded:

> Were the relations between an organism and its medium the most special, full and fit of their kind possible, action and reaction would be everywhere opposite and equal. There would be no passion then in the sense of suffering because there would be a perfect equilibrium between feeling and doing; an aggregate of perfect reflexes might function so exactly and completely on every occasion that consciousness would be swallowed up in the ... achievement of ideal perfection. [Such a man] would act perfectly from instinct without need of reason, his divinings being discoveries, his aspirations prophecies, his performances instincts: he might get a long way back towards the Paradise in which his first ancestor was before, eating the forbidden fruit of the tree of knowledge of good and evil, he obtained the fatal gift of consciousness.[115]

This is, of course, precisely the opposite of the psychoanalytic ideal of increased self-awareness as the means whereby to liberate the individual from the tyranny of unconscious forces (though not, perhaps, very far removed from a behaviourist utopia). For the psychotherapist, consciousness, and the bringing into consciousness of repressed ideas and feelings, constitute respectively the supreme values and goals of his healing art. But for the late-Victorian psychological physician, consciousness and its phenomena were at best epiphenomenal, and at worst actively detrimental to healthy and efficient mental action. As Maudsley put it:

> The interference of consciousness is often an actual impediment in the [correct] association of ideas. ... An active consciousness is always detrimental to the best and most successful thought.[116]

'Mental evolution' consisted in the progressive supersession of 'subject-' by 'object-consciousness'; and there was no place in this ideal for enhanced subjective awareness. Such a feeling was, indeed, an outmoded by-product of evolution, the outcome of imperfect psychological functioning, and in a highly civilized person almost to be regarded as symptomatic of mental disorder. However large the phenomena of 'subjective consciousness' might bulk in psychopathology, therefore, they could have no real value or significance outside purely diagnostic contexts. As they were virtually *defined* as symptomatic of *imperfect* mental functioning, they could scarcely have any part to play in concepts of normal mental functioning, nor could their analysis and manipulation find any place among the legitimate therapeutic resources of 'psychological medicine'.[117]

Notes

1 Sir Henry Holland (1839) 'On Dreaming, Insanity, Intoxication, etc.', in *Medical Notes and Reflections*, London: Longman, Orme, Brown, Green & Longman, pp. 213–41, on p. 240; reprinted in Sir Henry Holland (1852) *Chapters on Mental Physiology*, London: Longman, Brown, Green & Longman, pp. 109–44, on p. 143 (emphasis added). For brief historical commentary on Holland's medico-psychological writings, see Leslie S. Hearnshaw (1964) *A Short History of British Psychology 1840–1940*, London: Methuen, pp. 20, 22–3. For more detailed accounts of Holland's life and work, see Sir Henry Holland (1872) *Recollections of Past Life*, London: Longman & Co.; *Dictionary of National Biography* (hereafter *DNB*), vol. IX, pp. 1038–9; and William Munk (1878) *The Roll of the Royal College of Physicians of London* ... (hereafter *Munk's Roll*), London: Royal College of Physicians, vol. III, pp. 144–9.

2 See especially Aubrey Lewis (1934) 'Melancholia: a historical review', *Journal of Mental Science* 80: 1–42; Jean Starobinski (1962) *History of the Treatment of Melancholy from the Earliest Times to 1900*, Documenta Geigy, *Acta Psychosomatica*, no. 4, Basle: Geigy; Raymond Klibansky, Erwin Panofsky, and Fritz Saxl (1964) *Saturn and Melancholy: Studies in the History of Natural Philosophy, Religion and Art*, London: Nelson; Michel Foucault (1972) *Folie et Déraison: Histoire de la Folie à l'Age Classique*, Paris: Gallimard, ch. IV, 'Figures de la folie'; T.H. Jobe (1976) 'Medical theories of melancholia in the seventeenth and early eighteenth centuries', *Clio Medica* 11: 217–31; Michael MacDonald (1977) 'The inner side of wisdom: suicide in early modern England', *Psychological Medicine* 7: 565–82; Michael MacDonald (1981) *Mystical Bedlam: Madness, Anxiety and Healing in Seventeenth-Century England*, Cambridge: Cambridge University Press; Vieda Skultans (1979) *English Madness: Ideas on Insanity 1580–1890*, London: Routledge & Kegan Paul, chs 2 and 3; Roy Porter (1985) '"The hunger of imagination": approaching Samuel Johnson's melancholy', in W.F. Bynum, Roy Porter, and Michael Shepherd (eds), *The Anatomy of Madness: Essays in the History of Psychiatry*, London: Tavistock, vol. I, pp. 63–88; and Stanley W. Jackson (1986) *Melancholia and Depression from Hippocratic Times to Modern Times*, New Haven and London: Yale University Press, especially Pt II, chs 7 and 8.

3 John Reid (1816) 'On solitude', in *Essays on Hypochondriacal and Other Nervous Affections*, London: Longman, Hurst, Rees, Orme & Brown, essay VI, pp. 52–60. See also David Uwins (1822) '[Review of] John Reid, *Essays on Hypochondriasis* ... [2nd edn] London (1821)', *Quarterly Review* XXVII: 110–23; the phrase 'injuriousness of solitude ... [etc.]' occurs on p. 118. *Hypochondriasis* replaced *Hypochondriacal* in the title in the 1821 and 1823 editions. For Reid's life and work, see DNB vol. XVI, p. 874; *Munk's Roll*, vol. III, p. 14.

4 Henry Maudsley (1895) *The Pathology of Mind: A Study of its Distempers, Deformities and Disorders*, London: Macmillan, p. 72. For Maudsley's life and work, see especially Aubrey Lewis (1951) 'Henry Maudsley: his work and influence (25th Maudsley lecture)', *Journal of Mental Science* 97: 259–77, reprinted in Aubrey Lewis (1967) *The State of Psychiatry: Essays and Addresses*, London: Routledge & Kegan Paul, ch. 4; Hearnshaw, *British Psychology*, pp. 24–9; Alexander Walk (1976) 'Medico-psychologists, Maudsley and the

Maudsley', *British Journal of Psychiatry* 128: 19–30; Elaine Showalter (1987) *The Female Malady: Women, Madness and English Culture, 1830–1980*, London: Virago, ch. 4; and *Munk's Roll*, vol. IV, pp. 172–3.

5 Henry Maudsley (1874) *Responsibility in Mental Disease*, 2nd edn, London: Henry S. King & Co., p. 298 (emphasis added).

6 See below, especially pp. 77–80, 90–1. See also Michael J. Clark (1981) 'The rejection of psychological approaches to mental disorder in late-nineteenth century British psychiatry', in Andrew T. Scull (ed.), *Madhouses, Mad-Doctors and Madmen: The Social History of Psychiatry in the Victorian Era*, Philadelphia: University of Pennsylvania Press/London: Athlone Press, pp. 271–312; and J.P. Williams (1985) 'Psychical research and psychiatry in late Victorian Britain: trance as ecstasy or trance as insanity', in Bynum, Porter, and Shepherd (eds), *The Anatomy of Madness*, vol. I, pp. 233–54, especially pp. 233–4, 239–42.

7 See below, pp. 80–3.

8 William Bevan Lewis (1889) *A Textbook of Mental Diseases*, London: Charles Griffin & Co., p. 354. See also below, pp. 90–2. For Bevan Lewis's life and work, see especially his obituary by Sir James Crichton-Browne and J. Shaw Bolton (1930) in *Journal of Mental Science* 76: 383–8.

9 William Benjamin Carpenter (1874) *Principles of Mental Physiology: With their Applications to the Training and Discipline of the Mind, and the Study of its Morbid Conditions*, London: Kegan Paul, Trench & Co., p. 26 (emphasis in original). For Carpenter's life and work, see J. Estlin Carpenter (1888) 'William Benjamin Carpenter – a memorial sketch', in William Benjamin Carpenter, *Nature and Man: Essays Scientific and Philosophical* ed. J. Estlin Carpenter, London: Kegan Paul, Trench & Co.; *DNB*, vol. III, pp. 1075–7; *Dictionary of Scientific Biography*, vol. III, pp. 87–9. See also Hearnshaw, *British Psychology*, pp. 19–20, 22–4.

10 Robert Brudenell Carter (1855) *On the Influence of Education and Training in Preventing Diseases of the Nervous System*, London: Churchill, p. 139. For Carter's life and work, see especially (1930) *Plarr's Lives of the Fellows of the Royal College of Surgeons of England* (hereafter *Plarr's Lives*), Bristol: John Wright & Sons, vol. I, pp. 201–3; and Ilza Veith (1965) *Hysteria: The History of a Disease*, Chicago and London: University of Chicago Press, pp. 199–210.

11 Carpenter, *Mental Physiology*, p. 657 (emphasis added).

12 Maudsley, *Pathology of Mind*, p. 314 (emphasis added).

13 ibid., p. 83.

14 John Conolly (1830) *An Inquiry Concerning the Indications of Insanity, with Suggestions for the Better Protection and Care of the Insane*, London: John Taylor; facsimile reprint edn (1964) London: Dawsons, pp. 166–7. For Conolly's life and work, see Henry Maudsley (1866) 'A memoir of the late John Conolly, MD', *Journal of Mental Science* 12: 151–74; Sir James Clark (1869) *A Memoir of John Conolly, MD, DCL* ... London: John Murray; *DNB* vol. IV, pp. 951–4; *Munk's Roll*, vol. IV, pp. 33–4. See also Denis Leigh (1961) *The Historical Development of British Psychiatry*, Oxford: Pergamon Press, vol. I, pp. 210–70; Richard A. Hunter and Ida MacAlpine, 'Introductions' to Conolly, *Indications of Insanity*, pp. 1–35; John Conolly (1847) *The Construction and Government of Lunatic Asylums and Hospitals for the Insane* (facsimile reprint edn (1968) London: Dawsons), pp. 7–38; and (1856) *The Treatment of the Insane Without Mechanical Restraints* (facsimile reprint edn (1973) Lon-

don: Dawsons), pp. vii–xlvi; Andrew T. Scull (1984) 'A brilliant career? John Conolly and Victorian psychiatry', *Victorian Studies* 27: 203–35; Andrew T. Scull (1985) 'A Victorian alienist: John Conolly, FRCP, DCL (1794–1866)', in Bynum, Porter, and Shepherd (eds), *The Anatomy of Madness*, vol. I, pp. 103–50; and Showalter, *The Female Malady*, pp. 33–4, 42–50.

15 William Benjamin Carpenter (1855) *Principles of Human Physiology, with their Chief Applications to Psychology, Pathology, Therapeutics, Hygiene and Forensic Medicine*, 5th edn, London: Churchill, p. 779 (footnote).

16 These implications for the 'auto-prophylaxis' of mental disorder and for psychiatrists' conceptions of their role as 'moral entrepreneurs' and mental-hygienic propagandists are discussed at greater length on pp. 86–8 below.

17 Conolly, *Indications of Insanity*, p. 150.

18 John Abercrombie (1831) *Inquiries Concerning the Intellectual Powers and the Investigation of Truth* 2nd edn Edinburgh: Waugh & Innes, p. 174. For Abercrombie's life and work, see *DNB*, vol. I, pp. 37–8.

19 Abercrombie, *Inquiries Concerning the Intellectual Powers*, p. 174.

20 John Daniel Morell (1853) *The Elements of Psychology*, Part I, London: William Pickering, pp. 172–6; Robert Dunn (1863) *Medical Psychology*, London: Churchill, pp. 18–20. For Morell's life and work, see *DNB*, vol. XIII, pp. 899–901; for Dunn's, see *DNB*, vol. VI, p. 210. For brief historical commentary on Morell and Dunn's psychologies, see Hearnshaw, *British Psychology*, pp. 20–1.

21 Conolly, *Indications of Insanity*, p. 90.

22 Abercrombie, *Inquiries Concerning the Intellectual Powers*, p. 176.

23 ibid., pp. 175, 176–9.

24 Robert Brudenell Carter (1853) *On the Pathology and Treatment of Hysteria*, London: Churchill, especially chapter II 'Education and training', pp. 175–6; Carpenter, *Mental Physiology*, pp. 146–7, 153, 318–19, 332–3.

25 Daniel Hack Tuke (1878) *Insanity in Ancient and Modern Life, with Chapters on its Prevention*, London: Macmillan, pp. 214–15. For Hack Tuke's life and work, see *DNB*, vol. XIX, pp. 1223–4, and *Munk's Roll*, vol. IV, p. 237.

26 Theophilus Bulkeley Hyslop (1895) *Mental Physiology, Especially in its Relation to Mental Disorders*, London: J. & A. Churchill, p. 325. For Hyslop's life and work, see especially his obituary by W.H.D. Stoddart (1933) *Journal of Mental Science* 79: 424–6, and Stephen Trombley (1981) *'All That Summer She Was Mad': Virginia Woolf and her Doctors*, London: Junction Books, pt II.

27 See below, pp. 85–90.

28 Conolly, *Indications of Insanity*, pp. 90–1.

29 On the origins and historical development of the diagnosis of 'monomania' in Victorian psychiatry, and the legal and philosophical controversies which its attempted forensic application provoked, see especially Denis Leigh (1955) 'James Cowles Prichard, MD, 1786–1848', *Proceedings of the Royal Society of Medicine* 48: 586–90; Denis Leigh (1961) *Historical Development of British Psychiatry*, vol. I, pp. 163–6, 169–77, 181–5; Nigel Walker (1968–73) *Crime and Insanity in England*, vol. I of 2 vols, Edinburgh: Edinburgh University Press: (1968) *The Historical Perspective* pp. 93–4, 96, 99, 251; and Roger Smith (1981) *Trial by Medicine: Insanity and Responsibility in Victorian Trials*, Edinburgh: Edinburgh University Press, especially pp. 37–8, 95–6, 102, 128–9.

30 Holland, *Chapters on Mental Physiology*, p. 141.

31 Hyslop, *Mental Physiology*, pp. 301–2.
32 ibid., p. 303.
33 ibid., p. 302.
34 Carpenter, *Mental Physiology*, p. 293 (emphasis in original).
35 ibid., pp. 391–2 (emphasis in original).
36 ibid., especially chs XIV ('Of reverie and abstraction; electro-biology'); XV ('Of sleep, dreaming and somnambulism'); and XVI ('Of mesmerism and spiritualism').
37 ibid., pp. 297, 303, 311–12, 611–12, 683–5.
38 ibid., pp. 27, 251.
39 Carpenter, *Nature and Man*, p. 312.
40 ibid., p. 312 (emphasis in original).
41 See, for example, Carpenter, *Mental Physiology*, pp. 9, 25–6, 106, 147.
42 See Reid, 'On solitude', in *Essays on Hypochondriasis* (1821 edn), p. 81; and Uwins' (1822) review of Reid's *Essays*, p. 118. The quotation from Burton forms the last sentence (in English) of Robert Burton (1621) *The Anatomy of Melancholy* (emphasis in original).
43 Holland, *Chapters on Mental Physiology*, p. 36 (the phrase 'morbid solicitation' is his); Brudenell Carter, *Education and Training*, pp. 161, 163–4, 172–4, 178; Carter, *Pathology and Treatment of Hysteria*, p. 23; Carpenter, *Mental Physiology*, pp. 144–5.
44 Carter, *Education and Training*, p. 161.
45 ibid., pp. 163–4, 173, 224–5.
46 Holland, *Chapters on Mental Physiology*, pp. 36–7; Carpenter, *Mental Physiology*, pp. 144–5, 682–3; Carter, *Education and Training*, pp. 163–4, 173–4, 213–20; Carter, *Pathology and Treatment of Hysteria*, pp. 23–4, 57, 65–75; and Daniel Hack Tuke (1872) *Illustrations of the Influence of the Mind Upon the Body in Health and Disease, Designed to Elucidate the Action of the Imagination*, London: J. & A. Churchill, especially part I, ch. 2, and p. 334.
47 Bevan Lewis, *Mental Diseases*, p. 143 (emphasis in original).
48 ibid., pp. 133–4, 143–7.
49 ibid., pp. 116–22, 124, 125–6, 130–1, 133–4, 143–4; see also pp. 293, 303, 312–23, 353–6, 358–9.
50 ibid., p. 143.
51 Bevan Lewis, *Mental Diseases*, pp. 353, 354–9; 2nd edn (1899), pp. 466–7, 473. Compare Henry Maudsley (1870) *Body and Mind: An Inquiry into their Connection and Mutual Influence*, London: Macmillan, pp. 84–5; Maudsley, *Pathology of Mind*, pp. 1, 3, 22–4, 31, 78–81, 400, 551–2, 556; Charles A. Mercier (1902) *A Text-Book of Insanity*, London: Swan Sonnenschein, pp. 1, 10–11, 13–15, 96–7; Thomas Smith Clouston (1883) *Clinical Lectures on Mental Diseases*, London: J. & A. Churchill, pp. 484–6, 490–1, 546–7; (1892) 3rd edn, p. 684; Thomas Smith Clouston (1906) *The Hygiene of Mind*, London: Methuen, pp. 49, 68–9, 70, 143–4, 146. For Mercier's life and work, see *Munk's Roll*, vol. IV, pp. 463–4, and *Plarr's Lives*, vol. II, pp. 52–3. For Clouston's, see his obituaries in (1915) *British Medical Journal* I: 744–6 and (1915) *Journal of Mental Science* 61: 333–8. See also Sir David Henderson (1964) *The Evolution of Psychiatry in Scotland*, Edinburgh: E. & S. Livingstone, pp. 123–4, 138–43; and Margaret Sorbie Thompson (1984) 'The mad, the bad, and the sad: psychiatric care in the Royal Edinburgh Asylum, Morningside, 1813–1894', University of Boston PhD thesis, especially chs V, VI.

52 Horatio Bryan Donkin, 'Hysteria', in Daniel Hack Tuke (ed.) (1892) *A Dictionary of Psychological Medicine*, 2 vols, London: J. and A. Churchill, vol. I, pp. 618–27, on p. 620. For Donkin's life and work, see *Munk's Roll*, vol. IV, p. 273, and Charlotte MacKenzie (June 1985) '"The life of a human football?" Women and madness in the era of the new woman', *Bulletin of the Society for the Social History of Medicine* 36: 37–40. For Victorian medico-psychological attitudes to hysteria generally, see especially Veith, *Hysteria*, chs IX, X; Carroll Smith-Rosenberg (1972) 'The hysterical woman: sex roles and role conflict in nineteenth-century America', *Social Research* 39: 652–78; Showalter, *The Female Malady*, pp. 129–34, 137–8, and ch. 6, 'Feminism and hysteria'; and MacKenzie, '"The life of a human football"'. See also my 'Rejection of psychological approaches', pp. 293–8.

53 Donkin, 'Hysteria', pp. 623, 626.

54 See, for example, Brudenell Carter, *Pathology and Treatment of Hysteria*, especially pp. 53–8; Holland, *Chapters in Mental Physiology*, pp. 33–4; Carpenter, *Mental Physiology*, pp. 332–3; Maudsley, *Body and Mind*, pp. 79–80, 84–5; Maudsley, *Pathology of Mind*, pp. 135–6, 397–9; George Savage (1884) *Insanity and Allied Neuroses, Practical and Clinical*, London: Cassell, p. 85. For Savage's life and work, see note 83, below.

55 Carter, *Pathology and Treatment of Hysteria*, p. 55.

56 See, for example, Maudsley, *Pathology of Mind*, pp. 135–6, 397–9.

57 See, for example, ibid., pp. 389–96, 399–405; Bevan Lewis, *Mental Diseases*, pp. 340, 343, 353–4, 358–61.

58 See below, pp. 90–2.

59 See Alexander Walk (1954) 'Some aspects of the "moral treatment" of the insane to 1850', *Journal of Mental Science* 100: 807–37, especially pp. 817, 818; Kathleen Jones (1955) *Lunacy, Law and Conscience 1744–1845: The Social History of the Insane*, London: Routledge & Kegan Paul, especially pp. 30, 41–2, 60–1, 115; Foucault, *Histoire de la Folie*, pp. 164–75, 509–10; George Rosen (1968) *Madness in Society: Chapters in the Historical Sociology of Mental Illness*, Chicago: University of Chicago Press, ch. 5; pp. 164–71; Vieda Skultans (1975) *Madness and Morals: Ideas on Insanity in the Nineteenth Century*, London; Routledge & Kegan Paul, especially 'Introduction'; Michael Fears (1978) '"Moral treatment": the social organization of human nature', University of Edinburgh unpublished Ph D thesis, especially pp. 116–23; Andrew T. Scull (1979) *Museums of Madness: The Social Organization of Insanity in Nineteenth-Century England*, London: Allen Lane, pp. 62–6; 'Moral treatment reconsidered: some sociological comments on an episode in the history of British psychiatry', in Scull (ed.), *Madhouses, Mad-Doctors and Madmen*, pp. 105–18, especially pp. 106–10; (1983) 'The domestication of madness', *Medical History* 27: 233–48, especially pp. 233–8; Sander L. Gilman (1982) *Seeing the Insane: A Cultural History of Madness and Art in the Western World* . . ., New York and Chichester: John Wiley & Sons, especially pt 2; Michael J. Donnelly (1983) *Managing the Mad: A Study of Medical Psychology in Early Nineteenth-Century Britain*, London: Tavistock, especially pp. 36–7, 41, 44–5, 69, 71, 107–8, 120–1, 122; Anne Digby (1985) 'Moral treatment at the Retreat, 1796–1846', in Bynum, Porter, and Shepherd (eds), *The Anatomy of Madness*, vol. II, ch. 3, especially pp. 54–5, 68; Anne Digby (1985) *Madness, Morality, and Medicine: A Study of the York Retreat, 1796–1914*, Cambridge: Cambridge University Press, especially pp. 1–3, 5–6, 57–9;

and Janet Browne (1985) 'Darwin and the face of madness', in Bynum, Porter, and Shepherd (eds), *The Anatomy of Madness*, vol. I, ch. 6, especially pp. 151–3.

60 See, for example, Carpenter, *Mental Physiology*, pp. 658, 663; Hack Tuke, *Insanity in Ancient and Modern Life*, pp. 91–2, 93, 102; Maudsley, *Responsibility in Mental Disease*, pp. 220–1; Henry Maudsley (1883) *Body and Will: Being an Essay Concerning Will in its Metaphysical, Physiological and Pathological Aspects*, London: Kegan Paul, Trench & Co., especially part III, sections III–V; Maudsley, *Pathology of Mind*, pp. 1, 16; Mercier, *A Text-Book of Insanity*, pp. 6–7, 13–18; Mercier, 'Vice, crime and insanity', in Thomas Clifford Allbutt (ed.) (1896–9) *A System of Medicine By Many Writers*, 8 vols, London: Macmillan, vol. VIII (1899), pp. 248–94, especially pp. 258–60, 263–80; and Bevan Lewis, *Mental Diseases*, pp. 177–8, 191, 214–15, 251–3, 257–8, 289–90, 340, 341, 353–4, 356–61.

61 Clouston, *Hygiene of Mind*, p. 69. See also p. 49.

62 Maurice Craig (1905) *Psychological Medicine*, London: J. & A. Churchill, p. 22. See also p. 24. Compare George Fielding Blandford (1877) *Insanity and its Treatment*, 2nd edn, Edinburgh: Oliver & Boyd, pp. 377, 380–1; Bevan Lewis, *Mental Diseases*, 2nd edn, pp. 461, 466–7, 473; and Clouston, *Hygiene of Mind*, pp. 49, 69. For Blandford's life and work, see *DNB, 1901–1911*, pp. 176–7, and *Munk's Roll*, vol. IV, pp. 168–9. For Craig's, see *Munk's Roll*, vol. IV, pp. 474–5.

63 Craig, *Psychological Medicine*, p. 22.

64 William Henry Octavius Sankey (1884) *Lectures on Mental Diseases*, 2nd edn, London: H.K. Lewis, p. 390. For Sankey's life and work, see *Munk's Roll*, vol. IV, pp. 147–8.

65 Bevan Lewis, *Mental Diseases*, 2nd edn, p. 461.

66 Blandford, *Insanity and its Treatment*, p. 381. Compare Bevan Lewis, *Mental Diseases*, 2nd edn, pp. 466–7, 473; and Clouston, *Clinical Lectures*, 3rd edn, p. 684.

67 Blandford, *Insanity and its Treatment*, p. 380.

68 See below, pp. 90–2.

69 Francis Warner (1890) *A Course of Lectures on the Growth and Means of Training of the Mental Faculty*, Cambridge: Cambridge University Press, p. 94. For Warner's life and work, see *Munk's Roll*, vol. IV, pp. 297–8, and *Plarr's Lives*, vol. II, pp. 488–9.

70 Hack Tuke, *Insanity in Ancient and Modern Life*, p. 214.

71 Clouston, *Hygiene of Mind*, p. 143.

72 ibid., p. 128.

73 See especially Thomas Smith Clouston (1891) *The Neuroses of Development: Being the Morison Lectures for 1890*, Edinburgh: Oliver & Boyd, pp. 115, 123–4; Clouston, *Hygiene of Mind*, pp. 69, 143–4, 146.

74 Warner, *On the Growth … of the Mental Faculty*, pp. 138–9 (emphasis added). Compare Clement Dukes (1896) 'The hygiene of youth', in Allbutt (ed.), *A System of Medicine*, vol. I, pp. 457–75, on p. 462; Clouston, *Clinical Lectures*, pp. 36, 139; Clouston, *Hygiene of Mind*, pp. 115, 127, 130–1, 146.

75 Warner, *On the Growth … of the Mental Faculty*, p. 132.

76 ibid., pp. 138–9.

77 Clouston, *Hygiene of Mind*, p. 129.

78 ibid., p. 115. See also Clouston, *Clinical Lectures*, pp. 623–4.

79 ibid., pp. 623–4; Clouston, *Hygiene of Mind*, p. 130.
80 Bevan Lewis, *Mental Diseases*, p. 353. Compare Maudsley, *Body and Mind*, pp. 84–5; Maudsley, *Pathology of Mind*, pp. 542–4; Hack Tuke, *Insanity in Ancient and Modern Life*, p. 214; Clouston, *Neuroses of Development*, pp. 123–4; Clouston, *Hygiene of Mind*, pp. 167, 170–1.
81 Hyslop, *Mental Physiology*, p. 408.
82 Clouston, *Hygiene of Mind*, pp. 170–2.
83 George Henry Savage (1899) 'Mental diseases – introduction', in Allbutt (ed.), *A System of Medicine*, vol. VIII, pp. 179–97, on p. 182. For Savage's life and work, see *Munk's Roll*, vol IV, pp. 306–7; and Trombley, *'All That Summer She Was Mad'*, part II.
84 See above, pp. 83–4.
85 See especially E.H. Hare (1962) 'Masturbatory insanity: the history of an idea', *Journal of Mental Science 108: 1–25;* Alex Comfort (1967) *The Anxiety Makers: Some Curious Preoccupations of the Medical Profession*, London: Nelson, ch. 3; Thomas S. Szasz (1970) *The Manufacture of Madness: A Comparative Study of the Inquisition and the Mental Health Movement*, New York: Harper, ch. 11; H. Tristram Engelhardt, Jr (1974) 'The disease of masturbation: values and the concept of disease', *Bulletin of the History of Medicine* 48: 234–48; and Arthur N. Gilbert (1980) 'Masturbation and insanity: Henry Maudsley and the ideology of sexual repression', *Albion* 12: 268–82.
86 Hare, 'Masturbatory insanity', pp. 4–9, 11–15; Comfort, *Anxiety Makers*, pp. 76–77, 95–97, 107–11; Szasz, *Manufacture of Madness*, pp. 182–94.
87 See Richard P. Neuman (Spring 1975) 'Masturbation, madness and the modern concepts of childhood and adolescence', *Journal of Social History* 8, no. 3: 1–27.
88 Bevan Lewis, *Mental Diseases*, part II, 'Insanity at the periods of puberty and adolescence'; Clouston, *Clinical Lectures*, Lectures XIV, 'Insanity of masturbation' (pp. 482–92) and XVI, 'Insanity of adolescence' (pp. 534–53); Clouston, *Neuroses of Development*, pp. 114–30; Clouston, *Hygiene of Mind*, pp. 168, 169–73. See also Henry Maudsley (1868) 'Illustrations of a variety of insanity', *Journal of Mental Science* 14: 149–62; Maudsley, *Pathology of Mind*, pp. 400–14; Hare, 'Masturbatory insanity', pp. 6–7; Comfort, *Anxiety Makers*, pp. 77, 107–8; Szasz, *Manufacture of Madness*, pp. 189–90, 193, 308–9; Skultans, *Madness and Morals*, pp. 61–2, 86–94; and Skultans, *English Madness*, pp. 73–5.
89 Bevan Lewis, *Mental Diseases*, pp. 339–41, 354–9; Clouston, *Clinical Lectures*, Lecture XVI, especially p. 551; Clouston, *Neuroses of Development*, pp. 110–11, 114–16, 119–23.
90 Bevan Lewis, *Mental Diseases*, pp. 339–40, 343, 354–9; Clouston, *Clinical Lectures*, pp. 484–5; Clouston, *Neuroses of Development*, pp. 115–16.
91 Clouston, *Neuroses of Development*, pp. 115–16, 123–4; Clouston, *Hygiene of Mind*, pp. 172–3.
92 Clouston, *Neuroses of Development*, p. 124.
93 Bevan Lewis, *Mental Diseases*, pp. 358–9.
94 ibid.; and Clouston, *Clinical Lectures*, pp. 484–6.
95 Bevan Lewis, *Mental Diseases*, p. 359; Clouston, *Clinical Lectures*, p. 485.
96 Bevan Lewis, *Mental Diseases*, p. 354.
97 ibid., p. 358 (emphasis in original).

98 ibid., pp. 358, 359–61; Clouston, *Clinical Lectures*, p. 552.

99 Bevan Lewis, *Mental Diseases*, pp. 355, 360; Clouston, *Clinical Lectures*, p. 552; Clouston, *Neuroses of Development*, pp. 116–18.

100 See especially Comfort, *Anxiety Makers*, ch. 3; Szasz, *Manufacture of Madness*, pp. 192–3, 202–6.

101 See above, pp. 73–5.

102 Bevan Lewis, *Mental Diseases*, p. 360. Compare Clouston, *Clinical Lectures*, p. 484; Mercier, *A Text-Book of Insanity*, p. 3.

103 This aspect of medical attitudes to masturbation, contraception ('conjugal onanism') and other 'unproductive' sexual deviations has briefly been commented upon by Engelhardt, 'Disease of masturbation', pp. 247–8; Neuman, 'Masturbation ... and the modern concepts of childhood and adolescence', pp. 8, 14–17, 19, 21; and Gilbert, 'Masturbation and insanity', pp. 277–8.

104 See especially Thomas Laycock (1840) *A Treatise on the Nervous Diseases of Women: Comprising an Inquiry into the Nature, Causes and Treatment of Spinal and Hysterical Disorders*, London: Longman, Green, Brown & Longman, especially pp. ix, 85–6, 96, 101–3, 105–14; Thomas Laycock (1845) 'On the reflex functions of the brain', *British and Foreign Medical Review* 19: 298–311; Thomas Laycock (1860) *Mind and Brain: Or, the Correlations of Consciousness and Organisation* ..., 2 vols, Edinburgh: Sutherland & Knox, especially vol. II, pp. 140, 142–54; William Benjamin Carpenter (1846) 'Mr. Noble on the brain and its physiology', *British and Foreign Medical Review* 22: 488–544, reprinted in part as 'The brain and its physiology', in *Nature and Man*, pp. 159–63; William Benjamin Carpenter (1850) 'On the physiology and diseases of the nervous system', *British and Foreign Medico-Chirurgical Review* 5: 1–50, reprinted in part as 'The automatic execution of voluntary movements', in *Nature and Man*, pp. 164–8; Carpenter (1855) *Principles of Human Physiology*, 5th edn, especially ch. XI; Carpenter, *Mental Physiology*, especially book I, ch. II; John Hughlings Jackson (1931–2) *Selected Writings of John Hughlings Jackson*, ed. James Taylor, Gordon Holmes, and F.M.R. Walshe, 2 vols, London: Hodder & Stoughton, especially vol. 2, pp. 3–102; 116–18, 398–406; 431–3, 436–40.

See also Hearnshaw, *British Psychology*, pp. 20, 23 (Laycock), 19–20, 22–4 (Carpenter), and 70–3 (Hughlings Jackson); Richard J. Herrnstein and Edwin G. Boring (eds) (1965) *A Source-Book in the History of Psychology*, Cambridge, Mass.: Harvard University Press, section VII, pp. 204, 233–6 (Hughlings Jackson); Roger Smith (1970) 'Physiological psychology and the philosophy of nature in mid-nineteenth century Britain', University of Cambridge unpublished PhD thesis, especially chs 3, 6; Robert M. Young (1970) *Mind, Brain, and Adaptation in the Nineteenth Century: Cerebral Localization and its Biological Context from Gall to Ferrier*, Oxford: Clarendon Press, ch. 6; Kurt Danziger (1982) 'Mid-nineteenth century British psycho-physiology: a neglected chapter in the history of psychology', in William R. Woodward and Mitchell G. Ash (eds), *The Problematic Science: Psychology in Nineteenth-Century Thought*, New York: Praeger, pp. 119–46, especially pp. 121–2, 124–5, 128–33 (Carpenter), 124–8, 132–3 (Laycock); and L. Stephen Jacyna (1981) 'The physiology of mind, the unity of nature, and the moral order in Victorian thought', *British Journal for the History of Science* 14: 109–32, especially pp. 111–12, 115–17 (Laycock), 112–14, 118 (Carpenter); L. Stephen Jacyna (1982) 'Somatic theories of mind and the interests of medicine in

Britain, 1850–1879', *Medical History* 26: 233–58, especially pp. 236–7, 252–4 (Laycock).

105 See, for example, Maudsley, *Responsibility in Mental Disease*, p. 273; *Body and Will*, pp. 190–1, 193–4. Compare Holland, *Chapters in Mental Physiology*, pp. 67–8; Morell, *Elements of Psychology*, pp. 58–9; Robert Dunn (1858) *An Essay on Physiological Psychology*, London: Churchill, pp. 43, 47; Dunn, *Medical Psychology*, pp. 11–12.

106 Clark, 'Rejection of psychological approaches to mental disorder'.

107 See, for example, Maudsley, *Responsibility in Mental Disease*, pp. 287–8; Maudsley, *Body and Will*, pp. 130, 163–5, 171, 190–1; Mercier, *A Text-Book of Insanity*, p. 1; Thomas Smith Clouston (1882) *Female Education from a Medical Point of View*, Edinburgh: MacNiven & Wallace, pp. 19–20, 31; Clouston, *Hygiene of Mind*, pp. 68–9, 80, 90–2, 188, 199–200.

108 See especially Maudsley, *Responsibility in Mental Disease*, ch. IX, 'The prevention of insanity'; Hack Tuke, *Insanity in Ancient and Modern Life*, pt III, 'Auto-prophylaxis: or, self-prevention of insanity'; Clouston, *Hygiene of Mind*; and James Crichton Browne (1883) 'Education and the nervous system', in Malcolm Morris (ed.) *The Book of Health*, London: Cassell, pp. 269–380. Compare Warner, *On the Growth . . . of the Mental Faculty*, and Dukes, 'The hygiene of youth'. For an extended discussion, see Michael J. Clark (1983) '"The data of alienism"; evolutionary neurology, physiological psychology and the reconstruction of British psychiatric theory, *c.* 1850–*c.* 1900', University of Oxford unpublished DPhil. thesis, especially chs 7 and 8.

109 Maudsley, *Body and Mind*, pp. 84–5.

110 Maudsley, *Responsibility in Mental Disease*, p. 298.

111 Maudsley, *Pathology of Mind*, pp. 18–19.

112 See especially Herbert Spencer (1870) *The Principles of Psychology*, 2 vols (2nd edn) London: Williams & Norgate, vol. I, pp. 388–9, 495–6, 559–60; Carpenter, *Mental Physiology*, pp. 74–5, 228–9, 241, 341–4, 515–17, 718–19; Charles A. Mercier, *Sanity and Insanity* (London: Walter Scott, 1890), pp. 39–45, 57–8, 62. See also Bevan Lewis, *Mental Diseases*, pp. 119–26, 133.

113 Morell, *Elements of Psychology*, pp. 134–5; Dunn, *Physiological Psychology*, pp. 42–3.

114 See Spencer, *Principles of Psychology*, vol. I, pp. 382–3, 387–9, 403–4, 495–6, 559–60; Hughlings Jackson, *Selected Writings*, vol. II, pp. 68–9, 73, 93–7, 199–202, 212; Maudsley, *Pathology of Mind*, pp. 18, 24–5; Mercier, *Sanity and Insanity*, pp. 57–8; and Bevan Lewis, *Mental Diseases*, pp. 116–24, 132–4, 143.

115 Maudsley, *Pathology of Mind*, pp. 93–4.

116 Henry Maudsley (1867) *The Physiology and Pathology of Mind*, London: Macmillan, pp. 119–20.

117 Clark, 'Rejection of psychological approaches', especially pp. 277–92.

CHAPTER FOUR

Between soma and psyche: Morselli and psychiatry in late-nineteenth-century Italy

Patrizia Guarnieri
Translated by Terri Philips

From typologies to individuality

'There has been a time in which certain psychiatrists did not believe they were sufficiently "scientific", that is properly bound on the real, positive course, if all their scholarly activity were not taken up by the anatomical table, the microscope, or the laboratory.'[1] So announced a new psychiatric journal in 1914. Its editor was the illustrious, 62-year-old Enrico Morselli, alienist, anthropologist, and a lover of philosophy in Italy, who already had behind him a distinguished career, many publications, and wide experience in various subjects of study.[2] He received his degree in medicine in 1874 at the University of Modena – the city of his birth – at the time when several eminent personalities were teaching there: the zoologist Giovanni Canestrini, 'the most Darwinian among Italian Darwinists'; Carlo Livi, pioneer of forensic psychiatry; and the anatomist and anthropologist, Paolo Gaddi.[3] The latter induced his favourite student, Morselli, to devote himself to craniology which then seemed, because of its quantitative dimension, an objective and thus 'scientific' pursuit.

Immediately after his graduation, Morselli began practising medicine at the mental hospital in Reggio Emilia, which was then directed by Livi and considered one of the best institutions in Europe for the treatment and scientific investigation of nervous and mental disorders.[4] At the same time he won a post-graduate scholarship in anthropology at the Istituto di Studi Superiori in Florence, which claimed to provide the opportunity for close collaboration between philosophers and scientists without suffocating Darwinian inspiration in mere empiricism.[5]

The combination of medical practice – on the mad of Reggio Emilia, as well as on ordinary patients at the Florence hospital – and his training under Paolo Mantegazza, the leading anthropologist in Italy, proved decisive in Morselli's development.

At just 25 years of age he found himself directing and radically reforming the mental hospital of Macerata; in 1880 he left that southern town for Turin, where he worked at the Royal Mental Hospital and at the university, teaching psychiatry and anthropology. His lectures were eventually compiled in his *Antropologia generale; L'uomo secondo le teorie dell'evoluzione* (Turin, 1911). In the meantime he had written a well-received tome, which was also translated into English: *Suicide: An essay on comparative moral statistics* (1881; 1st edn, Milan: 1879), as well as *Critica e riforma del metodo in antropologia* (Rome: 1880), which examined critically the various methods of quantitative research applied to the human sciences.

In what had been Italy's first capital, Morselli founded the *Rivista di filosofia scientifica* (1881–91), which became the organ of Italian positivism.[6] He cultivated varied interests, never limiting himself to the confines of his medical specialization. In 1886 he subjected himself to the hypnotic powers of a Belgian, a former officer – his stage name was Donato – who performed in crowded theatres in Turin and other European cities.[7] This experience inspired Morselli to edit a treatise entitled *Magnetismo animale, la fascinazione e gli stati ipnotici* (Turin: 1886), which was later followed by the two volumes *Psicologia e spiritismo* (Turin: 1908). These latter volumes were concerned with Morselli's observations, made over the years, of the Neapolitan medium Eusapia Paladino, who even attracted the attention of the Society for Psychical Research in London.

Morselli's somewhat unorthodox attitudes often incurred the disapprobation of the scholars of Turin – for instance, Cesare Lombroso and Giulio Fano – just as his reforming ideas encountered strong opposition in the board of directors of the mental hospital. Therefore in 1889 Morselli decided to move to Genoa, where he remained until his death in 1929. During the forty remaining years his psychiatric experience embraced 'qualitatively different' types of patients: backward children from the Institute for the Handicapped in Nervi, the poor he visited free of charge at the neurology clinic of the Policlinico, the upper-class clientele – mostly female – who frequented his private clinic Villa Maria Pia, insane criminals whom he defended in many legal trials (some of which became famous) and, finally, patients suffering traumas from war experiences.[8]

Without a doubt, Morselli enjoyed a position of authority in Italian medical and scientific culture. He was an active contributor to the leading journals of scientific research and promulgation, to psychological, psychiatric, and neurological societies and conferences, and as an interpreter of the ideas of Haeckel and Darwin, of Morel and Quetelet, of Galton and Freud.[9]

The polemical judgement, mentioned above, that Morselli passed on the attitude of psychiatrists, and not only of them, provides an important clue to his own position. According to him, such an attitude was destined to appear periodically: there was a quest for an organic cause, preferably quantifiable, of all mental phenomena under examination, and an assumption that between mind and body there existed a causative mechanical relation. Thus the symptom would always correspond to a lesion; every mental function was established in a specific area of the cerebral mass, and when the one appeared disturbed, it could be inferred that the performance of the other would be impaired or defective. A methodology of the exact sciences was being extended to medicine: from the cellular theory of Schwann and Schleiden, further elaborated by Rudolph Virchow, it seemed that the organism was analysable into elementary units where morbidity occurred. If the body hid the causalities of sickness and of health, the corpse unveiled them. None the less the autopsy could level some unknowns: it was not rare to find no lesion at all. Of course the greatest difficulties lay in the origin and the history of mental disease; Morselli had not failed to mention this himself, principally when as an assistant at the Florentine medical clinic he dedicated himself to epileptics. He then decided not to sacrifice the complexity of those cases to salvage a theory – cerebral localization – that was often contradicted by evidence.[10] What happened then, when instead of having cadavers on the anatomical table, one had to face the mentally ill admitted to an asylum?

In Macerata, in February 1877, Morselli found a suburban institute, not large, but none the less well constructed and, in certain aspects, comparable with some of Italy's most renowned hospitals. Upon his arrival it contained 156 patients: 88 men and 68 women, mostly over 40 years of age. The women were for the most part housewives and spinsters; prevalent among the men were farmers and day-labourers, followed by landowners, artisans, and workers. In accordance with the national averages, celibacy was considered a predisposition to madness. Mania and insanity were the most common forms. Not much more than this was known about these patients.[11] The new director had searched in vain for the medical records; he found admission forms, but nothing more, as though no changes had occurred in any of the patients during their stay in hospital.

This circumstance, among others, threatened the philanthrophic spirit with which the Provincial Delegation intended to preside over the hospital. Morselli immediately condemned facts which, he added, 'my colleagues would never believe': a woman abandoned in a pile of hay for over a year, completely naked and fed like an animal; others bound in straitjackets; some confined in cells for eighteen months, for no apparent reason, or just on the 'whim of a sick mind', and without even a nurse coming near them. In the large rooms the patients were left all together, dirty and restless; this mixing of patients impeded occupation of any kind on the part of the less serious cases, and it provoked violent relapses. The institute possessed none of the instruments necessary for clinical tests. Morselli discovered instead a 'disproportionately large number of obstetric instruments, among which one could admire three forceps and even a drill for craniotomies (!!)'. But the worst scandals were provided by the personnel. Arriving unexpectedly, day or night, Morselli surprised ward guards gambling. Once, rushing to a courtyard from which frantic screams were coming, he saw one of the nurses of the section on a bench, fast asleep. Inclined to drinking and instigating brawls, attendants of both sexes made obscene, disgusting spectacles of themselves in front of the patients. They behaved 'as though they worked in a tavern or a brothel'.

Morselli intervened with severity: dismissals, punishments, and strict regulation, so that at least the personnel did not steal food or linen from the patients, and that they performed their duties without themselves deciding how to employ the instruments of constraint. At the beginning he imposed a quasi-military discipline. At risk were the financial returns of the institution, which was just like any other business – and the realization of its aims. Morselli did not want to see helpless persons placed in the care of the community outside the hospital.[12] He always upheld this opinion, defending it, at just 28 years of age, at a conference in 1880 in front of the most famous psychiatrists; he disputed with those who still conceived the mental hospital as 'a Place of Custody where the deranged were enclosed, denying them the means to act on whim of sheer, mad impulse, by which they could be damaging to society'. Among those who believed that the psychiatric institution should merely perform a function of social defence was the socialist Enrico Ferri. Morselli suggested that he should read an aphorism written by Quetelet: 'Society has the delinquents and the mad it deserves, because it is generally the material, intellectual and moral conditions of collectivism that generate the tendency in individuals towards delinquency and the lapse to insanity.' This responsibility obliged society, which also had the right to defend itself, to recognize its duty to eliminate the causes of evil and to cure its victims.[13] Hospitals were to be staffed with persons capable of providing not only custody, but assistance for the alienated individuals. Diagnosis and therapy were tasks to be performed exclusively by physicians. But even more important, for these disturbed people, was perhaps their everyday life in an environment which was supposed to cheer them up: 'the nurses in particular, for their close, constant and mutual contact with the ill, for the influence they could easily gain over them with time, for their care and surveillance, were even more able than the physician himself to influence the course and outcome of the mental disease'.[14]

For therapeutic reasons Morselli wanted to instil proper hygienic conditions as well as discipline. The less disturbed patients were separated from the more unruly ones, so as to avoid contagion; the 'dirty' patients were assigned to a separate ward under special supervision by the nurses: 'every two hours the nurses directed them to the lavatory and obliged them, with words and with gestures, to relieve themselves'. Proper behaviour on the part of the personnel should ensure that 'nothing, absolutely nothing could weigh negatively on the ideas, concepts, or cerebral activity of any individual patient, each, with a disordered mind, being highly susceptible to external influences, having to procure from another source the harmony missing within himself'. Even physical exercise was considered useful in achieving these goals. As far as drugs were concerned Morselli was not opposed to them as much as some of his colleagues were, though he did lament that few of them were actually effective. He believed that better results could be attained with showers, and he had them installed, adding to the 'beautiful balneary arsenal' of the mental hospital of Santa Croce.

But the real cure was to be found in a peremptory 'Everybody to work!' The invalids, instead of languishing in the corridors, could be doing something constructive; the dangerous patients, once removed from isolation and distracted from their obsessions, would be able to contribute to the institution's budget. And so, to improve the financial situation, Morselli devised ways to economize. 'Work raises the morale of the masses; idleness is demoralizing': the psychological axiom applied even more to hospital patients. Certainly, work was preferable to blood-letting, laxatives and coercion:

> We belong to the modern school, and believe that the alteration of the mind should be cured, particularly by those means which influence and act on the mind: thus we give great, and almost exclusive, importance to *work*. Given this, we do not want anybody who is capable of labour or adept for any of a number of trades, or amateur of any liberal art, to remain idle.[15]

In less than a month Morselli more than doubled the number of people employed in various occupations, among which there were an embalmer, an engineer for technical tasks, clerks, and of course gardeners, blacksmiths, labourers, and painters. With enthusiasm he inaugurated an agricultural colony – complete with a stall, granary, and storerooms – where even women could be employed. To support the course he was taking Morselli quoted his teacher Livi:

> If you suppress labour in a mental hospital you will be returning to the times of chains and whips and brute force of every kind. And what will be the result? You will have idleness, which is the father of corruption; you will have permanent disorder; patients who break and tear things, who scratch and dirty themselves; you will see the unleashing of the worse instincts, a greater perversion of the intellect, more slackening of the body.

Many 'methods of moral and mental treatment' were undertaken at Macerata as well: distractions, small compensations in the form of food and tobacco, 'informal dances and parties' with a group of musicians, and an amateur drama group, in which the doctor himself – though with little talent – performed, as he later recorded in his autobiography.

These were all therapeutic initiatives recommended by the experiences of other mental institutions, in particular at Reggio Emilia, with which Morselli was already familiar. They were initiatives guided more by good common sense and humanitarian spirit than by diagnostic precision or well-founded doctrine. It was not intended, however, to favour an empirical trend. From his close relationship with Livi and from his experiences in the Bufalini group in Florence, Morselli had learned that clinical medicine needed the support of 'theory', and to make use of the basic sciences.[16] At the same time there was, undeniably, a difference between successfully administered therapy – which tended above all to 'influence' the mind – and heuristic methods, which had to resort to somaticism in order to redeem insanity from the moralistic and sentimental mortgage. Morselli's continual contact with the patients (he saw how they passed their days and got to know the cases in detail) induced him to reconsider assumptions and notions. At the second congress of psychiatry he presented post-mortem evidence relating to 240 ex-patients, showing that not every form of morbidity had a specific anatomical-pathological equivalent. The data at hand contradicted the thesis that behavioural problems were rooted in an organic substratum. The president of the congress, Andrea Verga, observed that the speaker had presented cases mostly having to do with insanity and paralysis (with high frequencies of lesions) and he invited the participants to verify that other forms of mental disorder were even less 'materially' correlatable. An expert on corpses even more than on the living, Verga was sure that quite often the brain remained uninjured. On the same occasion Antonio Berti of the Mental Institute for Women of Venice argued the opposite.[17]

Morselli investigated those presumed causalities and concomitances, advising circumspection. For instance, the skin diseases of the mad were often mere coincidence (as Griesinger had already noted); sometimes the connection turned out to be the opposite of what had been imagined, as in the case of 'emotional dermatosis'.[18] The fact that the psychophysical relations were not univocal and fixed was recognized with the discovery of 'stigmas'.

The issue of craniology returned to centre stage. At the third congress of psychiatry, Morselli raised some questions about the matter: what, if any, utility was there in performing craniometric tests on the mad; which were the best methods; which points were significant for the psychiatrist. It was decided to set up a special commission to answer the questions, though Morselli had already offered a model: 'whoever tries to convince you that alienists measure the skulls of the mad to deduce whether or not they are disturbed in the mind, shows that he has learned to tell tall tales'. It was agreed that a poorly developed skull did not justify inferences about the mental inferiority of its bearer. Just as, in statistics, large sets reveal general properties and averages, though individual cases always deviate – not of course because they are 'free', but because they are under the dominion of single forces.[19] Thus rather than studying the sutures of the skull, it was more revealing to scrutinize the face and the gaze of the subject, attempting to record the expressions. Emotion could uncover important secrets. Mantegazza's research, Ettore Regalia's reflections and, of course, Darwin's name guaranteed the seriousness of physiognomy, a visual angle too often granted 'to philosophers, speculators of the eccentric, physiognomists and crazy psychologists'. Finally, it should have been clear 'how exaggerated the reaction against the psychological tendencies of psychiatry had been, and that normal or morbid, the mechanism of mental processes cannot be grasped without the most profound knowledge of everything concerning comparative psychology and anthropology'.[20]

The mad were not only those committed to mental asylums. According to Morselli's calculations, in Italy the number of mentally disturbed was three times the number of those actually in institutions. Andrea Verga had elaborated statistics on institutional data. At the congress of 1880, psychiatrists asked themselves if it were possible to draw a complete map of insanity. The general census was available; in 1871 it had even recorded idiots and crazy citizens, indicating their sex, though not their age, marital status, or profession. Otherwise a study narrowed down to a sample group of the population could be done – a special but none the less complete group. However, popular attitudes were an obstacle: shame at such misfortunes and a consequent inclination to hide them, the incompetence of the people in judging their own and their relatives' mental states, and finally fear of incurring government sanctions for eventual hospital care and upkeep of the alienated. Morselli felt it was best to limit the calculation to a group of conscripts unfit for military service because of weakness of the mind, between 1869 and 1878. The results showed that even in Italy there was a visible, real increase of neurotherapy, not owing only to a greater 'sensitivity' on the part of investigation.[21]

The majority of the mentally ill none the less escaped hospitalization and thus official controls and consideration as well. Anyone who looked around carefully in the places he normally frequented could recognize some 'rather odd fellows', *mattoidi* (as Lombroso would have said), or a few 'insane temperaments'. It would have certainly been convenient for science to be able to draw a clear-cut line between health and sickness; but the border was flexible and uncertain. The nature of man – so Henry Maudsley's work had taught Morselli – presented infinite and imperceptible variations. Some individuals, without being completely insane, had peculiarities of character and feelings and lived with a continuous threat of deterioration. They were 'the paralytics, the originals, the eccentric, the so-called "rational lunatics"', or those considered 'morally insane', and also 'the fanatic utopians, the inventors of absurdities, the superior intelligences'.[22] All these escaped the notice of the census, in which not even the number of hysterics was noted. Those women affected by irritability and nervousness, instead of being entrusted to the care of their doctors, were favoured by their relatives and especially by their unfortunate spouses, with whom Morselli sympathized.[23] With the above in mind, Morselli estimated that there was approximately twice as much mental illness in Italy as the statistics on the young conscripts showed, even though these were more precise than the general statistics. He was interested in counting what actually existed, that is 'alienated individuals, and not just insanity or its nosology'.

It was not a superfluous precision: alienists, rather than manipulating abstractions, should have recognized that madness 'consists in an alteration of the *psychic individuality* of man', and that they should therefore turn to the individuals.[24] The diseased, not the disease; the criminal and not the crime, as Lombroso would have said: a concrete claim that criminal anthropology, however, blunted with typologies. Morselli instead insisted on accenting singularity, which was immersed in a collective context (highlighted by the statistics), yet endowed with its own dynamic characteristics. In delineating the psychophysical and social personality of a subject it was right to use eclectic methods. And so, other than those already critically tested (craniometry, the physiology of the senses, pathologic anatomy), it was necessary to perfect new methods: hypnosis above all, some drugs, moral treatment. Diagnosis and therapy exchanged roles continually. With anamnesis greater attention would be given to environmental influences and predispositions. Child psychology, hallucinogenic states, induced sleep, emotional traumas seemed to provide further sources for better understanding of the mobility of the mind.[25] New experiences emerged, not wholly integrable with traditional deterministic models, or constitutive of a definite project. This lack underlined the urgent need to improve the models by accepting new suggestions.

The mental specific

When in 1881 Morselli moved from Macerata to Turin, he found he had to make an attempt to systematize theory. He had been given a twofold assignment: director of the insane asylum and lecturer at the Faculty of Medicine and Surgery. The combination brought on an incessant comparison of hospital practice and psychiatric teaching; the physician was forced to be both 'empirical' and scientific at the same time; to theorize on his actions; to cure, complete with a philosophy of alienation and a perfect science of mental health. These were the conditions that in the second half of the 1800s favoured the 'rebirth of clinical medicine'. Describing psychiatry as *clinical*, Morselli inaugurated his lectures at the University of Turin on 17 March 1881. In his opinion, the speciality incorporated two elements: the physiopathological, common to general medicine, and the psychological, peculiar to mental phenomena. How these two elements were connected depended on how they were defined. Which psychology was in discussion?[26] Introspection, originating in philosophy, offered some insights but also an insurmountable limitation. The observer could never overcome his own subjectivity and was consequently unable to understand truly another individual – whether that individual belonged to a mental world far from his own (the soul of a young boy or a black man), or whether it was a question of a different dimension (the unconscious). Breaking away from philosophy, 'objective' psychology was born – a system with naturalistic bases, complicated by specializations. Its basic principle was that mental evolution ran parallel to that of organic forms. Comparative psychology would run through a series of ascendant gradations, slowly assuming ethnographic, ethologic, and anthropological aspects. It was mindful of anatomy and morphology; in the light of the customs, laws, vices, and virtues of the people, modern psychology could not do without a historical dimension, which Morselli considered essential. Studying collectivity, individual differences came to the fore, these being biologically (sex, age, body structure) as well as sociologically definable (environmental conditioning and reactivity). Hence social psychology was concerned with man as part of a whole, and his actions in the mass. And finally, psychophysiology, which subjected mental phenomena, seen as products of the nervous system, to experimental testing. In its brief digression, the direction psychology was taking seemed to be returning it to the starting-point. Yet, Morselli added, the *quid* that distinguished psychiatry from medicine remained intact. 'Reducing consciousness to ordinary organic processes' was just a useful structure for further research, whose goals did not include the mere demonstration of that reduction. It could also be taken as an hypothesis, but without exaggerating its importance. To exhaust psychology in a physiology of the nervous system would have impaired its future progress and narrowed its frontiers.

The warning, had it been heeded, might have prevented the neo-idealistic accusations made by Benedetto Croce and Giovanni Gentile, who were fiercely opposed to experimental psychology. In 1906 Morselli defended it with dignity, showing how different it was from the image its adversaries painted of it. For instance, a systematic disdain of introspection was erroneously attributed. Before declaring the failure of scientific psychology – and of all science – thus raising once again the barrier between spirit and nature, the importance of the 'positive' contributions to the understanding of the mind should have been recognized.[27] In 1881 Morselli praised Angelo Mosso, a physiologist and colleague from his university days, for having repudiated the theory that the study of the brain, however detailed and exact, actually reveals the human 'soul'. Avoiding undue euphoria, or pessimism, one had only to exploit all the resources science offered. Just as the surgical knife finely sections interlaced tissues, the phenomenology of the mind seemed to be decomposable into simpler elements, when under the effect of morphine or curare, or when in natural or induced sleep: all operations which tend to 'anatomize' the psyche. The principle so dear to modern chemistry was also recalled: 'the more perfect a science is, the better it can reduce phenomena to quantities'. Weight, volume, blood pressure, etc., were all recorded during emotional reactions, whether to show how 'matter' varied with mental labour, or whether to draw attention to the fact that the labour of the mind, far from being pure spirituality, required special preconditions. Between the two worlds of body and mind – which did not escape the law of the conservation of energy – were causality and continuity, two principles already evoked by Mantegazza in his essay *La trasformazione delle forze psichiche*, which Morselli had very much appreciated.[28]

These more or less deterministic axioms lost their bite when the physician attempted to apply them in the hospital. There more than anywhere, an 'irreducible mental specific' prevailed. It seemed that 'scientific opportunism' had led to this problem of the interlacing of theory and practice. Morselli explained it as follows: psychiatry had had to fight to gain its standing, overcoming the 'psychicism' predominant at the beginning of the century (here he mentioned Johann A. Heinroth and Karl W. Ideler) with a 'somaticistic reaction' (he considered Maximilian Jacobi, Andrew Combe, and François Broussais its exponents).[29] The clinical approach was the proper exit from that antithesis; it was able to account for the 'intermediate' mental states. The 'semi-insane' presented bizarre symptoms which disappeared and reappeared; neurological tests could not grasp them, since the illness concerned above all a moral sensitivity. *Quality*, not just gradation, as in fact the so-called 'functional disorders' had already required.[30] And *individuality*, more and more declared the home of the mind:

> Each of us thinks and acts differently, partly because our brain structure is extraordinarily variable and the combinations of our traits innumerable, and partly because our education, family relationships and social life create, in each individual, a different source of sensations, emotions and feelings.[31]

The alienists should have considered all these elements rather than 'racking their brains in search of those supposedly characteristic boundaries, which nature never respects, between one case and another'. It was a mania for classification from which Morselli tried to liberate himself, pleased to be able to express his freedom from prejudice. He imagined the shock of his colleagues, who saw in his proposals a 'complete overturning of the dominant systems of our schools'.[32] After so much polemics on contrasting theories, his courage consisted in renouncing the adddition of yet another that claimed the same omnicomprehension. Instead of defending itself, Morselli wanted psychiatry to vindicate an image of non-determinism, which had origin in its object. Conditions of health presented so much variety that it was not possible to define morbid phenomenology. The symptoms, which were to be subjected to the most accurate tests, were of alterable intensity, alternate, exaggerated, and simulated, often latent behind disorders or seeming equilibria or both. The objective method faithfully recorded exterior manifestations; but gestures, language, expressions, and writing were elements that remained to be interpreted. The diagnostic procedures used to do so were, according to Morselli, insufficient: the 'direct' method pretended immediate deduction by observation; the 'semiological' one, which constructed a symptomatological scheme of the disease, attempted to recognize it by looking for its analogy among classic nosographic types. The most valuable method was the 'historical-genetic' diagnosis based on the history of the disease. In fact, the new clinical method was, above all, to reconstruct the process of mental alienation, employing the useful elements eclectically, case by case. It was characterized by the focusing on the subjective suffering of the patient, on the changes in his character and feelings, without at all neglecting the individual picture: '*every disordered person*', Morselli emphasized, '*must be studied and analysed singly and for himself*'. In other words, each individual mind, when in a morbid state, must be compared to that which it was or should have been in its normal state.[33] There was an inevitable resounding of Claude Bernard's lesson. It is important to note, however, that the tensions which had surrounded the project of 'experimental medicine' were at that point left aside.[34] The call for a unitary vision of sickness and health did not imply the idea that the only differences between them were in degree. Nor was a mechanical perspective on pathology necessary, since it derived from physiology.

The heart of the matter lay elsewhere. This was pointed out by a student of Richard von Krafft-Ebing, whom Morselli esteemed highly. In his *Klinische Psychiatrie*, Heinrich Schüle created an anthropological model, in neo-Kantian style, for psychology, which allowed for the recognition of an unsuppressible element in the tendencies of the individual.[35] The individual, whether sane or not, enjoyed and suffered his own mental existence, in relation to his hereditary constitution and his environment, and, beginning with a particular origin, developed uniquely. 'Character' had to be taken into consideration: the anomalous behaviour was not to be compared with the normal 'type', an ideal or statistic, but rather with its previous functioning, judged to be restorable. 'One cannot be called crazy, if one has not undergone a change in character, in affections, feelings and anxieties; this implies the necessity of knowing what the patient was like previously, how he thought and acted, what he loved and how he reacted to external stimuli.' Just as, in curing a case of pneumonia or a subject suffering from heart disease, it was important to check respiration and blood pressure, so for the mentally ill it was indispensable to know his *past*, his family, the environment he grew up in, any progressive illnesses and traumas he might have suffered, and his constitution.[36]

The first thing to uncover was heredity, which was sometimes of a degenerative character. It was useful to learn about the parents: if the child was conceived early or late in their lives, if it was the fruit of an embrace surrounded by moral apprehension, during illness or under the influence of alcohol. But research had to explore all family relations – ancestors, descendants, collateral relatives – given that the transmission of the germ did not follow any mechanical rule. No piece of information about the patient was irrelevant, beginning with his development in the womb (the relationship between foetus and mother being quite important), continuing through childhood and adolescence. An imbalance hidden for several years could derive from a trauma which took place long before. Physical development could give an idea of how much evolutionary energy the individual organism possessed. Frailty and sensitivity (sleep-walking or nightmare) undoubtedly attested to a weakness of the nervous system. The domestic and school environments were the seats of the incubation of the temperament: it was sometimes surprising to find there the stimuli to which the child had been subjected; his reactions, memorized, were the 'presumptive trail' to what he became, good or bad, as an adult. Morselli found it difficult to believe, but 'not a few alienists, in the clinical examination of a mentally ill patient, ignored these laws of general psychological evolution'. They did not even take into consideration the radical change that always took place during puberty, and which the American Stanley Hall was then successfully demonstrating. Often, during that period of growth, mental development preceded physical development; sexual awakening occurred in the mind, before it reached the testicles or ovaries. In these cases an extraordinary nervous excitability arose, mostly in unconscious manifestations of fantasized voluptuousness. All youth, shaken by the development of sexual powers, was subject to this perturbation. Some never reach a superior equilibrium, and these individuals continue to suffer the problems that began during their puberty.[37] Anamnesis should be able to provide a list of all progressive diseases to which adults were subject, particularly sexual disturbances which often prepared the groundwork for, if they did not actually sow the seeds of, insanity. Morselli was convinced, perhaps not completely correctly, that psychiatrists were indifferent to the perils of sexuality: masturbation, the contrivances of the libido, even forced abstinence and ejaculation during sleep, aggravated by the 'cerebralism' that invaded the erotic sphere. Among the secrets of sex, he intended to discover how the mental *constitution* of the individual developed: that is 'what the inherited nature of the brain, the education, previous lifestyle, social and domestic atmosphere, illnesses and vices, misfortunes and joys have formed in the development of the character and intelligence'.

On the basis of his patients' behaviour Morselli ventured a distinction between two opposing natures: 'expansive' and 'concentric'. He knew that Griesinger had considered it useful to propose, on mental paradigms, a doctrine of the temperaments. His devaluation of Jung's theory of psychological types is therefore somewhat surprising; in 1916 he would comment that distinguishing between introverts and extroverts was like talking about dogs and cats, or light and darkness.[38] In 1882 he professed his certainty that one's life was dominated by a mental form, evident in the individual's affections. Feeling and not reason – he had read in Schüle's manual – was the true catalyst of human behaviour, whether normal or not. Not even with insanity was the tonality of feelings lost. Though altered, it was still an indication of the uniqueness of the individual; it differentiated him even from those suffering the same illness.

These concepts, however, were not so ignored in Italy as Morselli had supposed. In 1885 he expounded them in his *Manuale di semejotica delle malattie mentali*, which enjoyed wide circulation among 'physicians, legal experts, and students', for whom it had been compiled. His insistence on individuality, *constitutio*, and retrospective investigation found support in 'morphological' clinical practice, proclaimed in Padua, in 1878, by Achille De Giovanni.[39] The two teachings had in common an interpretation of Darwin and Lamarck, monism à la Haeckel, a critical interest in Charcot and an anthropological conception of medicine deemed to be superior to empiricism. Exalting the notion of 'clinical medicine', both Morselli and De Giovanni attempted to anchor it philosophically, and protect it from the ramifications of specialization.

Morselli had no doubt that in this respect psychiatry would encounter the greatest difficulties because of the 'something else' of the mind. Mental illness tore the fine veil in which the most profound mysteries of the mind were wrapped, and allowed an invasion of the cocoon. This had been noted often; it was upheld by Livi and Tamburini when in 1875 they launched the *Rivista sperimentale di freniatria*. It was like a leitmotif: the mental imbalance that divested a man of his manners and social conventions amplifies certain aspects of his character, which it breaks down into elements, and whose 'spirituality it analyses', according to a Lombrosian formula.[40] Ten years after this psychiatric 'manifesto', the attitude had become more complex and prudent, and research on the symmetry of symptom and lesion less obsessive. In his *Manuale di semejotica* Morselli called for a concentration on those areas of knowledge that 'in particular, medicine could not nor would know how to teach'. He well understood that the 'average' or 'normal' man was an ideal created by poets and philosophers, or perhaps even the recent invention of scientists too preoccupied with generalities to concern themselves with the lives of individuals.[41]

The search for a new curability

'The investigation of the mental phenomenon constitutes the true, intrinsic aim of psychiatry.' Morselli affirmed this in polemic with whomever accused theory of having betrayed the experimental path and of falling into speculative abstractions. In his opinion the 'mental' path – as it was called – had responded to practical and theoretical needs raised by the rebirth of clinical medicine. Only to those who considered 'science' an accumulation of data could that path seem a digression. He claimed this in 1889 while commemorating Dario Maragliano, a friend of his who had had experiences very similar to his own: the assistantship at the mental hospital in Reggio Emilia, neuropathological research, hospital practice all over Italy, and finally the twofold assignment – university lecturer and director of an asylum in Genoa where, at 37 years of age, he died from a pulmonary disease.[42] Though on this special occasion, Morselli chose to state his views in precise detail, under other circumstances he hesitated to do so, manoeuvring himself instead between opposing parties. As the successor to Dario Maragliano, in 1890 in Genoa Morselli began a course on clinical psychiatry, evoking Morgagni, who had been the first to study corpses of the mentally ill in search of anatomical-pathological causes of disturbance. Later, that lesson having been forgotten, too much attention was given to the 'spiritual' element because of misleading, aprioristic psychologies. 'If one admits that mental disturbances are caused by anomalies or lesions of the nerve centres', then one cannot help but deduce that psychiatry is the most sophisticated chapter of neuropathology. It is doubtful that Morselli accepted the presupposition, let alone its logical consequence. Such affirmations, common within the psychiatric community, can be misleading when taken out of context.[43] In fact Morselli's lectures took quite a different tone. He suggested that around insanity – in the proper sense of the word – there opened up concentric and indistinct zones, each overlapping one another without distinct borders. Passing through all of them, it could be seen that only one limited area was common to the two sciences. Psychiatry, though bordering on neuropathology strayed from it a great deal. This autonomy, Morselli explained, was tenable not for practical purposes, but because it was backed by fact and was of scientific value. Enumerating the relations between the mind and the brain Morselli emphasized those of *quality*. Very common symptoms – hallucinations, fixations, personality changes – could not be adequately explained by the neuropathology of the nervous system. The examination of individual cases left the psychophysical relation an enigma to be resolved. Yet it was still helpful to fall back on the principle of the conservation of energy, one of the 'greatest conquests' of the nineteenth century. Faith in the future progress of science, or better yet in the monistic *Weltanschauung*, was preferable to Du Bois-Reymond's *ignorabimus*. It was believed that this formula provided 'the means to reconcile the differences and eliminate the dichotomy between the body and the spirit'; it was the saviour from the dilemma between materialism and idealism. Armed with this philosophy, the alienists were able to defend themselves. To charge them 'with being "metaphysicians" or with following remote paths outside the scientific and medical realms, because they are forced to consider the mental phenomenon above all, is simply the result of the great ignorance of many people, including even scientists and expert laboratory technicians, mainly in Italy, about the significance of mental phenomena, objective methods and the experimental progress of modern psychology'.[44]

In fact, psychology was unveiling wide possibilities in the exploration of the mind. Of greatest interest were the feelings, joys, and distresses of the human soul. The manifestations of the collective spirit – the language, knowledge, religion of a certain society and even the delinquency and moral code – revealed the co-ordinates on which, by the reflex of its course, each conscience, normal or deviant, was formed.

The second volume of the *Manuale di semejotica*, published in 1894, placed psychological examination at the centre of non-symptomatological study of insanity, that is, all illnesses and deviations of the personality. The work was finished nine years after the first volume because, as Morselli explained, he had hoped for so long to see the necessary reform of psychiatry. He had waited in vain. Thus the book reflected 'not only the author's uncertainties, but the transitory conditions of scientific matters as well'. Yet a few steps forward had actually been taken; in fact it might not be too long before – with the convergence of the clinical and experimental methods – diagnosis could be derived from the 'simple and rough observation of external forms and elementary functions'. At that time, with that false anthropological model – which 'provided no criteria whatsoever with which to judge' whether an individual is mad – the 'equation with a hundred unknowns, between organism and thought, between brain and consciousness, was easily resolved'. In more than 800 pages, dedicated to the students of Genoa, the professor showed how the criticisms, on the one hand, of such a downright 'dangerous' path (which did not even take into consideration the individual characteristics of structure and function) and the necessity, on the other hand, of the psychological foundation, were indispensable presuppositions for the 'new psychology'.[45]

Given this, Morselli did not consider it a contradiction when he called himself an 'organicist'. The same terms were used in the medical lexicon and in all educated circles in the nineteenth century, but with different meanings; this brought on a great deal of confusion between the protagonists of the day and the historians who succeeded them. Organicism was also a positivistic 'mania', though in some it expressed the choice of descending the labyrinths of consciousness and unconsciousness, by keeping to the 'unitary anthropological and biosociological concepts of personality'. It was not a coincidence that one of Morselli's works concerned *Neurosi traumatiche*. Traumatic neurosis was the consequence of a blow to the head, which none the less continued after physical recovery. He held that the causes were all 'psychological'; among them were fear, difficulty of reinsertion, auto-suggestion and even a hope of indemnity (there was an increase in cases of these neuroses, after accident legislation was introduced).[46] The above specification holds also for psychiatry and neuropathology. Skilful in 'acrobatics', Morselli sometimes placed the accent on affinities, at other times on discord. At the twelfth congress of the psychiatric society and at the second congress of Italian neurologists, five years later, he repeated an appeal for co-operation between the two disciplines. Each, however, was to maintain its autonomy, rather than seek together a singleness which would be contradicted by the facts: *folie à doute*, moral insanity, hysteria, and neurasthenia were bridges between the two sciences. They presented organic signs in sensation and movement, but proceeded along psychic axes. Morselli understood this well; he preferred the views of the school of Nancy on hysteria to the 'neurologism' of Briquet and Charcot: 'a monstrous polyp fixed to the rock of the constitutional disturbances of the ontogenesis and replacement of the nervous system, it casts its tentacles on the one side into the most amazing corners of neurology, and on the other, into the most obscure hiding-places of psychology'. Render unto Caesar that which is Caesar's. Once the neurologists took only what was rightfully theirs, everybody would benefit, including the alienists. Since the 1880s, there had been progress: in Pavia Camillo Golgi was probing cerebral histology; new hypotheses on the localization of language were surpassing Broca's; thanks to Ernesto Lugaro and Arturo Donaggio, important contributions came from the Reggio Emilia and Florentine schools.[47]

Obviously, psychiatry had to keep itself up to date on the progresses of other specialities; if it was in need of help, Morselli observed in 1916, it could turn to qualified experts in the various sectors, and thus it could finally concentrate on its theoretical and therapeutic tasks. He took as a good sign the fact that manuals on mental illness were devoting less space to neurology; in his second edition of the *Trattato di Psichiatria*, Leonardo Bianchi shortened the section on neurology by almost a hundred pages. Coming from a rare expert on nerve morphology, the abridgement was significant, not so much as a repudiation, but as a more mature psychiatric identity.

The pioneering enthusiasm having subsided and the 'positivist fetishisms' been overcome, some remaining obscurities could be conceded to that most 'complex' of human sciences. The recognition of such obscurities should not frighten researchers. Morselli proposed further investigation, which was, however, to be carried on with a certain equilibrium. Some foreigners were perhaps guilty of being rash: Freud, Jung, Adler; Eugen Bleuler of Zurich and Hans Gruhle of Heidelberg exaggerated their insistence on the psychic component.[48] So, neither shabby somatism nor evanescent psychologism. The question was anything but academic. For the most part it was a matter of therapeutic options even though, as has already been noted, there was no congruence between general trends and hospital practice. Moral treatment, hot and cold showers, high calorie diets, rest, electric treatment: all these did not seem justifiable by the same line of argument.

At the end of the 1870s, innovation in therapy was found in mechanical vibrations. Between 1877 and 1879 Morselli had observed the experiments of the Roman clinician Carlo Maggiorani, in which the anaesthetized limb of a hysterical woman was slipped into a large tuning fork attached to a resonance box. The rhythmic shocks given were to have such an effect as to eliminate – it was hoped – all muscular contractions. Something similar was being done at the Salpêtrière with equipment that the Englishman Mortimer Granville claimed to have invented; Charcot corroborated the method, claiming that the continual rhythmic action had a positive effect on the nerves. The director of the asylum in Turin was well acquainted with these various endeavours. He had a vibratory box built, to which he subjected his depressed patients; others (though never the excitable ones) underwent half an hour of the 'trembling armchair' or the 'shaking helmet'. There were effects, although he believed they were the results of *suggestion*; none the less a good reason for using the instruments. It was the same for hydrotherapy and other similar operations on psychotics, who proved to be easily influenced subjects.

The use of physical remedies continued long after the decline of faith in somaticism. Whoever still confidently attributed insanity to a lesion would naturally believe that operating was an effective therapy. Morselli used to tell the story of two French doctors, Gueniot and Lannelongue, who believed that craniotomies would bring on a 'sudden regeneration and transformation' in idiots. Horrors of science, condemned with greater severity by those who understood their absurdities. He did not neglect what Daniel Hack Tuke called psychotherapy. *The influence of mind upon body* explained how pressure on the body was beneficial; not by healing lesions or irritations (which were non-existent in any case), but by inspiring the trustful credulity of the infirm. For this reason Morselli preferred docile patients who put themselves completely in the hands of their doctor. With types like Ms T.V., a hysterical, intelligent, well-educated and insatiable 33-year-old who 'had the bad habit of arguing even about prescriptions', little could be done.[49]

According to Morselli, the first rule in healing was not to have set rules; he was convinced that suitable therapy could be derived only from personalized diagnosis. Even though he distrusted excessive classifying, he recognized that its complete dismissal would have meant a surrender to empiricism. In 1885, adducing a preference for an historic-genetic taxonomy rather than a morpho-physiological one, he said that in Turin he had adopted a criterion for distinguishing the principal groups: the *parafrenie*, or anomalies of constitutional development, and the *frenopatie*, or real mental derangement. The first were congenital psychopathies, resulting from hereditary degeneration or relating to critical periods in the subject's life; the second considered toxic encephalopathies, cerebropathies and psychoneuroses. The *frenastenie* formed a group in itself (idiocy, cretinism, imbecility), their cause being an arrest of development. This tripartite division, Morselli confessed, did not exactly satisfy him, and did not differ much from what Andrea Verga had proposed, which was accepted at the first congress of psychiatry and had been in use for some time, even though its limitations were evident. In Genoa Morselli changed his system: there were nine nosographical groups provided for the compilation of medical records, from encephalic irritations to functional disturbances.[50] The risk of misunderstandings concerning ideas and criteria was continuous, and it denoted the substantial problems of a young science, as Morselli noted. With Pinel, psychiatric nosography consisted principally of melancholy, mania, and dementia; Esquirol introduced the concept of the monomanias; Morel, the 'Darwin of psychiatry', was responsible for the transition from symptomatology to aetiology. Wilhelm Griesinger, who firmly connected the study of madness to medicine, introduced a reformation of similar importance; Emil Kraepelin advanced similar propositions, specifying among other things a new clinical class, *dementia praecox*.

Yet agreement among psychiatrists had still not been reached (and never really has been), and classification was discussed at various symposia: by Andrea Verga in 1874 and Augusto Tamburini in 1886 (regarding a project for international statistics on those with mental disorders). In 1889, at the tenth congress of psychiatry, a special commission, including Morselli and Leonardo Bianchi (for whom the use of classifications was totally alien), was formed. Sante De Sanctis, the chairman, wanted to know what the

Italian psychiatrists thought, and he sent questionnaires to forty–seven of them. When accepted, the taxonomies never coincided; everybody chose as they wished, following the outlines given by Krafft-Ebing or Schüle or Morselli.[51] In attempting to describe the heterogeneity of institutional nomenclature, even if it was important, the thread of the question is easily lost. What counted most, beyond the modernized and combined categories, was the choice of the parameters: anatomical-pathological, psychological, descriptive, or aetiologic.

Annotating the Italian edition of Gilbert Ballet's *Trattato sulle malattie mentali*, Morselli let it be known that he was not very pleased with the type of classification given by this student of Charcot. It seemed senseless to him to correct it in detail, though he did alter the French text a great deal. He did not miss the opportunity to emphasize the importance of the criterion for distinguishing mental alienation which corresponds to an arrest in development, from the changes in, or dissolution of, an already formed personality. In the second case the ontogenetic analysis of the mental functions, according to Ernst Haeckel's formula – 'ontogeny recapitulates philogeny' – could be useful.

Actual diseases fell into the other group; they were to be examined by the physician and compared to the patient's normal mental *individuality*. With a constitutionalist approach, Morselli cited James Sully's personality studies; reconfirmed the lesson of the 'most profound of the German psychiatrists', and praised Schüle, among other things for having introduced the therapeutic-pedagogic criterion, whose aim was to organize diseases according to their potential for re-education.

After so much pessimism about therapy, caused by somatistic inclinations and degenerative theories, once again there was talk of the 'curability of the insane'. More than a well-grounded humanitarian inspiration (the real remedy, in Morselli's opinion, was social prophylaxis), it was a guiding hypothesis, with which to face the more obscure aspects of psychiatry. Too often the incurable was the one who, in his illness, was not even 'understood'.[52]

Notes

This is a modified version of a chapter of my book *Individualità difformi: La psichiatria antropologica di Enrico Morselli* (Milan: Franco Angeli, 1986).

1 Enrico Morselli (1914) 'Ciò che vuole essere la psichiatria', *Quad. Psichiat.* 1: 1–13.

2 On Morselli (Modena, 17.7.1852–Genoa, 13.2.1929), see his autobiography in Onorato Roux (ed.) (1910) *Infanzia e giovinezza di illustri italiani contemporanei. Memorie autobiografiche* … III. *Gli scienziati*, Florence: Bemporad, pp. 315–63; and Patrizia Guarnieri (1986) *Individualità difformi: La psichiatria antropologica di Enrico Morselli*, Milan: Franco Angeli, with the bibliography of his works.

3 On Canestrini (1835–1900), see Giuliano Pancaldi (1983) *Darwin in Italia: Impresa scientifica e frontiere culturali*, Bologna: il Mulino, pp. 149–208. On Livi (1823–77), cf. Enrico Morselli and Augusto Tamburini (1879) 'La mente di Carlo Livi', *Riv. sper. Freniat. Med. leg. Alien. ment.* 5: I–XLVII and 6 (1880): I-XXXIII. On Gaddi (1805–71), see Giuseppe Favaro's biographical sketch (1949) *Enciclopedia Italiana*, Rome: 1st Enc. Ital., *ad vocem*.

4 V. Grasselli (1897) *L'ospedale di San Lazzaro presso Reggio nell' Emilia*, Reggio Emilia: Calderini. One of the main journals of Italian psychiatry came from the Reggio school; see Enrico Morselli (1915) 'Come nacque la Rivista di freniatria', and Augusto Tamburini (1915) 'Il primo quarantennio della Rivista sperimentale di freniatria', *Riv. sper. Freniat. Med. leg. Alien. ment.* 41: XXXVI–XLV and I–XXV respectively. To avoid bibliographical repetitions, for rich information and references on the background see Annamaria Tagliavini (1985) 'Aspects of the history of psychiatry in Italy in the second half of the nineteenth century', in W.F. Bynum, R. Porter and M. Shepherd (eds), *The Anatomy of Madness*, London: Tavistock, vol. II, pp. 175–96; but her point of view (unlike mine) insists on 'faith in organic accounts of mental illness' and on 'neurological emphasis'.

5 On Mantegazza (1831–1910) and the Florentine intellectual ambient, see Giovanni Landucci (1977) *Darwinismo a Firenze: Tra scienza e ideologia (1860–1900)*, Florence: Olschki.

6 Concerning Morselli's journal, see Patrizia Guarnieri (1983) 'La volpe e l'uva: Cultura scientifica e filosofia nel positivismo italiano', *Physis, Florence* 25: 601–36, and Maria T. Monti (1983) 'Ricerche sul positivismo italiano: Filosofia e scienza nella Rivista di filosofia scientifica', *Riv. crit. stor. filos.* 38: 409–40.

7 On Morselli and the Donato case, see Patrizia Guarnieri (forthcoming) 'Theatre and laboratory: medical attitudes to animal magnetism in late nineteenth-century Italy', in R. Cooter (ed.), *Alternatives: Essays in the Social History of Irregular Medicine*, London: Macmillan.

8 Among his forensic pleas for insanity, note, at least, the following: (1877) *L'uccisore dei bambini. Carlino Grandi. Studio medico-legale dei periti F. Bini, C. Livi, E. Morselli*, Reggio Emilia: Calderini; with Cesare Lombroso (1885) 'Epilessia larvata, pazzia morale', *Archo. Psichiat.* 6: 29–43; with Sante De Sanctis (1903) *Biografia di un bandito. Giuseppe Musolino di fronte alla psichiatria e alla sociologia*, Milan: Treves; and (1905) *Linda e Tullio Murri. Studio psicologico e psichiatrico*, Genoa: Libreria moderna. On this, see Patrizia Guarnieri (1986) *Misurare le Diversità*, in *Misura d'uomo: Strumenti, teorie e pratiche dell' antropometria e della psicologia sperimentale tra '800 e '900*, Florence: Istituto e Museo di Storia della Scienza Giusti, pp. 119–71, esp. pp. 127–33.

9 He translated Ernst Haeckel (1904) *I problemi dell'universo*, Turin: Un. tip. ed. tor., with an introduction *Sulla filosofia monistica in Italia*. On 'Carlo Darwin', see his significant paper (1881–2) in *Riv. filos. scient.* 2: 237–71. Morselli's (1926) *La psicanalisi. Studi e appunti critici*, Turin: Bocca, 2 vols, was the first Italian treatise on Freudian ideas and therapy.

10 Enrico Morselli (1887) 'Patogenesi dell'epilessia', *Sperimentale* 30: 259–89.

11 Enrico Morselli (1877) *Agli onorevoli sig. Presidente e sigg. componenti la Deputazione provinciale di Macerata*, in the pamphlet *Relazioni sul Manicomio di Macerata in Santa Croce*, Macerata: tip. Cortesi, pp. 11–87.

12 Enrico Morselli (1877) *Sul lavoro agricolo e industriale nei manicomi. Osservazioni*, Sanseverino Marche: tip. Corradetti, p. 3. At the psychiatric congress in

Reggio, he presented a paper (1880) on 'L'amministrazione e la scienza nei manicomi', *Archo. ital. Mal. nerv.* 17: 373–458.

13 La Direzione [Morselli] (1920) 'La funzione speciale del manicomio', *Quad. Psichiat.* 7: 133–8. Referring to the socialist Enrico Ferri's (1920) 'Organizzazione della giustizia nella Russia dei Soviet', *Il comunismo* 1, Morselli accused the criminal anthropologists of being concerned only with the punishment, rather than the redemption, of criminals.

14 Enrico Morselli (1878) 'Le scuole per gli infermieri nel manicomio' and 'Agli onorevoli', *Gazz. Manic. Macerata* 1.

15 ibid., 37, 53 and 25–47. In (1878) *Gazz. Manic. Macerata* 1, see the following papers by him: 'Ozio e lavoro nei manicomi'; 'Inaugurazione di una colonia industriale nel Manicomio'; 'La colonia industriale ...'. The experience in Gheel was a model; but Morselli was worried that the communitarian style oppressed the individual exigencies.

16 Morselli, 'Patogenesi dell'epilessia', 289, where he accused the so-called practical physicians, who confused their ignorance of physiopathology with a comfortable empiricism.

17 Morselli's paper, 'Sull'anatomia patologica della pazzia', was not published in the *Proceedings* of the second congress of the Società freniatrica italiana, but a summary of it appeared in (1877) *Riv. sper. Freniat. Med. leg. Alien. ment.* 3: 746.

18 Enrico Morselli (1879) 'Leucodemia parziale (vitiligo) degli alienati', *Riv. sper. Freniat. Med. leg. Alien. ment.* 5: 77–93, with some clinical cases examined in the asylum of Macerata. See also (1881) 'Alcune annotazioni sulla patogenesi del tifo pellagroso e sui rapporti coll'ileio-tifo comune', *Archo. ital. Mal. nerv.* 18: 455–77.

19 Enrico Morselli (1881) 'Le ricerche craniometriche nei loro rapporti con la psichiatra', *Archo. ital. Mal. nerv.* 17: 59–80. With him on the committee were A. Tamburini, A. Tamassia, A Verga and G. Amadei; by the latter, see (1881) 'Delle migliori misure craniometriche da prendere sugli alienati', ibid., 18: 268–79. Morselli prepared the instructions on the basis of Broca's.

20 Enrico Morselli [n.d., 1881] *Fisiognomonia*, in *Enciclopedia medica italiana*, Milan: Vallardi, vol. VIII, part II, pp. 383–7. The analogy between the expression of physical pain and of depression was a key to the analysis of the physiopathological symptoms. Also in Paolo Mantegazza (1879) 'Un problema di fisiologia. L'espressione del dolore', *Nuova Antologia*, s. II, 15: 558–70; and (1880) *La fisiologia del dolore*, Florence: Poggi; see also his (1890) *Physiognomy and Expression*, London: W. Scott. Cf. Ettore Regalia (1916) *Dolore e azione*, ed. Giovanni Papini, Lanciano: Carabba. For all of them, the main reference was Charles Darwin's (1872) *The Expression of the Emotions in Man and Animals*, London: John Murray, translated by G. Canestrini in 1878.

21 Andrea Verga (1877) 'Prime linee di una statistica della frenopatie in Italia', *Archo. stat.* 2: 5–47 and (1880) 'Dei pazzi che trovansi reclusi nei manicomi ed ospitali d'Italia alla fine dell'anno 1877', ibid. 5: 235–65. By Morselli (1881) 'Note sulla statistica e sulla distribuzione geografica delle frenopatie in Italia', *Giorn. Soc. ital. Igiene* 3: 241–64.

22 Morselli, 'Note sulla statistica', 253–6, and the conclusions (p. 364). In (1893) *Pazzia e ragione*, Milan: Insubria, he complained that the psychiatric terminology was inadequate to express individual varieties. The word *mattoide*, proposed in 1879 by Lombroso, meant a man who was normal in his daily behaviour, but

insane in his ideas. Henry Maudsley's *Responsibility in mental disease* was translated into Italian by Arrigo Tamassia in 1875; of this, Morselli wrote a review in (1875) *Riv. sper. Freniat. Med. leg. Alien. ment.* 1: 390–8.

23 Enrico Morselli (1887) '*L'idroterapia nell'isterismo. Osservazioni e note cliniche*, Turin: Roux. He hardly refrained from his irritation before patients so lacking in docility.

24 Enrico Morselli (1881) *Introduzione alle lezioni di psicologia patologica e clinica psichiatrica*, Turin: Loescher, pp. 92–3. He claimed he was the first Italian to stress the priority of sick individuals upon generic diseases; see his (1885) *Manuale di semejotica delle malattie mentali*, Milan: Vallardi, vol. 1, p. 9.

25 Enrico Morselli (1886) 'Fisiopsicologia dell'ipnotismo. Le modificazioni fondamentali del processo psichico negli stati ipnotici', *Riv. filos, scient.* 5: 449–78; with Eugenio Tanzi (1889) 'Contributo sperimentale alla fisiopsicologia dell'ipnotismo', ibid. 8: 705–29 and (1888) 'Le condizioni della sensibilità generale e della funzione visiva nella ipnosi', *R. Acc. med. Torino* 30 defending the Nancy school thesis. See also Enrico Morselli and Gabriele Buccola (1881) *Ricerche sperimentali sull'azione fisiologica e terapeutica della cocaina*, Milan: Bernardoni. On evolutionary psychology, see Enrico Morselli (1887) 'Una inchiesta psicologica sull'infanzia', *Riv. Pedag. it.* 2: offprint, Turin (1887). He worked also on abnormal children, cf. his paper (1880) *Le scuole per i fanciulli idioti ed epilettici*, Milan: Civelli.

26 Morselli, *Introduzione*, pp. 9–27.

27 Enrico Morselli (1906) *La psicologia scientifica positiva e la reazione neoidealistica*, preface to Adelchi Baratono, *Fondamenti di psicologia sperimentale*, Turin: Bocca, pp. V–XXXIX. A significant position in this dispute was taken by a professor of philosophy in Florence, who had had a psychiatric training in the Frenocomio of Reggio Emilia: Francesco De Sarlo (1901) *Studi sulla filosofia contemporanea. Prolegomeni. La filosofia scientifica*, Rome: Loescher, pp. 163–241. About this, see Patrizia Guarnieri (1984) 'Il morale e il normale. Sull'antideterminismo di F. De Sarlo', *Riv. di Filos.* 75: 251–71.

28 Morselli, *Introduzione*, p. 28 and pp. 34–7. About Mosso's stance, neither materialism nor spiritualism, note Claudio Pogliano (1982) 'Inquietudini dela scienza positiva', *Giorn. crit. Filos. ital.* 41: 207–21. The paper by Mantegazza appeared in (1887) *Nuova Antol.* s. II, 6: 100–21.

29 Morselli, *Introduzione*, pp. 48–9, with an historical sketch, pp. 38–43. On 'somatists' vs. 'psychists', see Klaus Doerner (1981) *Madmen and the Bourgeoisie: a social history of insanity and psychiatry*, Oxford: Basil Blackwell, pp. 245–62.

30 Morselli, *Introduzione*, pp. 44, 51 and 57–8. On functional disorders, with or without unknown anatomo-pathological substratum, sometimes he said that they existed only as unscientific prejudices, at other times he demanded that more attention should be given to them. Such an ambiguity reflected the constant oscillation between psychism and somatism.

31 ibid., p. 58. Aware that the studies on localization were different in their assumptions, methods, and results, he criticized the phrenology of Gall and Spurzheim, but he was interested in Broca's research on aphasia (ibid., pp. 63–5).

32 ibid., quot., pp. 58 and 69.

33 Enrico Morselli (1882) *Il metodo clinico nella diagnosi generale della pazzia*. I. *Esame anamnestico*, Milan: Vallardi, pp. 93–7.

34 Denying the qualitative difference between normal and pathological, Claude

Bernard (1876) *Leçons sur la chaleur animale*, Paris: Baillière. On this, see the critical analysis of Georges Canguilhem (1942) *Essai sur quelque problèmes concernant le normal et le patologique*, Paris: Clermont Ferrand.

35 The books of Heinrich Schüle translated into Italian were (1883) *Manuale delle malattie mentali*, edited G. Bini, Napoli: Jovene e Pasquale, and (1890) *Psichiatria clinica, patologia e terapia speciale della malattie mentali*, Napoli: Jovene e Pasquale.

36 Morselli, *Introduzione*, pp. 99ff. There is more about this subject in the second volume of his (1894) *Manuale di semejotica. Esame psicologico*, Milan: Vallardi, esp. pp. 70–124, a section devoted to five enquiries (inspection, questioning, material proofs, experimental tests, and witnesses).

37 On that subject he presented a paper (1910) at the Congresso Sanitario dell'Alta Italia, Trento e Trieste (Genoa); then Enrico Morselli [n.d., 1912] *La neurastenia degli adolescenti*, Milan: Vallardi. He found the main cause to be sexual abstinence, not excess.

38 Enrico Morselli (1916) review of 'Jung, C.G., *Contribution à l'étude des types psychologiques* ..., Geneva 1914', *Quad. Psichiat.* 3: 61–2.

39 Achille De Giovanni (1879) *Aspirazioni nel metodo dell'indagine clinica*, Milan: Bignami. His previous work in the asylum of Milan and a visit to the Salpêtrière convinced De Giovanni how important the influence of nervous energy was on individual physiopathological processes. See Giorgio Cosmacini (1981) *Medicina, ideologie, filosofie nel pensiero dei clinici*, in *Storia d'Italia. Annali 4*, Turin: Einaudi, pp. 1179–87.

40 Carlo Livi (1875) 'Del metodo sperimentale in freniatria e medicina legale', *Riv. sper. Freniat. Med. leg. Alien. ment.* 1: 1–10; Cesare Lombroso (1887) 'Le nuove conquiste della psichiatria', *Riv. filos. scient.* 6: 641–55. In the chaos of a disintegrated personality, the psychopathology had to establish the 'order of the disorder'; see Enrico Morselli (1913) *Sugli effetti schizofrenici delle allucinazioni. Note di psicologia patologica*, in *Ricerche di nevrologia di psichiatria e di psicologia*, a volume dedicated to Leonardo Bianchi, Catania: Gianotta, pp. 31–49.

41 Morselli, *Manuale* I, pp. 8, 15 and ch. III on the *Elemento obiettivo somatico*, esp. pp. 84, 95, 141.

42 Enrico Morselli (1890) 'Il Prof. Dario Maragliano', in *Annuario R. Univ. degli studi di Genova*, Genoa: stab. Martini, pp. 147–58.

43 Enrico Morselli (1891) *La psichiatria moderna nei suoi rapporti con le altre scienze*, Naples: tip. Riforma medica, pp. 2–22.

44 On the theoretical meaning of the energy conservation law, Enrico Morselli (1895) 'L'eredità materiale, intellettuale e morale del secolo XIX', in *Annuario R. Univ. degli studi di Genova*, Genoa: stab. Martini, esp. pp. 35–7.

45 On individual and collective psychology, see Morselli's intervention in the discussion with Venturi, Lombroso, and Enrico Ferri, concerning Silvio Tonini's paper (1897) at the ninth Congresso Frenol. ital. (Florence, 1896), in *Riv. sper. Freniat. Med. leg. Alien. ment.* 23: 144–6. See also Morselli, *Manuale*, II, pp. VIII, 10 and 1–21.

46 Even about his 'somatistic' statements, we must avoid any extrapolation from the context; note, for example, Morselli, *Il metodo clinico*, pp. 88ff. On functional diseases of traumatized people, he presented a paper at the Italian congress of labour medicine (Turin, 1981), enlarged in the notable book (1913) *Le neurosi traumatiche. Studio clinico e medico legale*, Turin: Un. tip. ed.

47 Enrico Morselli (1905) 'Neuropatologia e psichiatra', *Riv. sper. Freniat. Med.*

leg. Alien. ment. 30: 15–43; (1911) 'Problemi odierni della neuropatologia', his presidential introduction at the second congress of Italian neurologists (Genoa, October, 1909), Genoa: stab. lit. Ligure. See also *Manuale*, II, pp. 2–3 and cf. Camillo Golgi (1903) *Opera omnia*, Milan: Hoepli, 3 vols; and Ernesto Lugaro (1900) 'I recenti progressi della autonomia del sistema nervoso in rapporto alla psicologia e alla psichiatria', *Riv. sper. Freniat. Med. leg. Alien. ment.* 26: 92–147.

48 Morselli, 'Ciò che vuole', pp. 1–13, esp. p. 2. Compare what he said about Leonardo Bianchi's book and Eugenio Tanzi and Ernesto Lugaro (1914) *Trattato delle malattie mentali*, Milan: ed. Libraria, 2nd edn, in 'Due trattati italiani di psichiatria', *Quad. Psichiat.* 1: 202–14, with his review of E. Bleuler (1916) *Lehrbuch der Psychiatrie* (Berlin: Springer), in (1920) 'Due recenti trattati tedeschi di psichiatria', ibid. 7: 116–22. See also Enrico Morselli, *Prefazione* to L. Scabia (1900) *Trattato di terapia delle malattie mentali ad uso dei medici*, Turin: Un. tip. ed., pp. IX–XVI.

49 Enrico Morselli (1892) *Sulle vibrazioni meccaniche nella cura delle malattie nervose e mentali*, Milan: Vallardi; Morselli, *L'idroterapia*, p. 24 and (26 Aug. 1893) 'La cura chirurgica dell'idiotismo', *Gazz. degli Ospitali* 14: 1065–7.

50 Enrico Morselli, *Saggio di classificazione delle malattie mentali*, in his *Manuale*, pp. 429–38. Cf. Andrea Verga (1874) 'Proposta di una classificazione uniforme delle malattie mentali a scopo particolarmente statistico', *Archo. ital. Mal. nerv.* 11: 217–41.

51 See Sante De Sanctis (1902) 'Sulla classificazione delle frenopatie', *Riv. sper. Freniat. Med. leg. Alien. ment.* 23: 182–254. The main references were the books by Wernicke, translated into Italian in 1896, Krafft-Ebing and Kraepelin, translated in 1886 and 1885.

52 Cf. G. Ballet, *Le psicosi*, trans. V. Colla, revised and annotated by Morselli; vol. VI of (1892–7) *Trattato di medicina*, ed. J.M. Charcot, C. Bouchard and Brissaud, trans. B. Silva, with *Aggiunte e annotazioni* by several Italian writers, Turin: Un. tip. ed.; written by Morselli, *Le psicosi tossiche*, pp. 169–90 and *Le demenze*, pp. 237–48.

CHAPTER FIVE

Medicine and religion: on the physical and mental disorders that accompanied the Ulster Revival of 1859

James G. Donat

In 1859, the year most historians associate with Darwin's *Origin of Species*, a religious revival took place in Ireland during the months just preceding the publication of this famous work,[1] which had nothing to do with Darwin or the controversy over evolution. It occurred in the province of Ulster, primarily in the counties where the Protestants were in the majority (that is, the land area of twentieth-century Northern Ireland), and almost exclusively among the Protestant portion of the population. Yet because the revival in 1859 was a noisy affair, it became an object of notice for both the public press and the medical journals of the time.

It began quietly with a small prayer group in the village of Connor (County Antrim) and subsequently spread to other parts of Ulster. But in the process of its transmission a large number of people were overcome by a powerful 'conviction of sin', which in some instances resulted in individuals being stricken down (usually once) with a variety of physical and mental effects that were shocking and 'dreadful to see'. The following is a typical scene described by a witness to revival meetings in Ballymena (County Antrim):

> Suddenly the [religious] services are interrupted by a piercing cry. A man has fallen in agony. Every portion of his body shakes as with an ague. His eyes are closed, or roll about in a manner frightful to behold. His frame is convulsed with pain. His pulse is quick and feverish, and his face is bathed in perspiration, whilst all this time he continues to ejaculate the most fearful cries for mercy. A few of his friends and neighbours collect around him. They convey him home and endeavour to soothe his mental agony by singing and prayer. The paroxysm continues for 3 or 4 hours, and at the end of that time, exhausted by its violence, he becomes calmer, and falls into a kind of stupor. This continues for three or four days, during which he refuses food, and at the end of that time he is able to resume his ordinary avocation.[2]

Another witness from Ballymena described the cases more in the language of a loss of muscular power:

> When the conviction [of sin] as to its mental process reaches its crisis, the person, through weakness, is unable to sit or stand, and either kneels or lies down. A great number of convicts, in this town and neighbourhood, and now I believe in all directions in the north where the revival prevails, are 'smitten down' as suddenly, and they fall as nerveless, and paralysed, and powerless, as if killed by a gun-shot. They fall with a deep groan – some with a wild cry of horror – the greater number with the intensely earnest plea, 'Lord Jesus, have mercy on my soul!' The whole frame trembles like an aspen leaf, and intolerable weight is felt upon the chest, a choking sensation is experienced, and relief from this is found only in a loud, urgent prayer for deliverance. Usually the bodily distress and mental anguish continue till some degree of confidence in Christ is found. Then the look, the tone, the gestures instantly change. The aspect of anguish and despair is exchanged for that of gratitude, and triumph, and adoration.... Some pass through this exhaustive conflict several times; others but once. There is no appetite for food; many will eat nothing for a number of days. They do not sleep, though they may lie with their eyes shut. When partially recovered, they cannot use the requisite quantity of food, and hence, I presume, the continued weakness and incapacity, and consequent indisposition to work on the part of some, complained of by parents and employers.[3]

Later in the course of the revival, numerous instances of a temporary loss of sight, speech, or hearing made their appearance, and received much attention in the press. These cases also made their recovery in a matter of hours or days, and I should add, like the above cases, they did so with little or no medical attention.

As there were no serious statistics kept as to the total number of people involved in the revival, one can only say that by the standards of the time 'multitudes' were attracted to the movement. Of those crowds, only a small fraction was said to have been stricken. The *Belfast News-Letter*, a journal that was sympathetic to the awakening, set the figure at one in a hundred;[4] Samuel James Moore (1810–76), a Presbyterian minister from Ballymena who was himself deeply involved in the movement, claimed that it was one in twenty;[5] David Adams (1818–?), another involved Presbyterian minister, from Ahoghill (County Antrim), suggested that it was one in seven;[6] and John Chapman (1822–94), whose attitude could easily be described as anti-revival, estimated, from his writing-desk in London, that it was one in four.[7] But why should there be such a wide discrepancy in these estimates? Chapman was guessing from reports he had read in London and may not have known any better. Yet the Ulster estimates varied widely too. Ballymena was twenty-seven miles from Belfast and three miles from Ahoghill. Could the differences be attributed to variations in local experience? If there was in fact a markedly lower proportion of cases in

Belfast, this was likely to have been because many of the town clergy, although sympathetic to the revival, openly discouraged the physical phenomena, an attitude which tended to reduce the number of revival meetings in which the prostration cases made their appearance.

Regardless of what the actual figures for Ulster may have been, the 'strikings down' were spectacular events and they occurred often enough to typify the revival in the public eye. A flurry of publications followed the progress of the 'awakening', newspaper reports and letters to the editors, journal articles, tracts and pamphlets, almost all of which, in one way or another, had something to say about these 'physical phenomena'. Controversies ensued, with opinions of every hue in the air, and Ulster was cluttered with tourists who had come to see the events for themselves.[8]

On a larger scale the movement was characterized by a groundswell of popular sensitivity to religion. Religion and the awakening became endless topics for discussion. There was an upsurge of interest in religious meetings, ranging from reinstated family prayers, newly formed prayer groups, and newly scheduled congregational and non-denominational open-air meetings. Churches were filled to capacity, while open-air meetings in the country towns attracted crowds in their thousands[9] and 'monster meetings' in Belfast and Armagh drew tens of thousands,[10] with special trains or carriages added to accommodate the pilgrims from the other parts of the province.[11]

Curiously the revival did not follow in the path of any great charismatic personalities. To the extent that the movement was led at all, the leaders were clergymen and laymen with evangelical sympathies,[12] from a cross-section of the existing Protestant denominations in the north, i.e. Presbyterians, Anglicans, Methodists, Independents, etc., and by lay-converts (called 'convicts' in the vernacular of the time) from the revival itself.

Nineteenth- and twentieth-century historians who have focused on the Ulster Revival have traced the roots of the awakening in three directions: to the original prayer group in Connor; to other local factors leading to spiritual changes in Ulster, e.g. Sabbath School instruction, Bible classes, tract distribution, prayers for renewal, etc.; and to the 1857–8 revival in New York and Philadelphia.[13] But the physical manifestations that accompanied the movement in Ulster were not evident in any of the above. There is no record of anyone in Connor being stricken down, nor of anyone in connection with Bible classes or tract distribution, and the American Revival of 1857–8 was notable for being prostration-free.[14] Furthermore, when the Ulster Revival spread to other parts of the British Isles, the accompanying physical phenomena were rare in England and Wales, and Scotland had a very low incidence when compared to Ireland.[15]

There is, however, a noticeable difference between the above historians when it comes to accounting for the physical phenomena. The nineteenth-century writers, who were contemporaries of the revival, quite naturally used the descriptive language of the original controversies, which was primarily dominated by the medical concepts of hysteria, insanity, catalepsy, convulsions, and sudden losses of muscular strength, and secondarily by the psychological notions of mental and emotional stress, or occasionally Irish racial excitability; while the twentieth-century writers, if they went beyond the original historical documents, tended to reflect on the issue from the predominantly psychological perspectives of their own times, with medical considerations being reduced to a secondary role.

Frederick Morgan Davenport (1866–1956), for example, in his book *Primitive Traits in Religious Revivals* (1905) explained the physical and mental effects in Ulster[16] not in terms of pathology, rather as a feature of a lower stage on an evolutionary scale of social psychology.[17] He regarded a number of the Irish ministers who were involved in the movement as 'self-controlled and excellent',[18] but depicted the members of the original prayer group in Connor as primitive, an ignorant butcher, a blacksmith's boy, and a stonebreaker whose mother was the sister of a notorious pugilist. 'It was not remarkable, therefore, that from the outset there were physical manifestations, singular and violent. They acted like a shock upon the community and were imitated far and wide.'[19] In this assessment Davenport assumed a post-Darwinian doctrine of social and mental evolution wherein the least 'self-controlled' persons stimulated the social action of the others.[20] He believed the above assertion to be a law discovered in the newly emerging field of social psychology, behind which lay the thinking of Gustav LeBon (1841–1931) on crowd psychology.[21] In this respect, the 'Scoto-Irish Revival of 1859' was selected as a 'religious' crowd to demonstrate the point.[22]

Half a century later, in 1962, Alfred Russell Scott's evaluation took into account Davenport's views along with some writers from the psychology of religion movement,[23] such as William James (1842–1910),[24] Edwin Diller Starbuck (1866–1947),[25] and George Albert Coe (1862–1951),[26] who at the beginning of the twentieth century were preoccupied with the psychological dimensions of religious conversion. But in his personal explanations for the phenomena, Scott used a number of psychological or psychiatric ideas that were old enough to be employed without reference to their authors. For example, with regard to the striking down of a drunkard from Coleraine (County Londonderry) he applied a [kind of non-Freudian] concept of 'repression'[27] to the drinking stage of the story:

> The explanation from a psychological point of view would appear to be that any habitual vice, being abnormal, required the repression into silence and even unconsciousness of all the larger and nobler qualities of human character.[28]

He applied the [Jungian] concept of a 'complex'[29] to the recovery stage of another story, of 'the profligate nailer of Broughshane',

> so that with an almost explosive force the sentiment of love supplanted the lower and narrower instinct, and a buried 'complex' was exhibited.[30]

At another place he referred to the sudden conversion of persons who were unable to deal with their religious conflicts on a conscious level.

> Sometimes the underlying conflict grew too violent for resolution, and they became neurotic. This might take the form of dissociated physical symptoms – a splitting off from consciousness of certain ideas and their accompanying emotions – an hysteria.[31]

The above refers to a concept of dissociation in hysteria that is historically associated with Pierre Janet (1859–1947),[32] which Scott applied to instances of trance or bibliomancy (a divination procedure whereby a Bible was opened and passages selected at random):

> It would appear in cases such as these that there is a common factor of a state of conflict to be resolved with spasmodic violence either at the level of consciousness or in such hysterical cases below that level.[33]

But it is not the purpose of this chapter to promote a particular medical or psychological theory of the disorders encountered in the awakening, rather to review the controversies that these physical and mental effects stimulated amongst the numerous authors that make up the corpus of the Ulster Revival literature.

It was a situation where the morbid language of medicine dominated the controversies, but not the medical profession itself. Doctors, clergymen, in fact anyone could and did use it, revivalists and non-revivalists alike. The stricken people often perceived themselves as sick, and many were unable to work for several days. The revival moved from place to place, so some said it was spread by imitation or contagion. Many people were affected, so others described it as an epidemic. The symptoms were similar to those of other revivals in history, so some ascribed the disorders to a recurring bout of religious enthusiasm, excitement, or fanaticism. Some were hesitant to propose any particular pathological label for the theological fear of putting limitations on God's methods of bringing about conversions. Some saw the physical phenomena as pure disease, of no religious value, and something to be categorically avoided. Yet most observers who were open to the religious and moral potential of the movement, saw the phenomena as mixed blessings at best, and did not promote their occurrence.

With so many opinions about the physical phenomena to choose from, the door was left wide open for disputes over medical explanations. But because these disturbing phenomena also occurred in a religious context, the medical explanations were usually accompanied with some opinion, explicitly or implicitly expressed, as to the correctness or incorrectness of the religious practices involved.

The Lancet controversy

The revival had been news in the local Ulster press since the end of March 1859. Knowledge of it had reached Edinburgh by early May and London by late May. These early articles were cautious, sympathetic, and exploratory. By mid June, though, certain opponents of the movement had begun to make their opinions known. A cluster of biting anti-revival letters and editorials appeared in Belfast's liberal Presbyterian daily, the *Northern Whig*, in Dublin's Catholic press, and in London's prestigious medical journal, the *Lancet*. It was, however, the article in the latter periodical, entitled, 'A moral epidemic', that inadvertently set the debate over the physical and mental effects of the revival into motion. Its anonymous author had not been a witness to the events in Ireland, yet had accepted at face value the hostile attitude and descriptions contained in a pseudonymous letter to the editor of the above-mentioned *Northern Whig*,[34] and added some medical commentary of his own. He envisioned a scene of shameful 'excesses' and fanatical 'religious frenzy', in which the 'howls of the organizers' induced the 'diseased condition of body and mind'. From his received information, he confidently diagnosed a variety of disorders, epidemic hysteria, hysteria, violent hysteria, epileptiform convulsions, and was not surprised to hear that 'several persons have gone to lunatic asylums, and others are in restraint in their own houses'. To cure the disorders, he recommended a 'free and pitiless drenching with cold water'.[35] The article was widely reprinted in the public press, and accepted as authoritative by some. But the attitude of the article was so cynical and its content so full of brash pathologizing that it caused an evangelical backlash, which challenged the medical credibility of the *Lancet*. A Methodist writer, who was a witness, retorted:

> To accuse the ministers of Ulster of 'getting up' these affections is as rational as to suspect physicians of bringing an epidemic.[36]

The *Freeman* (Baptist) claimed that the *Lancet*'s description of the revival as an 'epidemic' was only plausible for 'half the facts'.[37] The *British Standard* (non-denominational evangelical/pro-homeopathic medicine) accused it of exercising 'the most baneful empiricism'.[38] The *Belfast News-Letter* charged that the *Lancet* had 'not got an accurate diagnosis of what it terms the *disease*, and its opinion is, therefore, valueless'.[39]

As the *Lancet* at this time represented the orthodox medical profession as a whole, its commentary on the revival also elicited a few irate responses from individual practitioners, who perhaps wisely registered their complaints in the form of pseudonymous letters. 'An "Elder" and MD' lamented that the *Lancet* had disgraced his profession in the 'eyes of the Christian public' and protested against the *Lancet* being made a 'vehicle of cynic scepticism at so glorious a work'. He further dared the author to 'avow his name'.[40] Another correspondent, 'Chirurgus', was more discerning. He chastised the *Lancet* for recommending as a remedy only 'a free and pitiless drenching with cold water'. If he had been serious about his diagnosis of 'violent hysteria', why hadn't he also suggested a 'long array of sedatives and anti-spasmodics'? Chirurgus's answer was that the *Lancet* failed to follow through with his prescription, not because his diagnosis was especially wrong, but because he was personally 'actuated by feelings of hostility to the disease' and cold water was the 'most pitiless remedy'.

Chirurgus concluded that his 'professional brethren possess but a superficial knowledge of the "epidemic"'.[41]

The *Lancet*'s reaction to this public attention appeared on 23 July, in an article entitled 'The physical phenomena of the revivals'. It acknowledged that it had been

> warmly abused for taking such a view of the phenomena. This is so far a matter of congratulation that it has served to attract attention in quarters where it was else little likely to reach. He had no intention of furnishing matter for pulpit oratory, but physical phenomena have been pressed so mischievously into the service of fanaticism, that we are glad to have furnished arms to the eminent divines of Belfast, with which they are successfully combating a great evil.[42]

It is evident from the foregoing critiques and response that the *Lancet* articles were not only motivated by an ill will towards the physical phenomena of the revival, but also against the kind of religious behaviour that the revival represented, which it termed 'fanaticism'. With respect to the latter, the *Lancet* articles are much more an example of vitriolic rhetoric from a particular religious point of view, than good medical analysis. In all fairness to the *Lancet*, though, this attitude was not at all unusual in the history of British medical psychology, where religion, albeit not 'true religion', was commonly recognized as a cause of insanity.[43] But most of the other medical writers who expressed that attitude towards fanaticism or religious enthusiasm did so in monographs on madness, and certainly not in the heat of an historical circumstance where the public or religious opposition could talk back.

The hysteria controversy

In 1859, at Ewart's linen mill in Belfast, 'twenty or thirty' women were stricken in one day. 'A medical man was sent for, and such was the confusion created, that the mill had to suspend working for the day.'[44] If this were an isolated incident, there would have been little nineteenth-century hesitation in calling it an outbreak of hysteria. Yet add to this the testimony of one of those women:

> I was standing working in the mill. My conscience had been exercised under a sense of sin, but my mind was not constantly dwelling on it. I was struck down, and that same day there were twenty or thirty struck down in the mill.[45]

And the testimony of the overseer who could also view the conduct of those women in the cottages attached to the mill:

> and all of them were walking as humble Christians, regular in all their worldly duties, and exemplifying in a most satisfactory way their Christian character.[46]

Supplement this with the common knowledge that in other places in the province both men and women of all ages had been stricken with a variety of symptoms, in the context of an ongoing religious movement, then the usual diagnosis of hysteria would, and did, come under careful scrutiny, especially from defenders of the movement who wanted to minimize the amount of disease associated with it.

Among one particular group of commentators, though, clergymen from the Established Church (Anglican), the hysterical explanation for the 'physical phenomena' of the revival was commonly accepted throughout the period when the revival was being discussed. It was an opinion that was found in the earliest Anglican tracts, letters, and sermon reports on the awakening, as well as in the latest, regardless of whether the individual were sympathetic or hostile to the revival movement, or whether or not he had witnessed any of the physical affections to which he was applying the label. For example, it was the explanation of Robert Bent Knox (1808–93), Bishop of Down, Connor and Dromore, who supported the revival movement but not to the extent that it promoted the physical phenomena,[47] and of William Fitzgerald, Bishop of Cork, Cloyne and Ross, who forbade his clergy to have anything to do with the movement.[48] And lest the hierarchical organization of the Anglican Church suggest that the hysterical diagnosis were a kind of policy handed down from the top, it was also an opinion expressed by the lesser clergy before the bishops, deans, and archdeacons had got their own statements into print.[49]

Although the hysterical theory for the physical manifestations of the revival could be considered a typical view in the Established Church in Ireland, outside Ireland that view was often associated with a particular individual, who was also a high official of that church. Edward Adderley Stopford (1810–74), Archdeacon of Meath, had travelled north to Belfast, in late July, to view the revival for himself. After observing the proceedings for ten days, he returned to his vicarage in Kells (County Meath) and penned a tract entitled *(To the Clergy and Parents) The Work and the Counterwork; or, the Religious Awakening in Belfast. With an Explanation of the Physical Phenomena*. Between 7 August and 4 November it went through six editions and was widely reviewed in the secular and religious press of Ireland, England, Scotland, and eventually even in the United States. For many readers outside Ireland, Stopford's view was the only one with which they had come in contact and the hysterical explanation for the physical phenomena of the revival became synonymous with his name.

Stopford was not completely unsympathetic to the revival. But when it came to the physical phenomena, he was decided – all of the cases which he had seen or heard about were expressions of hysteria. His thesis was favourably received, though not entirely without suggestions and corrections, by Britain's leading medical journals: *Lancet*,[50] *Journal of Psychological Medicine*,[51] *Journal of Mental Science*,[52] *Edinburgh Medical Journal*,[53] *Dublin Quarterly Journal of Medical Science*;[54] and by John Chapman, himself a medical doctor, in the *Westminster Review*.[55] Yet the controversy over the diagnosis of hysteria did not really arise out of the suggestions and corrections made by Britain's orthodox medical journals. Rather it came from local clergymen and doctors who were themselves witnesses to the events in Ulster.

Grumbling about it surfaced even before the appearance of Stopford's pamphlet, from a minority within the established church itself. At a breakfast meeting, on 26 July, called by Bishop Knox to discuss the matter of the revival, William M'Ilwaine of St George's Church, Belfast, championed the hysterical view, while another clergyman who was present at that meeting anonymously dissented from the majority on the grounds that the 'strong, robust, and healthy are equally affected with the ill-fed mill girl'.[56] Theophilus Campbell of Trinity Church, Belfast, who was also at that meeting, later wrote that he disagreed with the hysteria theory because in his experience 'young men arc chiefly the subjects of the revival'.[57]

But the real controversy over hysteria did not begin until late September, after Stopford's pamphlet had been widely reviewed in Great Britain and Ireland. In support of his hysterical theory, the archdeacon had presumed that the medical profession had no doubt about the diagnosis and that there was 'no difference of opinion among the medical men of Belfast'.[58] Ironically, the chief critics of the hysteria theory were medical doctors, albeit men whose practices were outside Belfast. There were four of them: John Motherwell (?–1873) of Castlederg (County Tyrone), James Jasper Macaldin (1812–80) and James Crawford Leslie Carson (1816–86) of Coleraine (County Londonderry), and Alexander Cuthbert (1835–76) of Londonderry (County Londonderry). They were all Presbyterians, all residents of areas in the north that had experienced the fervour of the awakening, and all witnesses to cases of the stricken. Yet their diagnoses of the resultant disorders varied markedly from that proposed by Stopford. The archdeacon had considered *all* of the stricken cases to be hysterical,[59] which left him logically exposed. It was therefore the task of the respondents to the issue to establish that there was a range of exceptions to the rule. Each presented his views on hysteria in the revival in the form of a letter or letters.

John Motherwell's letter was read before the Evangelical Alliance Conference, in Belfast, on 22 September, after which it appeared in various evangelical journals that reported on the meeting. Initially, 'like many other medical men, on reading the "cases", or hearing about them ... close rooms or meeting houses, exciting language, sympathy, imitation, etc.', Motherwell favoured the hysterical explanation. 'Observation, however, dispelled such an idea', since 'distinctive symptoms' were missing. He actually mentioned only one missing symptom, *globus hystericus* (or the 'ball in the throat'), which he assumed to be an essential feature of true hysteria. As Motherwell himself had provided a field in Castlederg for open-air revival meetings, he was in a position to observe 'dozens of cases'. Instead of hysteria, he envisioned a disorder of the heart and respiratory system that varied more in degree than in kind.[60]

J.J. Macaldin was also involved in the organization of the revival, as chairman of the committee in Coleraine which managed the 'Union Prayer Meetings',[61] that were inaugurated in response to the arrival of the awakening. But unlike Motherwell, Macaldin admitted, in his letter of 24 September, that there was 'somewhat of hysteria even here'. 'Hysteria rarely attacks an able-bodied man, does not give man nor woman a sight of their sins and lead them to surrender their hearts to Christ.' Although he gave no clear examples, he said that he could recognize it in the 'unreal character' of many prostrations, 'what is merely the effect of excitement, fear, sympathy, or imitation, from the genuine working of a broken and contrite heart'. For Macaldin, the cases of hysteria were those which mimicked the features of people genuinely affected by the 'Spirit' in the revival.[62]

J.C.L. Carson, besides being a physician and surgeon in Coleraine, was the son of a Presbyterian minister, a lecturer on phrenology, a religious controversialist, and from July 1859 to January 1860, the author of eight letters on the revival that provide a virtual catalogue of the medical controversies surrounding it. Carson estimated that his letters, through British and foreign reprints, reached half a million readers. His letters on hysteria were originally published on 1 and 15 October respectively.[63]

Carson, like Macaldin, admitted that hysteria existed in the revival districts, something to expect in times of excitement. Yet he denied that the revival was confined to these cases; moreover he claimed that the broader spectrum of cases was distinctly *not hysterical*. His method of arguing was remarkably akin to that of Stopford, who used medical authorities as a proof for his hysterical theory; only Carson used medical authorities to disprove the same. While Stopford was looking at the characteristics of the revival that were similar to medical descriptions of hysteria, Carson searched for features that were different or absent from the usual descriptions of hysteria. Instances of *globus hystericus* were missing, as were alternate laughings and cryings, and convulsive movements of the limbs. Hysteria was supposed to occur almost exclusively in females. However, Carson claimed that almost half of the revival cases were male. Stopford had cleverly got round this point by suggesting that the male convicts were 'effeminate',[64] whereas Carson referred to 'an immense number of instances in which the strongest, stoutest, most vigorous, most lion-hearted men in the country have been struck down like children, and have called, with the most agonizing entreaties, for mercy for their souls'. 'How could all this be hysteria?' he asked.[65] He commented on the other social features of hysteria, namely that it was supposed to be prevalent among the 'rich and unemployed', and commonly found in the larger cities. As he saw it, the vast majority of revival cases came from the lower to middle working classes, and from rural districts and country towns. Lastly, when hysteria did occur among females, they were supposed to be of a debilitated, nervous, unhealthy type. On the contrary, Carson depicted the stricken women of Ulster as being healthy and vigorous.

So which were the hysterical cases in the revival districts? Carson was careful not to define them, save the inference that they were not religiously genuine. But in this category of not coming from the Holy Spirit, he included all instances of blindness, dumbness, and the visions and prophecies that tended to result in 'new revelation'. Instead, he depicted these cases as resulting solely from the action of some physical agent on the brain and nervous system.

Alexander Cuthbert was the only one of these Presbyterian doctors to have his letter published in a medical journal. It appeared in the 5 November issue of the *Medical Times & Gazette*, as an 'Original communication' entitled – 'On the prominent features of the Ulster Revival'.[66] Like Macaldin and Carson, Cuthbert did not attempt to deny the existence of hysteria, but rather attempted to show that there was much less hysteria connected with the movement than imagined.

He argued his case on several levels, racial, moral, physical, and diagnostic. The racial charge was largely an English prejudice, namely that the excitable Irish were prone to hysteria. Cuthbert saw the people of his northern area as being a racial blend of 'Scotch coolness' and 'Irish temperament'. The component of 'Scotch coolness', he implied, made these people poor candidates for hysteria. The perverse mental and moral nature which Cuthbert associated with hysteria did not match up with the moral improvements he had seen in Ulster as a result of the revival, i.e. less drunkenness, blasphemy, lying, malice, etc. As hysteria expressed itself in physical symptoms, he was anxious to reduce the volume of these physical phenomena. He did so by stating that these 'physiological accidents' did not occur in all revival locations, and when they did it was only among a small proportion of those affected. Diagnostically, he saw the physical manifestations of the revival as resulting either from deep mental stress or hysteria. He rejected the notion that every physical effect of emotion was hysteric, and found that most of the revival cases were due to mental stress; people who were deeply remorseful over their lives, seeking relief in the consolations of religion. It was a state where the mental condition regulated the body; a state which was out of the province and control of medicine – whose acolytes like 'Shakespeare's physician' could not minister to a mind diseased – and a state in which little medical aid was sought on the part of the people. Most of the people who suffered from this mental stress were only stricken once.

A minority of the cases he found to be hysterical. They were of three kinds: those victims of sympathy and imitation who were struck, i.e. on the roads, in homes, in the fields, etc., without reference to religion; those who manifested visions and trances; and those whose nervous temperaments were easily habituated by the repeated occurrence of deafness, blindness, speechlessness, or paralysis. The former two kinds, he said, were more common in the Belfast area than in his part of the north, and all three kinds failed to show any sign of moral improvement after their convalescence.

All of the above medical doctors agreed with Stopford on one point, that hysteria was different from genuine religious experience. Its origins were natural and not divine. In the context of the Ulster Revival, then, hysteria represented those physical and mental phenomena that were to be theologically rejected. But where did hysteria begin and genuine religious experience end? Each of the above writers drew the boundaries at a different place, according to his own sense of religious tolerance.

Stopford assumed that all of the physical phenomena were natural and had nothing to do with religion, that the preaching of Christ and the Apostles did not produce disease, nor was there any 'trace of hysteria' on the day of Pentecost, the biblical event with which the revival had been most favourably compared by some. For Stopford the 3,000 people who experienced the 'period of conviction' at Pentecost demonstrated the 'highest exercise of ... moral and intellectual faculties', and not the wild cries of hysteria.[67]

By comparison, all four of the Presbyterian doctors saw far less hysteria in the physical phenomena than did the archdeacon. Motherwell changed his diagnosis from hysteria to an affectation of the heart and respiratory system only after viewing the cases and deciding that the stricken ones had been affected by a 'large outpouring of the Spirit of God', which had improved the 'moral and religious tone of the community in his district'. Apparently he found no instances of hysteria among the stricken and accepted the religious integrity of all the physical manifestations he encountered in his area of Ulster. Macaldin was slightly more limiting than Motherwell. Through observation he thought that he could differentiate between the cases, the real from the unreal. In the 'real' ones he saw the 'Divine Spirit operating on the mind, the mind on the brain and nervous system, and these on the whole physical organization'. He accepted almost all of the accompanying physical phenomena as divinely sanctioned 'accidents' in the history of the cases, which included those 'weakly nervous persons' who were 'stricken several times', and with less certainty those cases which 'the Spirit of God may make use of', those with 'visions, supposed revelations, prophesyings, deafness, dumbness, etc., to which weakly, nervous, and highly excitable individuals attach so much importance ... to impress seriously a hitherto dead carnal mind with a sense of things spiritual'. But he rejected as 'unreal' and hysterical those few cases whose features were not rooted in a 'genuine working of a broken and contrite heart'. For Carson, both the physical and the spiritual elements of the revival cases came from God. They were no mere accidents. However, he did limit the spiritual integrity of some cases by suggesting that in those a physical agent alone was at work on the 'brain and nervous system'. Hysteria fell into this category because it was thought to be responsible for the instances of temporary blindness, deafness, and speechlessness, and possibly for the visions and prophecies that would 'supersede the written Word', or the group of cases that Macaldin accepted with ambivalence. Cuthbert saw a 'blessed agent' in the revival too, because of the moral improvements in the community that were associated with it. Like Macaldin, he regarded the acceptable physical phenomena as no more than 'physiological accidents'. But he reorganized Carson's catalogue of unacceptable cases by subdividing the category into regular hysteria, which included the cases of those who were repeatedly stricken with deafness, dumbness, and blindness, and into 'cataleptic hysteria', which included the visionaries and prophets, then expanded Carson's list slightly by adding to it instances of paralysis, trance, and sleeping and waking at a specific time.

Hysteria, however loosely or strictly defined it may have been, was still considered to be a natural disorder, and theologically disapproved of by all of the above writers in the circumstance of a religious revival. And the fact that the Presbyterian doctors judged there to be less hysteria in the movement than Stopford, had to do with both medical and theological considerations; the chief theological consideration being their estimate of the extent to which God might intervene in the physical lives of those stricken in the awakening. While the Presbyterian doctors put their theological stamp of approval on the majority of the physical affections, Stopford put his approval on none. Either way, the persons who exhibited theologically unacceptable symptoms were judged to be suitable candidates for hysteria. Hysteria, however, was not the only medical category to be influenced by religious considerations.

The insanity statistics controversy

Insanity is another disorder that made its appearance in connection with the awakening in the north of Ireland. Although the great majority of the people stricken in the revival required no medical attention, the insane cases were the ones most likely to have come in contact with the medical profession in the process of being sent to the district lunatic asylums, or, if there were not space available, to the county gaols. According to the annual reports of Ulster's four district asylums (for the year ending 31 March 1860), there were 67 cases admitted with religion listed as the exciting cause (Armagh 11, Belfast 16, Londonderry 14, and Omagh 26).[68] It was assumed by some that all of these cases were caused by the recent religious revival. These hard numbers become less firm, though, when other mitigating factors are taken into consideration, i.e. the bias towards the revival of the person making the claim, whether the total included readmissions, whether the figures took into account the average number of 'religious excitement' cases admitted in non-revival years, and whether those admitted with religious symptoms had any contact with the revival whatsoever, etc. There is no doubt that there were a few genuine lunacy cases among those stricken in the awakening, a fact that was regrettably admitted by defenders of the movement.[69] But the controversy over how many or how few cases could be chargeable to the revival arose long before the publication of the above asylum statistics. It began in July 1859, in the Belfast press.

On 12 July, the *Northern Whig* (as mentioned before, a journal known for its anti-revival attitude) published the following statement:

> A Result of the Revivals. – It is a melancholy fact that, within the last couple of weeks, no less than seven individuals have been admitted into our District Lunatic Asylum, whose aberration of mind is distinctly traceabie to the excitement consequent on the religious preachings which are going on in the various districts round about us.[70]

Another newspaper in town, the *Banner of Ulster*, an organ of the Presbyterian General Assembly that was in sympathy with the revival movement, apparently found the *Whig*'s claim offensive. As the Belfast District Lunatic Asylum was a public institution with inspectable records, the *Banner* made inquiries. The results of its investigation appeared on 14 July:

> Revivals. – Errors Respecting Their Mental Effects . . . Our contemporary, the *Whig*, stated on Tuesday, as 'a melancholy fact', that seven individuals had been admitted into our District Asylum for the Insane, within the last two weeks, 'whose aberration of mind is directly traceable to the excitement consequent on the religious preachings'. We are, happily, in a position to show, still more distinctly, that the *Whig* has made a grave misstatement. Two of the 'cases' admitted into the Asylum, during 'the last two weeks', were women who had attended revival meetings; but their 'aberration of mind' is not chargeable to that fact, as both of them had been inmates of that institution before. A male patient brought in had been mentally ill ever since November last, and of course long previous to the 'awakenings' and no mention was made by any person as to his having at all come within their influence. Another patient admitted, who was supposed to labour under 'religious melancholia', is found to be afflicted with a very different phase of mental disease – 'acute mania'. A female patient, admitted during the period specified, had been present at a religious meeting where another female was 'stricken-down'; but she herself did not suffer from any such physical visitation. Not even one of these cases would, we submit, be set down, by any unprejudiced person, as 'distinctly traceable to the religious preachings'.[71]

With the arrival of the press on the scene, the wheels of the ordinarily quiet medical machinery of admission and discharge from a local asylum became exposed to the public eye as part of a raging social controversy. The *Whig* wanted to discredit the revival movement by pointing to the number of cases of insanity it brought about, while the *Banner* sought to exonerate the same movement by arguing that five out of seven of those cases were not attributable to the revival, with both sides of the debate looking to the asylum admission records for proof positive of their respective views.

The hard fact stands that seven persons were admitted to the Belfast asylum, in a period of two weeks, whose disorders may or may not have had anything to do with the then current religious excitement in the Belfast area. There were two basic interpretations of the revival's influence on insanity – a broad one and a narrow one. The broad view, supported by the *Whig*, assumed that any patient who had the least contact with the revival, or who manifested any kind of religious symptom, or was even admitted to the Belfast Asylum during the time of the awakening, was eligible to have his or her disorder attributed to 'religious preachings'. In contrast the narrow view, promoted by the *Banner*, looked at the history of each case in hopes of locating an original cause outside the revival.[72]

The next skirmish between these two newspapers over this issue began on 14 September when the *Whig* published this report:

> The Insanity of Revivalism. – We have it on good authority, that, since the commencement of the revival movement, there have been lodged in Belfast Asylum and County Jail, no fewer than twenty-two cases of insanity from Larne [County Antrim] and that neighbourhood alone.[73]

The implication of the report was that all twenty-two cases were attributable to the revival. So the *Banner* countered with another investigation:

> As regards the District Hospital for the Insane, only one solitary case of insanity, 'from Larne and that neighbourhood', has been admitted since the commencement of the Revivals. This was a woman; and it was specially remarked that she was first sent to the County Jail, and thence transferred to the Asylum. This item is, therefore, to be deducted from the account of the former. We defy the *Whig* to deny the perfect accuracy of what we affirm. We add, for the comfort of our contemporary, that whereas, last year, when 'revivals' in Ireland had not been heard of, eight persons were admitted into the Asylum, from insanity attributed to 'religious excitement'. The number entered upon the books this year, for so far, after all the excitement has occurred, has been no more than ten. It is not necessary for us to say that insanity from religious enthusiasm, fanaticism, and delusions, has been common long before the year of grace 1859, and when no revival whatever was in progress. As regards the County Prison, here is the exact state of the matters. There have been admitted, since the commencement of the revivals, only five insane persons, 'from Larne and that neighbourhood', the cause of whose malady is set down as 'religious excitement'. The precise nature of that excitement is not set down on any document, and may have been altogether unconnected with the revivals, for aught that is shown. Of the five persons so admitted, one (as we have mentioned) has been transferred to the Asylum; three have recovered – one of whom has been discharged; and there remains but one in the jail who is really mad.[74]

In spite of a wide difference in the number of cases of insanity reported by the two papers, the *Whig* twenty-two and the *Banner* five, the *Whig* offered no counter-investigation of its own, finding it sufficient to reiterate its claim of twenty-two cases based 'on authority that we have no reason to question'.

Simultaneously with the publication of the *Whig*'s report, the *Dublin Evening Mail* printed its own version of the Belfast gaol statistics from a person of 'good authority' (probably the same person who provided the *Whig* with its figures). During the last three months, the *Mail* claimed, sixteen persons from a single town had been committed to the Belfast gaol as 'dangerous lunatics' of whom 'no less than 12 were labouring under religious delusions', with the suggestion that the other four cases may have also fallen victim to the 'prevailing enthusiasm'. To add weight to this latter implication, the *Mail* further claimed that during the same period in the previous year there were only six lunatics committed to the same gaol, none of whom 'evinced similar [religious] delusions'.[75] The *Banner* replied to the *Mail*'s figures by confirming that the correct number of cases admitted to the gaol with religious delusions was seven, of which five had come from 'Larne and that neighbourhood'.[76]

But with the arrival of the *Mail* on the scene, the controversy over the statistics took another direction. The *Whig* and *Banner* were located in Belfast, in the midst of the revival ferment, while the *Mail* was based in Dublin, a hundred miles distant from Belfast and the other stirring scenes of the movement. While the *Whig* and *Banner* focused on the specific number of cases in the local lunatic asylum and county jail that were either caused or not caused by the awakening that was going on about them, the *Mail* presumed that the Belfast figures typified the situation in all of the revival districts. Unlike the *Whig* and *Banner* who, more or less, viewed the revival as the exciting cause of the cases of insanity in question, the *Mail* concentrated on the broader psychological notion of the latent mental disease. It was an idea that was held by some of the most famous alienists of the first half of the nineteenth century, i.e. Philippe Pinel (1745–1826),[77] J.E.D. Esquirol (1772–1840),[78] and Sir Alexander Morison (1779–1866),[79] who believed that the seeds of mental disease had been sown long before through inheritance and predisposition and were latently waiting for any excitement, usually religious or political, to turn these 'weak and sensitive minds' into full-blown lunatics. And in the circumstance of the Ulster Revival the prevailing excitement, which gave the disease its colour, was religious.

The *Mail* was also 'attached to the principles of the Church of England',[80] or the non-evangelical part of the church that understood the *'re-vival'* of religion in terms of a quiet reformation of moral character and the development of a sense of religious duty. And it pointed to the Belfast insanity statistics as a warning to the danger of attempting to *'re-vive'* religion outside the constraints of its own religious principles.

Meanwhile, *The Times*, in London, reprinted both the *Whig*'s and the *Mail*'s lunacy figures.[81] Ten days later, on 26 September, *The Times* followed up that report with an article that was in some ways similar to that of the *Mail*, which contained a more expanded version of the Ulster gaol statistics:

> it appears that the number of persons committed to the gaols in the counties of Ulster where the revival movement has been more than usually successful are to be taken as an index to the condition in other counties.... Taking the period between the first of June last and the present time, the number [of dangerous lunatics] committed in 1858 to the gaols of Belfast, Downpatrick, and Monaghan were in all 22; while in 1859 they amounted to 45. Of the 22 committed in 1858, only one appeared to have his mind overturned from religious causes, while in the cases occurring in 1859 the religious element largely predominates. Thus of the 19 committed to the Belfast gaol no less than 13 were certified by the medical officer to have been insane on the subject of religion, and the remaining six might perhaps be traced to a similar cause. The same observation may be safely applied to the other cases mentioned, but as the medical men in Downpatrick and Monaghan had not devoted as much observation as the Belfast doctors to the psychological bearings of the movements, the exact proportion of cases of insanity produced by such religious convictions and other causes cannot be actually ascertained.[82]

Like the *Mail, The Times* reflected the principles of the Church of England.[83] With respect to these principles the *Times* writer viewed the insane cases as brought about by the erroneous 'convictions' of the revivalists. It confirmed that religion based on the wrong principles, exciting, emotional, and out of clerical control, had led to an outbreak of insanity that was spreading like a contagious disease.

Unlike the *Mail* writer who rested his diagnosis on the notion of latent insanity, the *Times* writer put the revival into a larger social context, namely the increase of insanity in nineteenth-century society.[84] Thus the secularized titles of the two articles – 'Progress of Irish insanity' and 'Lunacy', and the emphasis on the housing of dangerous lunatics in gaols instead of asylums. In other words, there were more insane people than specialized places to keep them; the district asylums were full and there was still no prison for the criminally insane in Ireland. In the Ulster Revival, *The Times* had discovered yet another source for the increase of insanity. For while the *Whig* and *Mail* were content to show that the revival was an example of a religious fanaticism that produced cases of insanity the numbers of which would naturally subside when the excitement had passed, *The Times* saw these revival statistics as part of the general increase of insanity in Irish society.

The Times's overview of societal insanity, however, did not excuse it from its journalistic responsibility to get the facts and conclusions straight, on which, in the instance of the Ulster 'gaol' statistics, it did a questionable job. *The Times* looked at the Belfast 'goal' figures and assumed that the situation was also true for the other counties of Ulster, even if there was a shortage of supporting facts. When the Downpatrick and Monaghan 'gaol' statistics did not compare favourably with those of Belfast, *The Times* did not doubt its own assumption, rather the psychological judgement of the prison doctors in Downpatrick and Monaghan. The medical attendants at Belfast and Downpatrick were Thomas Henry Purdon (1805–86) and John King Maconchy (?–1892) respectively. Both men were graduates of the same medical school – Trinity College Dublin; both were life-long Anglicans associated with the High Church; both had extensive practices among the 'aristocracy' and the 'principal families' of their regions; both were political conservatives; and as gaol doctors they both had extensive opportunities to observe the character of 'dangerous lunatics'.[85] So there is probably little ground for *The Times* suggestion that the medical attendant at Downpatrick was less psychologically observant than his counterpart in Belfast, especially as Dr Maconchy was judged to be astute enough to be appointed as visiting physician to the Down District Asylum when it opened its doors in 1869.

Another possible explanation for this lack of statistical parity would be that there were fewer religious cases in County Down. For the Monaghan 'gaol', the answer is easier. Even though County Monaghan was technically part of Ulster, its population was 73 per cent Roman Catholic (as opposed to 28 per cent in County Antrim/Belfast and 33 per cent in County Down)[86] and the revival made very little headway in the predominantly Catholic counties.[87] So there may well have been no cases of persons 'insane on the subject of religion', at the time of the revival, in County Monaghan.

In the mid-nineteenth century it was commonplace for secular newspapers to advertise their religious inclinations. The *Northern Whig* represented liberal Presbyterian opinions (views which some conservative Presbyterians stigmatized as 'Unitarian') and the *Mail* and *Times* avowed their allegiance to the principles of the Church of England. All three journals viewed the revival, on religious and medical grounds, as a danger to mental health. And the *Banner*, with its conservative or orthodox Presbyterian principles, was sympathetic with the awakening on religious grounds, but did not deny the risk of insanity, albeit a lower risk than that alluded to by any of the other three newspapers. Rather the *Banner* was the only one of the journals in this controversy which was willing to investigate the statistics by examining the medical records of the alleged revival cases.

Religious bias in the interpretation of the statistics of insanity was not limited to the public press. Robert Stewart (1803–75) was the resident physician at the Belfast Lunatic Asylum at the time of the awakening. He was a staunch Anglican,[88] and in one of his anonymous reviews for the *Dublin Quarterly Journal of Medical Science* he envisioned the revival as a 'reign of terror' in which the 'pious ladies of Belfast would have combined to destroy the practice of a doctor who expressed a doubt of the divine origin of the prevailing visitation'.[89] He described the sixty-seven cases of 'Religious Excitement', that were admitted into Ulster's four district asylums for the year ending 31 March 1860, as a 'prostitution' of the name of religion.[90] His own institution's share of the sixty-seven cases was sixteen. He attributed all sixteen of those cases to the 'Great Ulster Revival', and further suggested that there were not a few 'struck' among those twenty-three cases whose insanity was charged to 'Grief, Disappointment, and Anxiety'.[91] But William Gibson (1808–67), a Presbyterian historian of the revival writing in 1860, pointed out that eight of those cases of 'Religious Excitement' were admitted before there was 'any talk of revivals'.[92] And it should be noted that from 1839 to 1873, there were 222 cases of 'Religious Excitement'[93] admitted to the Belfast asylum, an average of 6.3 cases a year, all during Stewart's tenure as resident physician.[94] Although sixteen cases is substantially higher than the annual average of such cases over a 34-year period, it is also apparent that Stewart made no attempt to differentiate between the revival cases and the usual intake of religious cases, and like the *Whig*, the *Mail*, and *The Times*, he emphasized the maximum negative effect of the awakening, largely for reasons of religious dislike.

By way of postlude, 1860 brought with it a change in revival defence tactics when it came to the insanity statistics. The above-mentioned historian, in arguing for a reduction, from sixteen to eight, of the cases of 'Religious Excitement' at Belfast, also remarked

> that all great crises in the history of the world, political as well as religious, have swelled the number of the insane; and I believe that the revival in Ulster has led to fewer instances of the kind than any similar movement on record.[95]

It is apparent that Gibson was making no attempt to deny that there were revival-caused cases of insanity; on the contrary, he seemed surprised, in 1860, that there were not more instances!

Conclusion

All of the participants in the preceding controversies addressed the problem of the physical, or the physical and mental, phenomena of the Ulster Revival. However, estimates as to the number of people stricken and/or the proportion of those stricken who had pathological labels applied to them varied. On the one hand, some of the diagnoses were subject to medical debate; on the other hand, religious considerations had a strong influence on the outcome of the diagnostic process.

The *Lancet* saw no redeeming features in the movement, viewing it instead as an exercise in 'fanaticism' and the direct cause of an epidemical outbreak of disease. But some journalists and writers, being in sympathy with the revival, were so offended by the *Lancet's* religious insensitivity that they challenged the medical credibility of that journal on the subject of the awakening.

Archdeacon Stopford's judgement on the revival was not as harsh as the

Lancet's. In fact he perceived some moral good in the movement, and this was in spite of his view that the physical phenomena were symptoms of hysteria, a disease that he felt God would never use in the 'conversion' of sinners. The Presbyterian medical opponents to the hysteria theory agreed with Stopford on this point, but differed from him when it came to designating which portion of the physical and mental phenomena ought to be considered hysterical. The archdeacon applied the label to all of the cases, while the doctors assigned it to a few. Although these medical practitioners argued on the grounds of medical logic, that significant features of the disease were missing, the deciding differentiation was religious. Because they perceived an improvement in the moral behaviour of their districts, these northern doctors were willing to accept that the great majority of stricken cases were genuinely religious. Where there was no sign of moral improvement and/or the religious content of their behaviour was disagreeable or lacking, the cases were deemed to be hysterical – a natural disorder that God would not use in the 'conversion' of sinners.[96]

In the insanity statistics dispute, those journalists and writers who were antithetical to the revival attempted to maximize, without critical assessment, the number of insane cases that could be charged to the movement, whereas those who defended the awakening attempted to minimize the figures by investigating the admission records of the individual cases. Both sides assumed that erroneous religion could cause insanity. The critics, however, included the revival in the category of erroneous religion, while the apologists believed in the genuine religious undercurrents of the awakening. For the former, all cases of 'religious excitement' were indicative of faulty religion, and the latter were obliged to accept the fact that the Ulster Revival did have a few serious mental casualties.

Notes

1 C. Darwin (1859) *On the Origin of Species*, London: John Murray. Darwin signed John Murray's terms of publication on 2 April and the volume was ready for the Book Trade Sale on 22 November (for interim details see M. Peckham (1859) 'Introduction', *On the Origin of Species, A Variorum Text*, Philadelphia: University of Pennsylvania Press, pp. 11–20). In other words, the religious revival in Ireland more or less corresponded with the period in which the first edition of the *Origin* was in the press.

2 *Belfast News-Letter*, 25 May 1859 [p. 3], 'The religious revival in Ballymena'.

3 S.J. Moore (1859) *Revival in Ballymena*, Stirling: Peter Drummond, p. 10.

4 *Belfast News-Letter*, 4 July 1859 [p. 2], Editorial.

5 Moore, *Revival in Ballymena*, p. 11.

6 D. Adams (1859) *The Revival in Ahoghill*, Belfast: William M'Comb; C. Aitcheson, p. 15.

7 [J. Chapman] (1860) 'Christian revivals', *Westminster Review* NS 17: 198; or J. Chapman (1860) *Christian Revivals*, London: George Manwaring, p. 34.

8 See J. Baillie (1859) *The Revival: or, What I Saw in Ireland* ... *The Result of*

Two Personal Visits, London: James Nisbet; J. Grant (1859) *Personal Visit to the Chief Scenes of the Religious Revivals in the North of Ireland*, London: John Snow; J. Weir (1860) *The Ulster Awakening ... With Notes of a Tour of Personal Inquiry*, London: Arthur Hall, Virtue.

9 For example, a revival meeting in the small town of Castlederg (County Tyrone), with a population of 637 according to the 1861 census, attracted a crowd of 2,500 on 10 July (see *Londonderry Standard*, 28 July 1859 [p. 2], 'Religious revival') and 4,000 on 28 August (see *Londonderry Standard*, 1 September 1859 [p. 1], 'Religious revival').

10 The first 'monster meeting' in Belfast drew between 35,000 and 40,000 (see *Banner of Ulster* (Belfast), 30 June 1859 [p. 1], 'Great Union meeting for prayer'); the second, on 16 August, attracted a more modest 20,000 (see Weir, *Ulster Awakening*, p. 153); and the third, in Armagh on 14 September, was attended by not less than 20,000 (see *Banner*, 15 September 1859 [p. 2], 'Great revival meeting in Armagh'). All of the above are optimistic estimates from sources that were sympathetic to the movement. For a more cynical view of one of these meetings see *The Times* (London), 20 September 1859 [p. 7], 'Monster revival meeting in Armagh'.

11 It was estimated that 15,000 arrived by rail for the first 'monster meeting' in Belfast (see *Banner*, 30 June 1859 [p. 1], 'Great Union meeting for prayer'), and 3,000–4,000 were said to have boarded, in Belfast, an abnormally long train bound for the Armagh meeting (see *Banner*, 15 September 1859 [p. 2], 'Great revival meeting in Armagh').

12 'Evangelical sympathies' is used in a broad sense to include all views favouring 'Gospel Christianity' with an exaggerated interest in biblical literalism, extemporaneous prayer, a religion of the 'heart' which may or may not require strict decorum in worship. But not all Evangelicals approved of the kind of 'revival' that took place in Ulster, especially with regard to the physical phenomena. In fact two of the chief critics of the movement, W. M'Ilwaine and E.A. Stopford, both considered themselves to be Evangelicals (see M'Ilwaine's brave speech before the Evangelical Alliance meeting, *Banner*, 24 September 1859 [p. 4]; and *Daily Express* (Dublin), 23 April, 1874 [p. 3], 'The late Archdeacon Stopford'.

13 Only two extensive histories of the revival have been written, one in an anecdotal style by W. Gibson (1860) *The Year of Grace*, Edinburgh: Andrew Elliot, and the other of more academic merit by A. R. Scott (1962) 'The Ulster Revival of 1859' Dublin University unpublished PhD thesis. There are also two shorter histories, one by I.R.K. Paisley (1958) *The 'Fifty-Nine' Revival*, Belfast: Publications Board, Free Presbyterian Church of Ulster, and the other by J.T. Carson (1958) *God's River in Spate*, Belfast: Publications Board, Presbyterian Church in Ireland. Of the latter two histories, Paisley's follows the anecdotal style of Gibson, with numerous unreferenced quotations and occasional inaccuracies, whereas Carson's rendition is reliably referenced. All of the above historians have considered the 'three roots' of the revival, but also, being Ulstermen, they have placed their emphasis on the local sources. In comparison to the above, J.E. Orr (1949) *The Second Evangelical Awakening in Britain*, London: Marshall, Morgan & Scott, overlooked the Irish spiritual momentum in favour of stressing the view that the movement was part of the 'Great Evangelical' wave which began in America and spread to Britain. Orr, on the other hand, was an American!

14 See W. Gibson (1859) 'Introduction', Young Men's Christian Association,

Pentecost: or, The Work of God in Philadelphia, AD 1858 Belfast: C. Aitcheson, p. ix; W.C. Conant (1858) *Narrative of Remarkable Conversions and Revival Incidents ... The Great Awakening of 1857–58*, New York: Derby & Jackson, p. 376.

15 Orr, *The Second Evangelical Awakening in Britain*, p. 172.

16 F. M. Davenport (1905) *Primitive Traits in Religious Revivals*, New York: Macmillan. The footnotes therein reveal that the author's sole source of information on Ulster was Gibson's *The Year of Grace*.

17 ibid., p. 220.

18 ibid., p. 87.

19 ibid., p. 88.

20 ibid., pp. 2–3.

21 ibid., pp. 25–6. See G. LeBon [1896] (1920) *The Crowd*, translated from the French, London: T. Fisher Unwin; and for a background on LeBon's thought, see R.A. Nye (1975) *The Origins of Crowd Psychology*, London: Sage.

22 Davenport, *Primitive Traits*, pp. 87–93.

23 See B. Beit-Hallahmi (1974) 'Psychology of religion, 1880–1930: the rise and fall of a movement', *Journal of the History of the Behavioral Sciences* 10: 84–90.

24 W. James (1902) *The Varieties of Religious Experience*, London: Longmans, Green.

25 E.D. Starbuck (1901) *The Psychology of Religion*, 2nd edn, London: Walter Scott.

26 G.A. Coe [1900] *The Spiritual Life*, New York: Eaton & Mains.

27 See S. Freud (1856–1939), 'Repression' [1915], translation from the German edited by James Strachey, in [1953–74] *The Standard Edition of the Psychological Works of Sigmund Freud*, London: Hogarth Press, XIV, pp. 143–58; also the word 'repression' in the index to the *Standard Edition*. I have employed the expression 'non-Freudian' because of Scott's unusual use of the concept. In the ordinary Freudian sense of the word, disagreeable ideas or memories (usually of a sexual nature) are repressed; whereas Scott had envisioned a state where the 'nobler [presumably non-sexual] qualities of human character' were repressed into the unconscious. But it is logically possible. Why couldn't the 'nobler qualities' be deemed disagreeable to some people?

28 Scott, 'The Ulster Revival of 1859', p. 283.

29 See C.G. Jung (1875–1961), 'The psychology of dementia praecox' [1907], translated from the German by R.F.C. Hull, in [1950–76] *The Collected Works of C.G. Jung*, Princeton: Princeton University Press, III, pp. 1–151.

30 Scott, 'The Ulster Revival of 1859', p. 284.

31 ibid., p. 288.

32 P. Janet (1901) *The Mental State of Hystericals,* translated from the French by C.R. Corson, New York: G.P. Putnam. For a confirmation of this point, see I.R.C. Batchelor's (1969) revision of the 10th edition of *Henderson and Gillespie's Textbook of Psychiatry*, London: Oxford University Press, p. 157.

33 Scott, 'The Ulster Revival of 1859', p. 289.

34 A Clergyman [probably Catholic] of the County of Derry, 'Extravagances of the "Revival" Movement in Coleraine', *Northern Whig*, 13 June 1859 [p. 2].

35 *Lancet*, 25 June 1859: 635, 'A moral epidemic'.

36 W. Arthur (1859) *The Revival in Ballymena and Coleraine*, London: Hamilton, Adams, p. 5.

37 *Freeman* (London), 6 July 1859: 391, 'The revivals in Ireland'.
38 *British Standard* (London), 1 July 1859: 204, '"Lancet" divinity'.
39 *Belfast News-Letter*, 4 July 1859 [p. 2], Editorial.
40 An 'Elder' and MD, '"Lancet" Divinity', letter to the Editor, *British Standard*, 8 July 1859: 213.
41 Chirurgus, 'Medical opinions on the revival', letter to the Editor, *Banner of Ulster*, 3 September 1859 [p. 2].
42 *Lancet*, 23 July 1859: 94, 'The physical phenomena of the revivals'.
43 J.G. Donat (1986) 'British medicine and the Ulster Revival of 1859', University of London unpublished PhD thesis, appendix E, pp. 526–30.
44 R. Baxter [1859] *Revivals of Religion*, London: Hamilton, Adams, p. 21.
45 ibid.
46 ibid.
47 For references to Bishop Knox's sermon, in which he described the physical affections as 'chiefly hysterical' and discouraged their occurrence, see *Ballymena Observer*, 9 July 1859 [p. 1], 'The religious revival', and *Belfast Morning News*, 13 July 1859 [p. 3], 'Opinions of the clergy on the physical manifestations'.
48 Bishop Fitzgerald forbade his clergy to participate in extemporaneous prayer meetings, a common feature of the revival. It was a controversial move which he defended on the grounds of ecclesiastical law, in his (1860) *Letter to the Laity*, 2nd edn, Dublin: Hodges, Smith. For his opinion of the physical phenomena, especially hysteria, see his (1860) *Thoughts on the Present Circumstances in the Church of Ireland*, London: John W. Parker, pp. 27–9, 39–41.
49 Cf. R. Oulton (1859) *Religious Revivals*, Dublin: Hodges, Smith, pp. 17–18; E. Metcalf (1859) 'The revival movement', *Christian Examiner and Church of Ireland Magazine* NS 1: 166–7; C. Seaver (1859) *Religious Revivals*, Belfast: George Phillips, p. 21; E. Hincks (1859) *God's Work and Satan's Counterworks*, Belfast: George Phillips, p. 11.
50 *Lancet*, 17 September 1859: 'The work and the counterwork, by E.A. Stopford'.
51 (1859) *Journal of Psychological Medicine* 12: 612–13, 'Hysteria in connexion with the Belfast revival'.
52 E.S. (1860) 'The work and the counterwork, by E.A. Stopford', *Journal of Mental Science* 6: 167–78.
53 (1860) *Edinburgh Medical Journal* 5: 654–62, 'Religious revivals'.
54 [R. Stewart] (1860) 'Reviews', *Dublin Quarterly Journal of Medical Science* 58 NS 30: 400.
55 [Chapman], 'Christian revivals', pp. 197–9.
56 *Revival*, 6 August 1859: 15, 'Opinions of the Irish clergy as to the revival'.
57 T. Campbell, 'Revival at Trinity Church, Belfast', in W. Reid (ed.) (1860) *Authentic Records of the Revival*, London: James Nisbet, p. 66.
58 E.A. Stopford (1859) *The Work and the Counterwork*, 3rd edn, Dublin: Hodges, Smith, p. 12.
59 ibid.
60 J. Motherwell, 'Letter' [read by W. Gibson, Moderator of the Irish Presbyterian General Assembly, to the members of the Evangelical Alliance], *Banner of Ulster*, 24 September 1859 [p. 4]. For his presence at a revival meeting on his field in Castlederg, see *Londonderry Standard*, 1 September 1859 [p. 1], 'Religious revival'.

61 See Carson, *God's River in Spate*, p. 41; Paisley, *The 'Fifty-Nine' Revival*, p. 95. For Macaldin's identity as a Presbyterian, see S. Gwynn Jr (1859) *The Ulster Revival*, Coleraine: S. Eccles, p. 27.

62 J.J. Macaldin, 'Letter, on the revival, to the Rev. H.G. Guiness', *Coleraine Chronicle*, 24 September 1859, p. 4.

63 J.C.L. Carson (1859) *Three Letters on the Revival in Ulster*, Coleraine: S. Eccles; letters II and III were originally published in the *Coleraine Chronicle*, 1 October, 1859 [p. 4] and 15 October 1859 [p. 4] respectively. His other five letters were also published in the *Chronicle*, but are more conveniently collected in *Additional Letters on the Revival in Ireland*, which was later bound together with another of his works (1877) *The Heresies of the Plymouth Brethren*, London: Houlston, pp. 425–62. For biographical information, including his Presbyterian connection, see the *Chronicle*, 5 June 1886, p. 4. 'Death of Dr Carson JP, Coleraine', and 12 June 1886, p. 8, 'Funeral of the late Dr Carson, JP'. The British Library has an extensive collection of his publications.

64 Stopford, *The Work and the Counterwork*, pp. 39–40.

65 Carson, *Three Letters*, p. 9.

66 A. Cuthbert, 'On the prominent features of the Ulster Revival', *Medical Times & Gazette*, 5 November 1859: 293–4. That author's Presbyterian affiliation is mentioned in the *Londonderry Standard*, 4 March 1876 [p. 2], 'Death of Alexander Cuthbert, Esq., MD, of Waterside, Derry'.

67 Stopford, *The Work and the Counterwork*, pp. 13–14.

68 W. M'Ilwaine (1860) 'The religious aspects of the Ulster Revival', *Journal of Mental Science* 7: 65.

69 J. Morgan, 'The awakening in the north', letter to the Editor, *Saunders's News-Letter* [p. 3], was sad to hear that a fellow Presbyterian minister 'was out of his mind from overwork'; Moore, *Revival in Ballymena*, pp. 13–14, knew of three 'poor creatures' whose minds had given way; and Adams, *The Revival in Ahoghill*, p. 15, admitted that with one exception none of the 'awakened have gone astray in their mind'.

70 *Northern Whig*, 12 July 1859 [p. 2], 'A result of the revivals'.

71 *Banner of Ulster*, 14 September 1859 [p. 2], 'Revivals – errors respecting their mental effects'.

72 For an example of another nineteenth-century religious movement, in America, in the 1840s, that faced a similar controversy over insanity, see R.L. Numbers and J.S. Numbers (1985) 'Millerism and madness', *Bulletin of the Menninger Clinic*, 49, pp. 289–320. The chief value of the Numbers' study is that they evaluate the case records of those who were admitted to asylums, whose derangement was allegedly due to the excitement of Millerism. In most cases, Millerism turns out to be one of many factors involved, but rarely the sole cause of the person's disorder.

73 *Northern Whig*, 14 September 1859 [p. 2], 'The insanity of revivalism'.

74 *Banner of Ulster*, 15 September 1859 [p. 2], 'The revivals – The 'Whig's' statements on "good authority"'.

75 *Dublin Evening Mail*, 14 September 1859 [p. 2], 'The religious revival'.

76 *Banner of Ulster*, 17 September 1859 [p. 2], 'Falsehoods respecting the revivals'.

77 Reference to Pinel in J.E.D. Esquirol (1845) *Mental Maladies*, translated from the French by E.K. Hunt, Philadelphia: Blanchard & Lea, p. 47.

78 Esquirol, *Mental Maladies*, p. 47.

79 A. Morison (1848) *Outlines of Lectures on Mental Diseases*, 4th edn, London: Longman, Brown, Green & Longmans, p. 312.

80 (1860) *Newspaper Press Directory*, London: C. Mitchell, p. 100.
81 *The Times*, 16 September 1859 [p. 7], 'Progress of Irish insanity'.
82 *The Times*, 26 September 1859 [p. 4], 'Lunacy'.
83 *Newspaper Press Directory*, p. 17.
84 See Donat, 'British medicine and the Ulster Revival of 1859', appendix C, pp. 513–16; A. Scull (1979) *Museums of Madness*, London: Allen Lane, pp. 222–33.
85 For biographical information on T.H. Purdon, see *Medical Directory of Ireland, 1859*, p. 142; *Alumni Dublinenses*, p. 686; *Belfast News-Letter*, 9 August 1886 [p. 5], 'Death of Dr T.H. Purdon', and *North Whig*, 9 August 1886 [p. 8], 'Death of Dr T.H. Purdon'. Likewise for J.K. Maconchy, see *Medical Directory for Ireland*, 1859, p. 123; *Alumni Dublinenses*, p. 542; and *Down Recorder*, 30 January, 1892 [p. 3], 'Death of Surgeon Maconchy'.
86 'Census of Ireland for the year 1861, part IV, report and Tables relating to the religious professions, education and occupations of the people', *House of Commons* 60 (sess. 1863): 479–82.
87 In Gibson's *The Year of Grace*, 72 of his 437 pages were devoted to the revival in County Antrim (pp. 17–89); 53 to Belfast (pp. 90–143); 51 to County Down (pp. 166–217); and only *seven* pages to County Monaghan (pp. 292–8)!
88 *Northern Whig*, 7 April 1875 [p. 3], 'Death of Dr Robert Stewart'; 10 April 1875 [p. 5], 'Funeral of Dr Robert Stewart, MD'.
89 [Stewart] (1859) 'Reviews', *Dublin Quarterly Journal of Medical Science* 56 NS 28: 370. Stewart was quoting an anonymous author on the revival (see note 51) in his capacity as lunacy literature reviewer for the *Dublin Journal*, a position which he exercised from 1850–61 (see *Medical Directory* 1865, p. 829).
90 [Stewart] (1860) 'Reviews', *Dublin Quarterly Journal of Medical Science* 58 NS 30: 432.
91 ibid., 427–8.
92 Gibson, *The Year of Grace*, p. 395. Gibson was quoting an anonymous official, possibly one of the Board of Governors at the asylum. John Edgar (1798–1866), who was sympathetic to the revival and a professorial colleague of Gibson's at the Belfast Theological Institute, was also a member of the board (1836–66). He, for example, could have been that 'official'.
93 'Religious excitement' was Stewart's preferred label for cases with religious symptoms. In this respect he was consistent with the practice of the majority of asylum doctors of his time. But the psychiatric vocabulary of the mid-nineteenth century was also fluid, in a minority of instances, with this type of case. In the 1840s, Stewart himself used, on the odd occasion, the terms 'enthusiasm' (10th report, 1839–40, p. 4), 'Strong religious feelings' (12th report, 1841–2, p. 6), or 'Perverted views on religious subjects' (14th report, 1843–4, p. 8). For consistency's sake, I have listed these variant expressions under the rubric of 'Religious Excitement' in my compilation of the Belfast totals.
94 These figures were summarized from those printed in the 10th to the 43rd annual reports of the Belfast Asylum, which were all written by Stewart himself.
95 Gibson, *The Year of Grace*, p. 395.
96 Although the four Presbyterian medical men gave no religious credibility to the bona fide cases of hysteria in the revival, theirs was not the only Presbyterian opinion on the market. S.J. Moore, a Presbyterian minister whose tract, *Revival in Ballymena* [30 July], appeared prior to the publication of the doctors' letters, was theologically less restrictive with regard to the cases of the physically stricken:

We may call them *Hysteria*, and know as little of their cause as before. . . . may not God, as in ordinary times, send the affliction of body to rouse to consideration, to fear, to prayer to Christ for pardon and life? Cannot God work by means or without them? Is it not the glorious *number*, not the *nature*, of the cases that puzzles? Hitherto we have not thought it strange that affliction should be made the occasion by God of a wanderer's beginning to love God and to keep His law; and why should not God, when He pleases, as now, make it so for multitudes? (p. 11)

CHAPTER SIX

Henry Maudsley: psychiatrist, philosopher, and entrepreneur

Trevor Turner

> Comical, almost pitiable at times, is the ludicrous display of vanity by men of great eminence ... they leave behind them carefully preserved letters and elaborate memoirs of what they thought and felt.[1]
>
> *Religion and Realities* (1918)

On 2 August 1870, at the annual meeting of the Medico-Psychological Association (MPA), Dr Henry Maudsley was elected president.[2] He was 35 years old, had been joint editor of the association's *Journal of Mental Science* (*JMS*) since 1863,[3] physician at the West London Hospital since 1864, lecturer on insanity at St Mary's Hospital since 1868,[4] and in 1869 had become Professor of Medical Jurisprudence at University College, London, as well as a Fellow of the Royal College of Physicians.[5] While this metropolitan advancement might simply have been due to John Conolly's coat-tails – Maudsley had moved into Lawn House, Hanwell, Conolly's small private asylum, having married his youngest daughter Anne a month before Conolly's death in early March 1866[6] – Maudsley's innate talents were considerable. His 'clutch' of ten gold medals as a student[7] and some thirty published articles since 1860 were evidence of his excellent memory and literary energy. His book *The Physiology and Pathology of Mind* had received wide acclaim when published in January 1867[8] (a second edition came out in 1868, and German and Italian translations in 1870), and his European pre-eminence was sealed in the same year. Along with Griesinger and Morel he was named as one of 'a consultation of eminent European alienists', who were to 'assess the mental state of the (Habsburg) Archduchess Charlotta, Empress of Mexico'[9]. It is no wonder that Thomas Clouston, one of his proposers for the presidency of the MPA, was fulsome in his praise. The minutes of the 1870 annual meeting report him as saying: 'We do ourselves honour by electing Dr Maudsley to a much greater extent than we honour him.... His reputation is European, he is a man who has done more than any living Psychologist in this country for our science. He is our President in fact and we ought to make him so in form.'[10] And his reputation, then at its apogee, has largely remained intact. The *Popular Science Monthly* in March 1875 described him as 'among the foremost men in the branch of medicine to which he devoted himself'.[11] In 1910 Sir Bryan Donkin called him our 'now renowned Fellow',[12] while a 1918 reviewer referred to his 'lamp of true doctrine'.[13]

Yet if we look at this 'shadowy figure of the Victorian past',[14] what is the basis for his apparent influence? Why is there no biographical study of any detail? Apart from Aubrey Lewis in his 1951 Maudsley lecture, and Peter Scott in a 1956 article which focused on his criminological contributions,[15] little has been done to evaluate the Maudsley story. It is as if his own strictures on the value of biography have paralysed any progress or research. Certainly the available material is very scanty and the assumption has been made that he arranged for the disposal of his private papers before or at his death, although there is no direct mention of this in his will. There is a bibliography, unpublished, drawn up in 1947 by an American publisher and admirer, Oscar Aurelius Morgner.[16] This lists ten books and some eighty other papers, lectures, and pamphlets. There is a brief autobiography, dated as written in 1912, nine-tenths of which describes his life before his coming to London in 1862. There are recorded meetings of the MPA published in the *Journal of Mental Science*, his first attendance being noted also in 1862.[17] A few letters, mostly routine,[18] the obituaries and reminiscences after his death in 1918 (largely written by Mott and Savage),[19] and memoirs in the first two Maudsley lectures,[20] add a little to the picture. Serendipitous findings of accounts of his doings fill out the perspective,[21] as do his answers to the 1877 Select Committee on Lunacy Law[22] and his three annual reports (1858–9, 1859–60, 1860–1) from the Manchester Royal Lunatic Asylum near Cheadle.[23]

Given this voluminous literary output and parsimonious personal detail, how should the tempted biographer proceed? Is there some value in equating the poverty of our sources with something important about Maudsley himself? Because the period of his 'extended' presidency, as the 'model for the psychiatrists of his age',[24] coincides with a deadening decline in the whole atmosphere of the speciality. An LCC committee of 1889 unanimously agreed that 'knowledge about . . . insanity is not commensurate with that regarding other kinds of diseases . . . mainly due to the circumstances that the patients have been withdrawn from ordinary methods of investigation and treatment'.[25] The asylums hailed as the source of cure were silting up with chronic cases and ever-expanding numbers were filling Scull's 'museums of madness'.[26] Ernest Jones, recalling his days as a young doctor in the early 1900s,[27] described how hard it would be for modern psychiatrists to 'form any picture of the low level at which their branch of medicine subsisted'. He quotes a friend as suggesting that alienists 'read papers on an improved variety of Chubb lock', and an asylum superintendent (looking for someone to fill a vacancy on his staff) as stating: 'I don't expect him to be interested in insanity, but he must be able to play cricket with the patients.' An MPA committee, considering the status of British psychiatry, reported in 1914 'in frank and damning detail' the many faults of the situation.[28]

None of which is Maudsley's fault, but it clearly provided a motive for his most significant contribution to modern psychiatry, namely £30,000 for the establishment of a hospital for the 'early treatment of curable mental illness and for research and teaching in psychiatry'.[29] Thus the cliché of 'the debt' owed to him and thus, too, the eponymous hospital that prolongs the memory of his name, in contrast to the anonymity of most of his contemporaries. His bronze bust, by Isaac Rosen, darkly surveys the staircase of the Institute of Psychiatry. But that £30,000 was an astonishing sum, given that his near-contemporary George Savage left a mere £16,000, and Maudsley still had £60,000 spare when his final estate was published.[30] One must presume he obtained this by 'getting such practice in lunacy as I could',[31] assisted perhaps to a lesser extent by his book royalties, and clearly he had an extremely successful private practice. The evidence of the 'Archduchess Charlotta', and known patients of his at the plush Ticehurst Asylum, suggests that he was very much the aristocrat's alienist. But allied to this is his known reserve and unsociability. The word 'cynical' unites all his obituarists. There is evidence of a break with the MPA over the impending 1890 Lunacy Bill.[32] The 1870 president, it seems, subsided into an increasingly isolated position. 'He abandoned the teleological platform on which we both started', states Crichton-Browne in his 1920 inaugural Maudsley lecture,[33] 'and advanced into scientific materialism and agnosticism, where I could not then follow him.' His books and writings become increasingly obscure, receiving variable reviews both scathing and dutifully admiring. And what of his influence? Kraepelin does not refer to him, nor does Bleuler include him in the many references in his 1911 *Dementia Praecox or the Group of Schizophrenias*.[34] Interestingly, Bleuler does refer to Clouston, the fulsome proposer at Maudsley's election, who was knighted in 1912, an honour never accorded to Maudsley.[35]

By examining the career of a man dubbed 'the young philosopher' by Bucknill,[36] by reviewing his ideas and philosophy, taking note of the absences as well as the available data, I hope to clarify some of the factors leading to the decline of psychiatry in Britain. Myths about great men can also throw light on those wishing to preserve them, and the sceptic, as Maudsley so proudly was, might suggest he and his heritage had something to hide. This is far too incomplete to be considered as biography. Rather it seems useful to look afresh at a man whose scorn for 'the fatuity of egotistic optimism'[37] contrasted so sharply with his younger zeal on behalf of those who had become 'victims of the most pitiful of diseases'.[38]

Early life

His 1912 fragment of autobiography[39] (some 4,000 words in length and as yet unpublished), outlines the details of his schooling, family background, and early career, and these are uncontroversial. Born on 5 February 1835 at a farmhouse called 'Rome' near Settle in Yorkshire, he described his stock as 'yeomen' farmers, owning buildings and land. There is some detail of the Maudsley family tree and familial characteristics, with references to his paternal grandfather being nicknamed 'the old philosopher', to the general reticence of Maudsley males, and to the 'sombre and dreary years' of his early schooldays at Giggleswick. Emphasis on inherited characteristics is constant. 'I owed much to the emotional quality of my maternal stock' while his sound arteries bespoke 'my paternal texture'. There is the much-quoted statement that 'the paternal and maternal were never vitally *welded* in me, but only *rivetted*' (cf. Crichton-Browne's lecture)[40] and Maudsley's father apparently described him as 'like a woman, belonging to a varium et mutabile genus' on the occasion of his resigning his appointment at Cheadle Royal. 'I became restless and desirous of change . . . and threw myself on London' writes the son, but the details of this transition are otherwise most obscure.

Prior to this Maudsley's early medical career had been characterized by serendipity, a photographic memory, and considerable neglect of regular study. The encouragement of his aunt, Elizabeth Bateson, had got him through Oundle, the matriculation examination at London University, and a medical student apprenticeship. Initially apprenticed to a Mr Glover who was preoccupied 'in quickly building up a private practice for himself outside the hospital' (University College Hospital), Maudsley was, it seems, 'assertive and stubbornly rebellious against all control, *as I have always been*'. He gained prizes, ten gold medals in all, despite abilities that he 'has chosen to throw into the gutter', according to one professor. Savage recalls him saying that 'he felt rather a fraud in winning prizes, for he simply wrote out what he visually recalled from the textbooks'.[41]

The journey back to London was then relatively direct. Nine months as a locum – assistant medical officer at Wakefield Asylum – apparently to gain experience before joining the East India Company, led to his becoming assistant medical officer at Essex County Lunatic Asylum, Brentwood.[42] In this capacity he makes his first appearance in the MPA list, being elected a member at the annual meeting of 28 July 1858 as 'Maudsley Hy, Co. Asylum, Essex'.[43] But in comparison to his 'congenial Yorkshire countrymen' he found the 'character of the Essex people sly, secret and insincere'.[44] He moved very soon, in late 1858, aged 23, to become superintendent of the Manchester Lunatic Asylum at Cheadle, where his three years and three annual reports are seen to exhibit a 'mature and conscientious outlook' according to Aubrey Lewis.[45] Maudsley himself merely notes: 'It turned out fairly well, for I had an indulgent and considerate committee.'[46]

The committee minutes support this. After one year in the post his salary was increased from £200 to £300 per annum; he was active in improving the hospital's amenities, such as laying on gas to the farm buildings; patient numbers increased from sixty-six to eighty-two, with demand outstripping supply; the resolution of appreciation on his departure recorded 'their high opinion of his professional talents, his moral conduct, his administrative abilities, and his uniform courteous demeanour'.[47]

His reports vary. The first two (1858–9, 1859–60) are rather wordy, quoting Esquirol, referring to marriage preventing madness, stressing hereditary factors and the need for asylum care. His third is by contrast very brief (three pages as compared to fifteen and twenty).[48] His interests seem to be moving elsewhere, and it was also at this time that he was starting to write seriously. 'The correlation of mental and physical forces' was his first publication, appearing in the *Journal of Mental Science* in 1860.[49] The opening words are prophetic: 'Philosophy arrives at strange conclusions', and the subsequent twenty-five pages of rambling discourse do not clarify matters much further.

The essence of his early history is, however, much clearer. Here was an intelligent and well-read young man, of independent temperament, who had leapt into the expanding psychiatric profession of the mid-nineteenth century. How much he saw this as a vehicle for philosophy rather than committed therapeutic action is uncertain, but the seeds of his 'hypercritical nature' (viz. the Essex folk), of his understanding of private practice as the key to an income (viz. Dr Glover), and of his literary output are all present. This tendency, to prefer the rich interests of a philosophical psychopathology to the more detailed clinical task of describing symptoms (as Hughlings Jackson was to do in neurology and Kraepelin in psychiatry) persisted throughout his life. More important still, the scepticism that he was to ally to the degenerationist theories of Morel accompanied a dreadful paralysis in the profession as a whole. His relations with the MPA, his very private, probably aristocratic, practice and his increasingly obscure and outdated philosophizing are all evidence of this. It is by the first of these, the MPA, that his career was most closely defined.

Maudsley and the Medico-Psychological Association

One of the best documented areas of Maudsley's life is his relationship with the Medico-Psychological Association. In fact it may have been he, in 1865, who suggested this title, which replaced the cumbersome 'Association of Medical Officers of Asylums and Hospitals for the Insane'. Such at least is the *Lancet*'s version[50] as printed also in the *JMS*.[51] 'The Association . . . has done wisely in adopting Dr Maudsley's resolution, proposed at its recent annual meeting, and changing its name to that of the "Medico-Psychological Association".' But there is no such formal resolution actually recorded in the minutes of the meeting. Instead, the committee appointed to revise the laws of the association (set up in 1863) includes this change of name as rule I and there is a debate concerning membership during which Maudsley (who was *not* on that committee) states: 'I propose that we should retain the title Medico-Psychological.' Perhaps the *Lancet* is merely reporting hearsay that Maudsley instigated the term and conflates this knowledge with its report of the debate. Whatever the truth, it is interesting how the tale has been used to garland the Maudsley legend, by Walk, for example. Walk also stated that this new title must have been in imitation of the French 'Société Medico-Psychologique' and 'that it was good, nevertheless, to have a title indicating the spread of psychiatry beyond the bounds of institutional care'.[52]

Whatever the reasons, the pages of the association's *Journal of Mental Science*, published quarterly, are invaluable to those looking for the less formal side of Maudsley's nature. They provide the minutes of the MPA's annual meetings (and the quarterly meetings from their initiation in 1868) with lists of those attending and details of the discussions that ensued. Maudsley is prominent in these from his first recorded participation at the 1862 annual meeting,[53] and reminiscences of him usually insist on his concern for the MPA in general. Thus Mott declared: 'Dr Maudsley felt a great interest in this Association. His earlier work was intimately connected with it, and he had not forgotten it ... a large sum of money had been left to this Association. Therefore members ... would be extremely grateful to him ... and had Dr Maudsley been alive he would have extended a warm welcome to the members.'[54] Crichton-Browne, in his first Maudsley lecture of 1920,[55] reckoned that 'in this lecture ... he has devised a much-needed means of maintaining and extending the scope and usefulness of the Medico-Psychological Association, for the building up of which he did so much, and of conveying to those who stand outside our speciality and to the public generally some little knowledge of the work it is accomplishing'. In fact, it becomes an opening commonplace for the Maudsley lecturer to make some generous tribute to the benefactor. Aubrey Lewis (1951) and Hubert Bond (1931)[56] – whose speech oddly enough was not published and apparently is lost – actually devoted their whole lectures to his memory.

Yet if one reviews this involvement, a more ambiguous picture emerges. The early concern with active participation is undoubted. He was an editor of the journal from 1863 to 1878,[57] bringing out sixty-three quarterly issues (numbers 43–106) and contributing many articles and reviews. He was president in 1871, on committees, attending meetings and arguing against infiltration of the MPA by laymen (1865) and against a takeover by the Royal Medical and Chirurgical Society (1870).[58] But by the late 1870s rumblings of discontent could be heard. He resigned the editorship amidst an obscurely acrimonious debate. After 1881 he rarely attended meetings, annual or quarterly. In 1890 his name was suddenly absent from the list of members published annually, and one has to assume that he has resigned. But no reasons were given, no official notice was published and no mention was made of the event in any obituary. Walk[59] incorrectly states that he 'never resigned, nor, as might be expected, was he ever elected an Honorary Member', yet in 1912 (the year in which his fellow psychiatrists

Savage and Clouston were knighted)[60] Hayes Newington proposed him for this very honour, in words which hint at the underlying dissensions that presumably had to be papered over.

> One need not describe Dr Maudsley's qualifications for the receipt of this honour. There was nobody more worthy of it, and no one would be accorded the honour more readily. He thought it would be well that, in order especially to mark the occasion, the nomination should receive the strongest possible support, namely, that of every living ex-president and every officer of the Association. He was pleased to say that everybody concerned fell in with the idea at once, and the resulting list of names was one of which anybody might well feel proud to have behind his form of proposal. Such *strength of nomination was not obtained because it was thought it would be required, but simply in order to enhance the honour which it was sought to confer.*[61]

Such circumlocutory reinforcement of the proposal (which was unanimously accepted) bears all the hallmarks of the psychoanalytic mechanism of denial; something very strong was apparently required to bury this particular hatchet. Just as, in 1912, the flourishing psychology of Freud might tell us more about such statements than the sterility of 'brain mythology', so the silence about Henry Maudsley can give us an alternative version of his dealings with the MPA. Despite the gloss of the late reconciliation, he had virtually abandoned the commonality of alienists for his own lonely philosophy. Why did he do this?

Perhaps the answer partly lies in the tone of some of his contributions. Thus on his first attendance in 1862 he withdrew his paper because of lack of time to deliver it, remarking that 'the members would be more generally interested' in one by Robertson on the utilization of asylum sewage. In fact Robertson did 'not propose to trouble the meeting with a paper', simply producing a ground plan as a basis for discussion.[62] Deferring to a senior was polite, but perhaps necessary for other purposes (*vide infra*). In 1865, as joint editor of the *JMS* and a committee member, he exhibited another, absent, member's 'instrument for feeding' via the nostrils. Admitting 'it is rather large for the nostril, but it is intended for that', he mentioned an episode of 'near-asphyxiation' from his own experience so that 'since then I have never fed anyone except by a stomach pump'. Such criticism of someone else's device, at the same time as being its official exponent, went on to an implicit mockery, which seemed to be taken up by other members present.[63] In 1868, at the annual meeting, Maudsley was defeated in a proposal that London, again, be the venue for next year's meeting and withdrew a motion for lengthening the presidential term of office.[64] Although a dominant figure, it seems that his personal convenience – he several times suggested London for the meeting and often did not attend when provincial venues were used – may have annoyed certain members of the association.

Furthermore, the trait of cynicism that all his obituarists mention is apparent in many of his statements of the period. 'The history of human thought is the history of human delusions' intoned the 28-year-old prodigy in his 1863 paper on 'Delusions',[65] while Clouston greeted the 1871 presidential address on 'Insanity and its treatment'[66] as one 'of utter and entire scepticism'. Maudsley's rejoinder, quoted with relish by Aubrey Lewis ('Such a sceptic we do well to honour'), insisted that 'scepticism is nothing more than doubt, and doubt leads to enquiry, and enquiry leads to understanding'.[67] But he then put the question – not quoted by Lewis – 'My dear friend, are you sure you are quite right in your belief?', a question that rings with condescension. At the same annual meeting – 3 August 1871 – he warned against admitting interested laymen to the association, describing them as 'a peculiar class of members', and mentioning letters from 'Swedenborgians and Spiritualists and people of that class', so his rudeness was not confined to his medical peers. The multidisciplinary team would have been anathema to him. His absence from the November 1870 and April 1871 quarterly meetings was actively regretted – he would be expected to attend as president – but a remark of his at the 1874 annual meeting perhaps best sums up his attitude to the MPA and his acknowledgement of their attitude to him. For after the presidential address of that year he carefully stated that he 'did not rise for the purpose of criticism, but simply to propose a vote of thanks'.[68] Praise does not seem to have been in Maudsley's armamentarium, so that even after his death a reviewer (of *Religion and Realities*, published posthumously in 1918)[69] had to record: 'It has been said that Dr Maudsley was a destructive critic, and that he suggested no constructive system of philosophy.'[70]

Notwithstanding these ambivalences, the central aspect of Maudsley's relationship with the MPA probably lay in his role as editor of the *Journal of Mental Science* (*JMS*). Maudsley was a writer, a prolix and weighty wordsmith; his early articles attracted the attention of Conolly; his reputation was founded on his books; his love of Goethe and Shakespeare and philosophy informed all his opinions.[71] He himself described the impact of his article on 'Edgar Allan Poe'[72] as 'exciting a good deal of attention at the time and making me favourably known among the subscribers to that Journal'[73] (the *JMS*). Crichton-Browne supports this with enthusiasm. 'Maudsley was revealed to me in a brilliant essay on Edgar Allan Poe ... so rich in insight, originality and happy similitudes as to betoken unmistakably "the lighting of another taper at heaven", which was at that time Maudsley's way of describing the arrival of a new man of genius on the scene.'[74] Whatever the quality of this piece (*vide infra*) it is certainly lengthy, and prior to his formal appointment as co-editor with Lockhart Robertson in 1863 he had already published eight articles in the journal.

But while the process of his becoming editor was overtly serendipitous, it is worth examining some of the details. The years 1862 and 1863 were momentous ones for Maudsley, embracing as they did his sudden departure from Cheadle, his first attendance at the annual meeting of the association[75] (the best attended meeting in its brief history), his meeting with Conolly (and presumably thereby his future wife) and the foundation of his London career. In his own words he 'became restless and desirous of change, resigned my appointment and threw myself on London',[76] but is it not equally likely there was some method in his madness? After all, Maudsley was a Yorkshireman and very gifted. His later memoir of Conolly criticized the great man for 'troubles, shirked at the time', requiring 'at last some convulsive act of energy, in order to disperse them'.[77] Certainly Maudsley was not consistent in his notions ('consistency signifies prejudice and stagnation')[78] but John Bucknill's appointment as Visitor in Lunacy in 1862 meant that a new journal editor was bound to be needed. At a Special General Meeting of the association, in September 1862, Bucknill's recommendation for the editorship, C.L. Robertson – also a prolific contributor – was duly elected. He did, however, announce: 'I have received from Dr Maudsley, a man that I am quite sure every gentleman who reads the Journal will appreciate, the promise of his co-operation during this period.'[79] Given that Robertson was also busy as superintendent of the asylum at Haywards Heath, it is not surprising that Maudsley joined him formally as (junior) co-editor in October 1863. Nor is it surprising that two of Conolly's pet themes, *Hamlet* and *Middle-Class Hospitals*, should have been two of the topics that Maudsley chose to write about in this interim period, the one in the January 1863 *Westminster Review*, the other in the October 1862 *JMS*.[80] In fact a coherent view of these events would suggest that Maudsley – who had never previously attended an annual meeting – saw his window of opportunity and shrewdly aimed at the job.

Nor should it be assumed that the post was uncontested. A printed circular, dated 10 September 1862, was sent to all members of the association by J. Stevenson Bushnan, proprietor of Laverstock House, Salisbury, a private asylum.[81] Offering himself as candidate for the editorship, Bushnan cited his experience as editor of the *Medical Times*, his numerous publications (both the April and July issues of the *JMS* in 1862 contained articles by him)[82] and the need for a single editor. He was proposed for the post at the Special General Meeting[83] by a Dr Burnett 'in consequence of receiving Bushnan's circular' and as 'a much superior man to Dr Robertson'. The need for a private proprietor to take over – taking turns, so to speak, with public asylum physicians – was also expressed, but such a notion was rejected by Harrington Tuke, among others, and Burnett's proposal was not supported. Robertson became temporary editor but was 'prevented from formally associating Dr Maudsley's name (with his) as joint editor', although he gave notice of his intention to move this proposition at the next annual meeting.[84] There may also have been more than influence at stake. At the same year's AGM (3 July 1862) Bucknill stated his resolution that 'the surplus funds should be devoted to payment for assistance in my editorial work ... I propose now to engage the regular services of a sub-editor.'[85] A regular stipend was the first necessity of a physician newly arrived in London and trying to establish himself. Maudsley may well have needed some extra income, like his contemporary and fellow-

Yorkshireman Hughlings Jackson who lived off medical reporting during his early days in town.[86]

Certainly the business of editorship was in keeping with Maudsley's perceptions of medical psychology, stressing as he did throughout his life the need for a powerful philosophical basis to clinical practice. It also gave him the contacts he needed to build up his practice, a sounding-board for his own ideas, and a practical method for honing his textbook. Papers on 'Delusions' (1863), 'Classification of the sciences' (1864) and *On Some of the Causes of Insanity* (1867) (which ends with the phrase the 'foundations of a true physiology and pathology of the mind') as well as detailed reviews of *Syphilitic Disease of the Brain* (July 1864) and *Recent Metaphysics* (January 1865) were clearly precursors to the larger work.[87] In a more general sense, the very role of editor was in itself a new means for advancing scientific careers, and it was a real foresight of Maudsley's to realize this and take on the job. Again, the influence of Conolly may have been significant. At the July 1863 annual meeting Conolly described the journal as 'a publication of extreme importance, as containing the expression of the opinions of the Association; and it depends almost entirely on the conduct of the Journal whether the Association maintains its character'.[88] Organizing and encouraging papers was probably unpopular among his fellow practitioners – 'I ask you not to make any very great alterations . . . as we shall have endless expenses – I am sorry that we are obliged to appear so parsimonious'[89] – but the increasing importance of the medical press can be seen in the number of journals that were soon being regularly exchanged, some twenty-three being listed in the April 1866 issue of the *JMS*.[90] Yet it is also clear that Robertson was the senior partner. Books for review, pamphlets, and exchange journals were sent to him, his name was always printed first, and he seems to have provided most of the abstracts of foreign literature that were a new and admired feature of the journal (features attributed by Aubrey Lewis to the sole influence of Maudsley, though clearly introduced by Robertson).[91]

Maudsley continued as editor until October 1878, contributing some two to three major articles a year in the 1860s, about one a year in the 1870s, and doubtless many of the unattributed 'Reviews', items in 'Notes and News', etc. He was always re-elected unanimously, was singled out (along with Robertson) by Westphal in 1868 for special thanks for 'successful endeavours to further the objects of my scientific journey'[92] and became senior editor in 1870 after Robertson's resignation. His new partner, Dr J. Sibbald, resigned in 1872, and Maudsley successfully requested Clouston as co-editor. Clouston greeted his appointment with the remark, 'If any will stimulate me to do my duty it will be my association with him',[93] and stayed in harness with Maudsley until the latter's resignation. It was this period as editor that also saw the publication of *The Physiology and Pathology of Mind* in 1867, *Body and Mind* – the Goulstonian lectures – in 1870 and *Responsibility in Mental Disease* in 1874.[94] Maudsley attended every annual meeting of the association between 1862 and 1878 (except for that of 1869), usually attended one or two quarterly meetings every year, was on the committee for asylum statistics which first reported in 1867[95] and on another committee (of five members) formed to consider a 'Tuke Prize' in 1874.[96] There is little doubt that he was fully at the centre of things, dominating the MPA with his written and spoken presence. For example, in a letter to the young Dr Bastian in 1865 he hinted that 'the next vacancy will be at Colney Hatch', and warned that 'committees are very prone to the absurdity of estimating the standing of a man by his age'.[97]

But there were signs of dissent. After the editor's re-election 'by acclamation' at the Annual Meeting of August 6, 1873, a Dr Boyd complained that "no encouragement was given by the editors to superintendents of asylums to publish the facts that came before them"'. Maudsley replied that 'the editors would be only too glad to publish them, but were obliged to give it up in the past as so little responded'.[98] This seems to indicate that editing in those days was more a matter of filling up than paring down. Yet nervous, would-be authors were not easily welcomed by their formidable 38-year-old senior editor. In 1877 an even more unseemly debate ensued[99] when Harrington Tuke – also married to a Conolly daughter, and said by Crichton-Browne to have been socially close to Maudsley ('in a restaurant in Soho, where over frugal meals, he and I and Lockhart Robertson, and Broadbent and Harrington Tuke . . . held high discourse and adumbrated projects for the future of lunacy')[100] – suddenly insisted on a letter from Dr Bucknill being read, 'in the event of the resignation of Dr Maudsley'. He continued: 'I am not satisfied with the way the Journal is at present conducted', and, although he admitted the editors' great literary abilities, said that 'there were certain doctrines taught there, certain tenets, which are contrary and repugnant to me, and I may say, to some others here'. Tuke went on to insist that 'the present editor or editors of the Journal in their doctrines do not represent the majority of the Association' and concluded: 'I understand that Dr Maudsley proposes to resign next January.' This embarrassing speech was strongly supported by a Dr Lindsay who stated:

> The Journal has not done for the Association what it might have done, what it ought to have done and what it was expected to have done. It has not advanced our interests, not been of that practical use we have looked for . . . I regret to say its weight has not been very much felt in high quarters, if we may judge from the results.

Quite what this is all about is most uncertain since the 'doctrines' and 'interests' referred to were not further detailed in the minutes. Walk[101] suggested it may have been Harrington Tuke's religious convictions bridling at some of Maudsley's insouciance towards theology. Perhaps there was a rift between private practitioners and public asylum doctors; perhaps Maudsley's grinding and persistent forays against 'metaphysics'[102] had started to weary those attempting to explore the psychodynamics of mental illness; perhaps people were just fed up with his cynicism and apparent contempt for so many of his fellow-practitioners.

Whatever the truth, it was a watershed in Maudsley's career. Offering to resign on the spot – 'I am entirely in the hands of the Association' – he also stated: 'I am not in the least anxious to continue the job.' There was a muddled debate concerning who should be editor and how many editors – at one stage four are proposed – there should be, but eventually Maudsley and Clouston were re-elected by twenty-eight votes to nine, accompanied by Harrington Tuke's barbed comment that he hoped it might be a lesson to them 'to amend the future as to some of ... the opinions expressed there'. By the next annual meeting, 26 July 1878, Maudsley was insistent on resigning. Harrington Tuke anyhow 'thought it his duty ... to object to the re-appointment of the former editor, Dr Maudsley'. Even though Bucknill urged him to reconsider, Maudsley declared that 'during the past year his own editorship had been almost nominal', proposed new editors (who were accepted) and resigned.[103] He did not attend the 1879 meeting, and was only recorded as present at three more annual meetings (1880, 1881, 1887) before leaving the MPA altogether. Apart from February 1880 he was also absent from quarterly meetings, until a late burst in 1888 when he came to hear Hughlings Jackson, in February, talk on post-epileptic states, and himself presented a paper, 'Remarks on crime and criminals', in May.[104] At this latter event Dr Hack Tuke commented: 'Although Dr Maudsley will probably not care to be associated with angels, there was one particular in which they bore a certain resemblance, Dr Maudsley's visits to the meetings of the Association were like theirs, few and far between. They were therefore all the more indebted to him for having come to this meeting and read a paper.'[105]

Other negatives also abound. He was not on the parliamentary and statistical committees, did not contribute to the Eames Memorial Fund (for the widow of a colleague), saw his book *Body and Will* (1883) reviewed in the *JMS* as 'a hymn for pessimism',[106] and was not reported as attending the Antwerp (1885) or Berlin (1890) congresses on psychiatry. Between 1877 and 1909 he published only three papers in the *JMS*, that of 1888 (see above), one on 'Criminal responsibility in relation to insanity' (1895),[107] and one on 'The new psychology' in 1900.[108] This latter effort he surprisingly read at an MPA meeting (by invitation?) in London on 10 May, and the discussion following it was critical (e.g. Mercier 'criticized the matter of it as inconsistent and unduly depreciative of the labours of others'). Most important of all, he did not even mention the MPA in his autobiographical fragment, and, of course, he does seem to have been unique in actually leaving the association altogether in 1890. There was no stated reason for this, although the act fits in with the evidence presented indicating his increasing distance from his colleagues. Perhaps his disenchantment with the MPA's attitude towards the 1890 Lunacy Bill – as recorded at the 1887 'poorly attended' annual meeting[109] – was the key, for then he is quoted as saying that 'their parliamentary committee might have perhaps taken a strong post . . . they should have refused to take any responsibility on it'. He went on that 'early treatment of insanity in its present sense would be practically abolished . . . during the last two years he had seen restraint practised which he had never in his life seen before'. This was quite an understandable complaint from Conolly's son-in-law and torch-bearer, but did learned philosophical tracts and an élite private practice have any relevance to the dreadful contemporary problems of massive asylums (the LCC was starting to plan a group of asylums for 10,000 persons on the Horton Manor estate), relapsing public concern, and a fossilizing system of care for lunatics generally?[110]

Whatever the answers to the queries thrown up by these MPA dealings, the overall course of events is apparent. Maudsley actively used the MPA and editorship as a springboard for his own career. He certainly did his best to nurture the association, but once spurned he soon divested himself of much involvement. Instead of attempting to rescue it from its turn of the century inadequacies he concentrated on articles for *Mind* – the new philosophy journal – and became a celebrated recluse, firing off postcards and watching cricket.[111] But this process has close parallels in the development of his psychiatric philosophy, which needs to be more fully examined.

Maudsley's psychiatric philosophy

As we have seen, it is clear that the written word was the basis for Maudsley's extremely successful career. 'He has been for a quarter of a century one of the foremost medical men of London and in the world of science is in the front rank' proclaimed Clark Bell in 1910.[112] Writing predominantly for the *Journal of Mental Science* until the mid-1870s, Maudsley then concentrated more on his eleven books (see table 6.1), which largely reflect and expand upon the theories laid down in the early papers. In all, this is a voluminous body of work, and a detailed review would be out of place here. However, an outline of his ideas, their sources and their impact, can be sketched in, although his style is somewhat diffuse and heavy-handed.

Certainly his attitudes to psychiatric practice were not consistent. He lost faith in the use of tranquillizers, the role of asylums, and even the causative role of self-abuse.[113] But no doctor can be blamed for changing his opinions in the light of clinical experience. By contrast the progress of his underlying philosophy follows a distinct and coherent path, matching his social remove from busy professional activity in the MPA (with its concerns for practical matters to do with the business of insanity) towards the well-known reclusiveness and concentration on ideas *per se*. Thus after a British Medical Association address in 1895, described as an 'intellectual treat' by the meeting's president, a Dr Nicholson said 'this was an occasion on which to be congratulated at Dr Maudsley coming out amongst us once again'.[114] Whether his work does repay reading, as Aubrey Lewis suggested it would, in the late twentieth century, is an open question, but it surely represents a body of theory that cannot be ignored in assessing the status of psychiatry in his time.

Among the earlier articles, his piece on 'Edgar Allan Poe'[115] is perhaps most instructive, not least because of its contemporary impact (*vide supra*). Prior to this is only the review, 'The correlation of mental and physical forces; or, man a part of nature',[116] in which he described metaphysics as 'the vanity of vanities' in the course of an eulogy to the progress of science. It seems there had apparently been 'an increase in practical morality; and this, not as the result of any supposed exacerbation of moral principle, but as the simple and inevitable result of the progress of science'. As a result there was appearing 'the claim of a social science'. He saw the progress of the intellect as 'owing to the progress of man's acquaintance with the laws of nature' and asked, 'What does the history of the created universe tend to if not to show that mind has been the gradual resultant of ages on ages of previous operations?' This Darwinian optimism, ending in impressive quotations from Carlyle and Goethe, was reached via sardonic references to the creationist P.H. Gosse (father of Edmund and author of *Omphalos*, and probably better known and loved now because of his son's work) as 'the strangest specimen of human ingenuity' and a display of impressive quotes and references to Bacon, Spinoza, Comte, Leibniz, etc. What the humble asylum officers thought of all this (the books reviewed were by Grove – 'a book which will probably be one of the most notable in the history of science' – Carpenter, Oersted and the Rev. B. Powell) is difficult to say. Certainly the following article, 'On general paralysis' (by Harrington Tuke),[117] beginning 'It is with reluctance that I attempt any definition', comes from a different version of scientific writing.

But 'Edgar Allan Poe'[118] carried on and expanded this air of youthful intellectual certainty. Aged 25, Henry Maudsley (MD London, medical superintendent of the Manchester Royal Lunatic Asylum) was fearfully well read, but this long and circumlocutory piece seems by any standards unpleasant in its tone and banal in its truisms. Inveighing against 'stuccoed man . . . worldly prosperous, with a wife who looks upon him as a hero . . . and happy in children who are the most wonderful children in the world; capable, moreover, of a decided opinion upon all things under heaven', he went on to a wordy discussion of the contrasting habits of men of genius. Concluding that 'in fact, a Shakespeare or a Goethe is rather a rare phenomenon in this universe of ours' and that 'the plausible hypocrite passes muster with commendation', he proceeded to a dismissive and condescending assessment of the life and work of Poe. The basis for this was often moralistic, but the influence of degenerationist ideas is unmistakable. Bemoaning Poe's father's marriage he declares: 'It was bad, irrecoverably bad, David Poe, for are not the sins of the father visited upon the children unto the third and fourth generation?' But such biblical platitudes are soon stated as scientific facts. Thus 'we may rest assured of this, that infirmities of mind are transmitted from parent to child by a law as sure and constant as is any physical infirmity', and in a more ambitious strain he goes on: 'Before the child is born it is certain that its after-constitution may be seriously affected by its mother's state of mind.' All of which fitted with contemporary notions, but did not sit well on the crowned head of scepticism. Likewise his tribute to Poe's 'quick intellect' was soon put in place by a remark on 'skill in fencing, swimming and all such feats – not incompatible elements with immorality in a character, as too many examples every day prove'. But degeneration ruled ('the eternal laws exhibit their warning in disease and deformity; and if such be disregarded, the end soon comes') and he went on to a denunciation of Poe's 'self-feeling', 'insincerity of character', and 'malignant and cynical' personality. He was cruel about alcoholism – 'Edgar Poe, a teetotaller!' – insisted that 'few people have lived upon this earth as miserable as was Edgar Poe' and concluded weightily that the 'highest development of scepticism can in the end but arrive at this conclusion, that sin is ignorance; and if a man have the capability of knowledge in him, is he not responsible for such ignorance?'

Such a combination of moral certainty and 'scientific' analysis was clearly a potent brew in 1860. The Maudsley of cynicism and 'hypercriticality' was well on his way. While his acquaintance with Darwinian ideas was both detailed and admirable,[119] the uses to which these were put are very much of his (Victorian) time. Thus his essay on 'Delusions'[120] wanders from 'the meditations of the philosopher' (after quotes from Shakespeare, Plato and Goethe) to a paean on the 'holiness of Endurance', and 'the sermon which more than eighteen hundred years ago was preached from the Mount of Olives near Jerusalem'. And in the middle of this bio-psycho-moralism, not only have we to follow 'the gradual course of mental degeneration' via 'far too much feeling of self' and 'morbid egoism', but we have to accept that 'delusion is the certain companion of extravagant development of self'. It is tempting to transpose the question, 'Quis custodes custodiet?' Furthermore, not only was the degeneration theory held across generations – 'the habitual passion of the parent becomes the insanity of the child' – but this 'gradual degeneration of mind through morbid passion, delusions, and dementia to extinction, frequently takes place – is, in fact, the *regular* course of insanity – in an individual life'. The examples of several saints were given as instances – 'their follies have been the symptoms of an insane selfhood which identified itself with religion' – and there is real virulence in Maudsley's remark that 'the aping of humility by religious pride makes it the more odious'. It was perhaps this unpleasant edge which started the rift with the significantly religious Harrington Tuke, because their obscure row terminating the editorship (*vide supra*) may well have derived from Maudsley's increasing agnosticism. Of like tone is the line that 'few things are more irritating to the temper than an attempt to reason with the self-constituted wreck which the persistent onanist is'; it gives us a glimpse of Maudsley's notoriously difficult manner in individual dealings, and leads into an area of psychiatric aetiology about which he was strikingly eloquent.

Amongst the mass of material from this 1860s editor is a paper read before the Harveian Society of London on 5 March 1868 entitled 'Illustrations of a Variety of insanity';[121] the author spoke of 'that kind of insanity which is brought on by self-abuse'. Developing Skae's[122] theory with considerable force, there is a detailed and actually interesting description of what might today be described as 'hebephrenic schizophrenia'. This is not to claim any primacy or greater correctness for that label, rather to acknowledge Maudsley's ability to combine ideas, metaphor and case histories in a coherent presentation. The needs of a crowded lecture hall seem to have removed much of the otiosity required of a potentially unfilled journal,[123] but again the sentiments expressed were hardly those one would expect of a detached 33-year-old scientist. Havelock Ellis referred[124] to 'his vigorous, picturesque manner' in this piece, but the details have a darker edge.

Describing 'the miserable sinner whose mind suffers by reason of self-abuse', he used such phrases as 'vicious habit', 'utter moral perversion', and 'degenerate beings ... who, as regards moral character, are very much what eunuchs are represented to be – cunning, deceitful, liars, selfish, in fact, morally insane'. He gave an example of one of these 'degraded beings' whose 'plan ... was to masturbate every morning into a tumbler of water and then to drink it', so as to be 'strengthened by the nourishment afforded to his brain'. Lambasting this 'mind enervated by vicious practices, dwelling continually on sexual subjects', Maudsley found it 'curious' that such individuals 'will actually defend their vice on some pretence or other'. There seems no hint here that perhaps he was dealing with an hallucinated psychotic, no hint of the mental physiologist searching for the organic substrate to crazy behaviour. Yet having decided that 'the sooner he sinks to his degraded rest the better for himself, and the better for the world which is well rid of him', he went on to a peroration decrying the 'vain' and 'fruitless' results of studying mind from 'the psychological point of view', and demanding that it be studied 'inductively ... from a physiological and pathological basis'. Leaving aside the tempting speculations as to why Maudsley showed such religious zeal in hounding mad masturbators (after all, he himself wrote in 1863 that 'conscious formation for unconscious action is a law of mental development'),[125] it is clear from this appeal why his first and most influential book was titled *The Physiology and Pathology of Mind* (1867).

That this work made his name seems undoubted. Darwin quoted from it extensively[126] (as did Maudsley, incidentally, from Darwin – one good turn deserves another), it was widely translated,[127] went quickly to a second edition, achieved mitosis as *The Physiology of Mind* in 1876 and *The Pathology of Mind* in 1879[128] (both also much republished) and was well reviewed. A *Saturday Review* article on it (25 May 1867) was actually reprinted in the 'Notes and News' section of the *JMS* for July 1867,[129] which may reflect a certain entrepreneurial spirit in the then co-editor. Described overall as an 'original enterprise' undertaken with 'courage' and executed with 'skill', the second part (Pathology) was regarded as a 'most judicious summary', a 'moral study', marked by the 'stamp of wide experience' in that Maudsley had apparently traced the causes of increased insanity 'to the varied excitements of English life'. Although there was no index, the sources quoted are certainly extensive and it is clear that Maudsley packed the book with a mass of learning both recent and ancient. Acknowledging his debt in the preface to Bain, Herbert Spencer,[130] Drs Laycock and Carpenter, he also used Goethe, Bacon, Spinoza, Hobbes, Hume, Montaigne, Comte, Hartley, Berkeley, Whytt and more, to illustrate his physiological case and no less a parade of psychiatric writings (Pinel, Morel, Moreau, Esquirol, Griesinger) in the 'pathological' treatise. A quotation from Swedenborg as a note to chapter IX on 'Memory and imagination' was perhaps less impressive given Maudsley's subsequent description of this man as a 'learned and ingenious madman'.[131]

That its influence may have been more in the sociological and philosophical field than in clinical psychiatry is also apparent. In a review of a later work, *Organic to Human*,[132] in 1917, Maudsley's 'mastery of all the available knowledge of the structure and functions of the human nervous system, no less than his signal capacity for thinking scientifically' was acknowledged in reference to *The Physiology and Pathology of Mind*. But the reviewer also suggested that the earlier work 'drew the attention of philosophical thinkers more than that of practising medical men', and its study was 'recommended by the late Walter Pater to a candidate for classical honours as a help to straight thinking'.[133] Earlier in the same year, another reviewer in the *JMS*[134] suggested that 'Dr Maudsley, had he lived in the good old persecutory days, would scarcely have survived the publication of the *Physiology and Pathology of Mind*. Probably the title alone would have caused the powers to invoke the assistance of the common hangman. Probably also the author would have been roasted on a funeral pyre of the first edition.' Stoddart wrote to Aubrey Lewis in 1948, 'My impression is that Maudsley was a philospher rather than a psychiatrist or physician.' Lewis himself admitted that, comparing the third edition with Kraepelin's second edition, it was a 'treatise as compared to a textbook'.[135]

Of course it was not all plain sailing. A more critical *BMJ* review led to space being found in the subsequent *JMS*[136] for a detailed rebuttal, the reviewer being chided for his ignorance of Prochaska's work on the 'Sensorium Commune'. There is little that a modern commentator can usefully say in all this, although one may doubt the *Saturday Review's* assertion that Maudsley 'will not advance beyond ascertained facts'. For once more that seminal theme, self-abuse, accompanied not uncommonly by 'sexual excess', is aetiologically apparent. Case 4,[137] ' a conceited cockney', imbued with 'offensive dissenting zeal' and 'hopelessly addicted to masturbation', suffered from the 'disagreeable form of mental derangement following such cause'; likewise case 49's 'extreme moral perversion' and 'extravagant conceit' were flatly attributed to 'self-abuse'. Paradoxically the same author goes on to inveigh against the public outcry when 'some poor madman who has committed homicide in a paroxysm of his frenzy is permitted to pass the remainder of his unhappy life in confinement instead of being hanged forthwith!' And throughout his life Maudsley fought an admirable battle against the hanging of lunatics, strangely unwilling to postulate a parallel between violence and masturbation, that both might be secondary to mental illness. But inconsistency was his hallmark, as he proudly asserted in his autobiography, so it is again not surprising that he should be actively critical of treating the insane in 'overgrown and overcrowded asylums', having asserted in his Manchester Royal Lunatic Asylum annual report of 1860 that 'repeated experience has shown it to be really a rash folly, if not a positive cruelty, to send them forth into the trials of life, when they are utterly unable to encounter them'.[138] Modern views would see this as a progressive change in outlook, but his asylum experience was actually very limited. Of his 'twenty years' experience' announced to the 1877 Select Committee,[139] only a little over four years had been spent in asylum work, and that largely in the middle-class (and small) hospital at Cheadle.

However, by 1871, when he came to give his presidential address on 'Insanity and its treatment',[140] it was not inconsistent with the themes apparent so far that his discussion of prevention, the use of asylums or private houses, and the use/abuse of sedatives should conclude with Macbeth's fearful lines about 'sound and fury, signifying nothing'. Clouston was amazed at this 'utter and entire scepticism', but we should not be. Faust-like Maudsley had gorged at philosophy's table, his photographic memory recording page upon page and line upon line in his search for an understanding of the causes of madness. He had seen the asylums start to fossilize, the limitations and dangers of bromide and chloral and digitalis, the limits of knowledge in dealing with intractable diseases. His moral nature could not detach itself from the follies of patients, colleagues, the public. He dominated the MPA, his medical honours were outstanding, but what directions were now open to him?

If we look at his published work it is clear that criminology became increasingly important, with his 1874 *Responsibility in Mental Disease*[141] achieving acclaim and reprints. The review by the chaplain of Bristol Lunatic Asylum commented on the 'fearlessness' with which Dr Maudsley proposes his opinions and 'beautiful passages that will long linger in our memory', while admitting that he (the reviewer) 'differed always with regret'.[142] Work on heredity, the increase of insanity, hallucinations and medical education also followed,[143] but the profound themes of philosophy increasingly absorbed his time. *Body and Will* (1883), *Natural Causes and Supernatural Seemings* (1886), *Life in Mind and Conduct* (1902), *Organic to Human: Psychological and Sociological* (1916)[144] were the major works, with articles for *Mind* and latterly, again, for the *JMS* filling in the intervening years. Much of this is difficult to read today, since it doggedly follows a rather banal materialism, repeating the same themes of organic influence and metaphysical absurdity, in language even more otiose (if possible) than his earlier work. 'It reveals a dignified if rather forlorn figure, watching beside a flag which it has kept waving for half a century, grim, unflinching, and unafraid', wrote the reviewer from the *Oxford Magazine* in reference to *Organic to Human*,[145] and the pessimistic degenerationist of the 1860s certainly seems like someone caught in a philosophical cul-de-sac.

Of course, it is not all downhill. His earlier influence continued to obtain residual respect. In 1890 Havelock Ellis, in a piece on 'The criminal', referred to him as an 'artist as much as a man of science, master of a solemn and weighty style, illumined by vivid flashes of imagination, and by his numerous works popularising new ideas'. He was 'justly regarded abroad as a distinguished pioneer of criminal anthropology'.[146] Max Nordau's extraordinary anthem *Degeneration*[147] referred to him in the context of 'Borderland dwellers – that is to say, dwellers on the borderland between reason and pronounced madness', as well as in association with 'moral insanity'. Yet at around the same time Maudsley was trying to move away from the more apocalyptic versions of degeneration theory. In his 1895 discussion on *Criminal Responsibility of the Insane* he insisted 'I do not see why crime should necessarily be degeneracy', and went on to ask

> 'Has not the theory of degeneracy been abused of late? As used by Morel the term has scientific meaning and value, but much has been done to rob it of definite meaning by stretching it out to cover all sorts and degrees of deviations from an ideal standard of thinking and feeling ...' [Thus] 'the meaningless name has been converted into a quasi-metaphysical something, so that many persons think, when the word degeneracy has been spoken, that all has been said that need be said, though nothing actually has been said'.[148]

Later reviews also delineated his contemporary role. Gladly welcoming 'yet another book' (*Heredity, Variation and Genius*, 1908), a *JMS* reviewer summarized Maudsley's Lamarckian position, and his concern for the 'wise conduct of life' and the need for 'the terrestrial mortal' to 'imbibe the wholesome material spirit of the earth to sustain the virile strength of the race'. The concluding quote from Descartes – 'that if mankind is to be perfected the means of perfecting it must be sought in the medical sciences' – was seen as an 'incitement and an encouragement'.[149] In the same journal Hubert J. Norman reviewed *Organic to Human* some eight years later with similar admiration.[150]

> Any work which deals with such subjects as ethics, psychology, and sociology from a biological point of view must, at the present time, necessarily be iconoclastic. The breaking of popular idols is, when not actually fraught with danger, certainly a thankless task. Dr Maudsley has not been deterred by any considerations of this kind. As one reads his trenchant criticisms of many vague theories and baseless speculations which pass for axioms, Nietzsche's phrase of 'philosophy with a hammer' recurs as an appropriate description of the process. The blows are

not, however, given in the crude manner which such a phrase implies. His hand has not lost its cunning any more than its force.

The reviewer went on to quote approvingly Maudsley's lines about 'subtle physico-chemical sympathies and synergies of motions and rhythms' and his insistence that the 'introspective ego, be it ever so acute, expert and free, is tied down by material bonds'. In an exchange of letters with Sir Bryan Donkin (in 1917) Maudsley thanked him for an appreciative review in the *Lancet*, and lamented the coming period of 'spiritual recrudescence'. He wrote that 'science is claimed as having validated spiritualism and cranks of all sorts', and it is clear that whatever his shortcomings in respect of scientific method, Maudsley could be deemed to fulfil Lewis's portrait of him as a symbol of positivism and empiricism.[151]

Whatever the later role, the process of isolation undoubtedly began with his resigning the editorship of the *JMS* in 1878. Instead of laudatory reviews reprinted, the 1879 volume carried significantly critical pieces on *The Pathology of Mind* (3rd edition) as well as on *The Physiology of Mind* reprinted that year.[152] 'Dr Maudsley fearlessly, in a paragraph, settles questions that have puzzled wise men since the world began. He calls it a nonsense that a man can love God ... he has the personal hatred of the religionists to everything that is opposed to his own creed', wrote one anonymous reviewer. Another, a certain 'OXON', suggested that 'Dr Maudsley has here no theory of life that does not end by speciously denying the patent facts it started to describe'. There is also a report[153] of a Dr Herzen interposing 'in a controversy between Dr Maudsley and Dr G.H. Lewes' concerning consciousness accompanying the activity of nerve centres, but all these difficulties were as nothing compared to the reactions to *Body and Will* (1883). Again OXON is the reviewer[154] and he is clearly amazed at this 'hymn of pessimism'. Humanity it seems would be 'new and degenerate varieties with special repulsive characters – savages of a decomposing civilisation', and 'all that which is past is a dream: and he that hopes will depend upon Time coming, dreams waking'. No wonder OXON regarded it as 'the Ultima Thule of pessimistic scepticism'.

More wounding than these puzzled regrets was a review in *Brain*,[155] a journal edited by Bucknill, Crichton-Browne, Ferrier, and Hughlings Jackson. Despite several learned neurological articles, as one on aphasia,[156] Maudsley never wrote for – or his articles were never accepted for? – this particular journal. The review in question was by Charles Mercier, who insisted that it 'would be presumptuous in me to offer an opinion upon a book of Dr Maudsley's, and I have not ventured to make any critical observations' ... 'the issues are largely questions of fact, and the verdict must be left to the voice of the public'. But this was his last paragraph. The preceding twelve so cruelly and brilliantly exposed Maudsley's avowed aim to be 'intelligible' and 'practical' that it is difficult to know what to leave out. Quoting with relish the tortured description of the 'Physical basis of conscious identity' Mercier found that 'the body is an ego', then a few pages further on that 'the ego appears to be shifting its ground from the body to the mind', and then that the 'ego is both body and mind'. He was forced to conclude that 'Dr Maudsley commits himself to the opinion that the individual and the organism are identical, and are not identical', and was left gently reminding his readers that 'practice cannot be founded upon contradictions'. Moving on to the issue of intelligibility – 'beyond question the chief aim of his (Dr Maudsley's) book' – he quoted the author's discussion of the sensations which the ego represents (p. 80): 'These sensations themselves representing the sum of multitudes of activities that are going on below the threshold of consciousness, and which, albeit unperceived and unfelt immediately, vibrate subtilely (*sic*) in the most intimate and intricate interactions of organic depths, and in the result affect deeply the tone of consciousness.' Mercier now writes:

> It is not certain from the context whether it is the sensations or the activities that vibrate, but let us follow Dr Maudsley's directions and try to realise the vibration of a sensation or an activity. Having got a definite notion of that, let us add the quality of subtileness, and imagine them vibrating subtilely. Now go a step further, and imagine this vibration occurring in an interaction. Again, imagine an organic depth; and yet again, get a firm grasp of the notion of the interaction of organic depths. Now combine all these notions together, and imagine an activity or a sensation vibrating subtilely in the interactions of organic depths. If the reader finds in this expression exact terms and phrases, and can gather from it clear and definite ideas, Dr Maudsley has succeeded in his object.

Subsequent paragraphs continued in this vein, ridiculing Maudsley's language – 'an all-pervading mentiferous ether', his syntax – 'There is a scarcity of verbs in this sentence', and contradictory philosophy. As for following 'Dr Maudsley's treatment of the various subjects considered in this book', Mercier simply had to list them to reveal the pretensions of the work. They included, among many others,

> the question whether animals have souls, the invention of lucifer matches, the use of Christianity, the Exodus, the fall of man, the origin of dermoid cysts, the morality of science, the doctrine of the atonement, the habits of ants and the possible nature of their religion, the immortality of the soul, the failure of the Christian morality, the belief in God and the existence of the Devil. It is a book de omnibus rebus et quibusdam aliis

(a book about everything and then some).

Such mockery in a scientific journal, in a journal devoted to neurology, to the organic aspects of cerebral function that Maudsley had presumed himself to champion, cannot have left him unscarred. He was now an outsider and further criticisms followed him. In the *JMS* of 1896[157] a review of the latest edition of *The Pathology of Mind* described his philosophy as 'frequently unsound, his psychology prohibitive of truth, and his sociology repulsive and unsuited to average humanity'. 'One reads and wonders how much of Dr Maudsley's vivid descritpions of mental states emerges from the subject and how much from the author himself' – a barbed line indeed. His ideas were felt to be 'out of sympathy with the general tenor of recent research and philosophical thought'; it was not surprising that his old adversary, Mercier, should also criticize his 1900 paper to the MPA (on 'The new psychology') as being 'inconsistent and unduly depreciative of the labours of others',[158] nor was it odd that his reputation as a recluse should flourish. That the BMA should, however, have him give the address in medicine at their seventy-third annual meeting[159] in 1905 is somewhat strange, and one would like to know whether perhaps a snub was intended towards the MPA. This was of course the era of 'Chubb lock psychiatry' as Ernest Jones recalled it.[160] Whatever the background, Maudsley's speech was traditionally weighty. He had taken on board some eugenicist ideas,[161] and asked 'might not the ultimate costs to the commonwealth be greater were these persons (consumptives) to go living and breathing in it?', but the power of Morelian degeneration still informed his final perspective.

> Moral deterioration in the parent is pretty sure to be visited somehow upon the mental constitution of the children and the children's children . . . and it is I believe the moral or affective, not the intellectual nature – the tone of feeling infused into the forming germ – which counts most in human heredity.

Perhaps the strangest aspect of Maudsley's philosophy is the sheer difficulty of providing an adequate summary. Showalter[162] has summarized him as representative of 'Darwinist, determinist, evolutionist psychiatry, which claimed a new social authority as experts on the laws of heredity and the operations of the mind'. Maudsley claimed to 'treat all mental phenomena from a physiological rather than from a metaphysical point of view' (1867),[163] so that by 1876 he could describe 'sound morality' as 'being like the connective tissue of an organism'.[164] He felt that 'when we take the most decided forms of human wrong-doing, and examine the causes and nature of the moral degeneracy which they evince, we find that they are not merely subjects for the moral philosopher and the preacher, but that they rightly come within the scope of positive scientific research'.[165] Such emphasis on the physical basis of mental illness and its hereditary origins even extended to a form of reverse Morelian doctrine, insisting that 'education by the scientific method does demand and therefore strengthen certain qualities of the moral nature'. By his later years, though, his insistence on 'the principle of the unity of the human organism and its continuity with the rest of Nature's processes'[166] had become a rather glutinous word-soup, wherein 'all so-called causes are effects and all so-called effects causes'. He was also, *malgré* Showalter, a convinced Lamarckian, holding that 'mental organisation has been evolved by the successive registration of individually acquired ideas'. In some strange way he represented the dark, negative side of Freud, claiming science where there was often only pseudo-science, obsessionally seeing causality in everything, and paralysed by the frightful demons that could ambush every act. Unlike Freud he failed to generate a therapeutic method to fight off the shadows of degeneration, heredity, and immutable human weakness.

His last works do not alter one's view of this philosophy, but do set the seal on the blighted pessimism of his outlook. Under the magnifying lens of an aged isolation, that openly longed for death once his wife had died, the long-haired prophet *manqué* shrouded himself in a depressive ideology. 'If death be the "last enemy" of the individual mortal and nation, it has always been, is now, and ever shall be the best friend of the race.'[167] 'Of all the consoling illusions . . . none is perhaps more wildly irrational than that of a complete regeneration of human nature.'[168] There was still the dense prose, the 'subtile bodily motions', the truistic materialism, and the final 'quasi-prophetic warning' of 'War psychology: English and German', published posthumously because 'exception was taken by the censor to certain passages' when originally submitted in 1916.[169] Concluding with the words 'the pilgrimage of labour and sorrow which reason teaches that human life is, a lesson which the lust of life joying to live prevents man from ever really minding', it provided a suitable epitaph to a chronic purveyor of leaden prose and pessimistic views. It seems fit that only a world war could stop the repetitive productions of his melancholy genius, the same war that curiously demanded a new psychologism in dealing with its victims. Shell-shock, the impact of impossible living conditions on ordinary young men, as opposed to the abuse of the good English life by degenerate perverts, could not be contained by Dr Maudsley's philosophy.

Maudsley – man and doctor

Given all these achievements, writings, ideas, given his MPA dealings and eventual wealth, what sort of a man, as a friend or physician or family member, can be glimpsed behind the camouflage of words and actions? Terms like entrepreneur, sexual puritan, depressive, quickly come to mind, but are they sufficient?

The most striking fact is the lack of information, apparently due to the destruction of all his private papers.[170] There are extant some letters, mainly of clinical interest, although larger collections may well be available. At the 1931 Maudsley lecture[171] given by Sir Hubert Bond – and entitled 'Maudsley: testimonied in his own bringings forth' but never published – a Dr Vernon Briggs from Massachusetts stood to support the vote of thanks and stated that 'he had at home about a hundred of Maudsley's letters'. Apparently one of these expressed Maudsley's 'annoyance and irritation that people were not interested in the subject of psychiatry' and another told of his never having 'known anybody to go into psychiatry and afterwards leave it'. Briggs described these letters overall as a 'revelation of the working of the mind of a big man who was struggling to bring about help to the unfortunate and to prevent their breakdown'.

Another recipient of Maudsley's correspondence was G.H. Savage, who described him as having 'a Gladstonian habit of using postcards'. He went on: 'I have a collection of these, which I have headed "Maudsley's Fire". I shall never forget some of those, in which he criticised either something I had written, or some opinion I had given.'[172] Whether or not this fiery collection survives is uncertain, but there are several letters in the Ticehurst case books and at the Institute of Psychiatry. One sent to F.W. Mott in 1915 is somewhat poignant. Returning a book, the third edition of *Natural Causes and Supernatural Seemings* (1897), he wrote: 'With it I present you with a copy of a book which you have never probably seen or heard of – what the writer might think or say of what he wrote so many years ago – he cares not to enquire. Don't trouble to acknowledge – I am instructing my publishers to destroy all unsold copies of my books – and reserve two or three.' Not for him those 'ludicrous displays of vanity' by which 'men of great eminence . . . leave behind them carefully preserved letters . . . and elaborate memoirs of what they thought and felt'.[173] Not only would his private papers not see the biographical light, but unwanted books also. (In 1907 he had sent Mott a copy of *Physiology of Mind*, of which, he said, 'there are yet more on hand than are ever likely to be sold I imagine'.)[174]

Of course, being Maudsley, it is not difficult to find less jaundiced attitudes towards biography. Thus in 1867[175] he wrote: 'It is plain that biography which estimates both the individual and his circumstances, and displays their reactions, can alone give an adequate account of the man. . . . It is in fact the application of positive science to human life.' His own attempt, 'under editorial obligation', to provide a 'memoir of the late John Conolly, M.D.'[176] also displayed little restraint in the matter of personal factors. Conolly was thus chided for being unable 'heartily to recognise or accept the stern and painful necessities of life'; as not being 'unamenable to flattery which made things pleasant'; as having a mind 'of a feminine type'; and for liking 'enjoyment without a liking for paying the painful cost of it'. The final eulogy was grand – 'his public life has been the gain and honour of mankind' – yet the mixture is somewhat bewildering. Maudsley's ambivalence about this whole topic is in the end the central theme – 'the impossibility of speaking sincerely is a bar to all true biography' – and are there personal hints in his concern for 'the secret and mortal struggle with the traitorous and hidden weaknesses of one's own character'?

Whatever the realities behind these selected jottings, or his relationship with his father-in-law, Conolly, the very paucity of solid biographical data on Maudsley still begs for some sort of explanation. We have seen his eventual professional isolation from the MPA, and how it reflected the development of his personal philosophy. Could his 1879 decision 'to concentrate entirely upon the responsibilities of a large and important practice as a psychiatrist'[177] have had any bearing upon the matter? For this practice was noteworthy for having been, if nothing else, extraordinarily lucrative. The evidence of his last will and the Maudsley bequest is unequivocal on this[178] (some £100,000 in all, perhaps equivalent to £1 million or more today?), and he did not come from a rich family, nor did his wife bring much in her dowry if the Clark memoir – 'he did not die rich, it was far otherwise' – of Conolly is correct.[179] This points strongly to the likelihood that Maudsley's practice was at the very top end of the market, the aristocrats and very rich, and there is reasonable evidence to support this.

One strand relates to Ticehurst House, the expensive private asylum in Sussex run by the Newingtons.[180] For Maudsley was linked to at least eight patients there, three of them from the peerage. There are several letters extant concerning a Lady D—, and he was called in for consultation on a number of occasions as well as signing certificates. Ticehurst was the most lavishly equipped of private institutions, with extensive grounds, private carriages, numerous attendants and servants, and facilities for golf, hunting, and cricket. Maudsley's regular contact bespeaks equally lavish consultation fees. Nor should we forget that it was Hayes Newington, who ran Ticehurst from the early 1870s, who made the convoluted 1912 proposal[181] that Maudsley be granted honorary membership of the MPA.

There are also letters from a Dr Reginald Stilwell,[182] who recalled being put in charge of '2 or 3 single cure cases in various places, where I had some very good times'. It seems these cases 'were wealthy people and where I enjoyed some excellent shooting, golf, etc. – those were the days and I was young!'. If we add the comment of Crichton-Browne,[183] that Maudsley's life was 'prosperous and uneventful', and consider that he took over the running of The Lawn, Conolly's small private asylum, in 1866, (not giving it up until 1874),[184] it seems clear that in 'getting such practice as he could' Maudsley did very well financially. Perhaps the key was the already reported 'consultation of eminent European alienists'[185] concerning the mental state of the Archduchesss Charlotta, the Habsburg Empress of Mexico. Her embarrassing tour through Europe was something of a *cause célèbre*, and aristocratic notice of Dr Maudsley would have been considerable. Given his handsome appearance – Savage described him as such, with a 'healthy amount of conceit', and as being 'carefully dressed and scrupulously careful of his hands'[186] – and his impressive bearing, such that he 'gave the world assurance of a man',[187] he must have made a considerable personal impact. Is he perhaps the archetype of the philosopher-alienist as seen in T.S. Eliot's *The Cocktail Party*, combining this role with that of Wodehouse's Sir Roderick Glossop, who knew all there was to know of hidden insanity in Wooster's aristocratic world?[188] In fact it may be that his separation from the MPA enhanced his élitist practice. For what self-respecting peer would like to be consulting with a man involved in the messy business of public asylums and a stigmatized medical group? All of which may also explain the enormous lacunae of his life. For the essence of keeping such a clientele would have been absolute discretion and the guaranteed disposal of any damning documents or notes. The secrets of the mad rich proved safe with Henry Maudsley, in his time and our own.

Arguing against such a position, however, is the evidence of Maudsley's 'hypercritical' and 'cynical' personal manner. Would this not have militated against the courtier-like qualities required of aristocratic psychiatry? Such tartness may have been a reason for his failing to get the post as resident physician at Bethlem in 1866 despite references from Conolly, Bucknill, Griesinger (!), Lawrence (surgeon to the Queen) and Jenner (physician to the Queen).[189] W. Rhys Williams's appointment was announced in the *BMJ* on 17 March, two months after Maudsley's marriage and two weeks after Conolly's death. For not only was Maudsley 'rather scathing' about most of the 'men he used to know in the profession',[190] but 'he was rather abrupt in his manner to some of his old patients'. In a letter to Newington about a Lady D— he wrote of her 'mood of perverse action' that was so 'evidently and instantly assumed that it confirmed the opinion of her real mental power beneath all the manifestations of derangement'. Musing as to a 'way to arouse in her a motive to wish and try to recover her natural state', he offered the hope that she 'will take to lawn tennis when the time comes, for good vigorous exercise of that sort would probably do a vast amount of good' – contrast the fencing and swimming said to have contributed to immorality of character in Edgar Allan Poe – and suggested that 'the steady improvement of the habits is of good augury'.[191] Unfortunately this proved inaccurate. Three months later he wrote describing her as 'afflicted with hallucinations of hearing' that 'are of serious significance not only because they are so often permanent in their nature, but also because of the sudden, incalculable and sometimes violent acts which they are apt to instigate'. The available clinical notes confirm this, and Lady D— remained in the asylum with a severe, chronic psychotic illness, not the outcome suggested by Maudsley's first letter.

But clinical acumen has never been shown to be the first necessity of fashionable medicine. A certain style and manner, compliance with the habits and wishes of patients, and a silent tongue have always been the vital accomplishments. Another letter in Lewis's archive describes Maudsley as 'getting the diagnosis completely wrong, of course',[192] implying that this did not really matter. Physical and social damage limitation – as so assiduously practised by the Newingtons of Ticehurst – may have been more important when dealing with the often recoverable mental states of psychiatric illness. Of interest in this regard is the brief glimpse of his earlier practice at Lawn House given in his evidence to the 1877 Select Committee on Lunacy Law. He had conversations 'night after night . . . at first' with the difficult (and hallucinatory) patient Mrs Lowe, his wife accompanied her on walks and he discharged her because she kept running off and was 'not an agreeable inmate of one's house'.[193]

Nevertheless, Maudsley was by all accounts a difficult man to get on with. Vernon Briggs[194] described him as 'very energetic', a 'man of decided opinions', who 'had very clear thoughts'. Crichton-Browne[195] commented on the 'very small circle of his intimates' and 'a dash of gloom and austerity of Wuthering Heights', describing him as 'cynical and sententious betimes, but the tartness of his tongue was belied by his genial smile'. Savage[196] in his obituary notice also called him 'cynical and rather unfriendly', and stated that at times he 'showed his critical side, and was not personally popular'. Apparently he (Savage) 'once told him he seemed to be so absorbed in his love for humanity that he had no affection to spare for the individual man'. But in the next sentence he does admit to Maudsley's 'strong feelings' about the treatment of the insane, and to his being 'very jealous of any return to undue control being used over them'. Forcible feeding, for example, he regarded as 'degrading' to both doctor and patient.

Mott's reminiscence for the *Lancet* likewise admitted to his 'satirical and cynical attitude towards mankind generally', but insisted that he 'found an extraordinarily kindly nature' once he got to know him intimately. In both this memoir[197] and in a parallel piece for the *British Medical Journal* he described spending the evening with him and coming away 'humbled but always mentally refreshed', but the latter also contains references to the 'hypercritical manner', the pessimism (ascribed as partly due to his having no children) and the cynical/satirical side. Other obituaries agreed. 'Childless and with a somewhat difficult temperament, Dr Maudsley was not of the type which readily inspires affection' intoned the *American Journal of Insanity*. The *Journal of Nervous and Mental Diseases* felt he had been 'feared as a materialist', while eulogizing his other achievements. Savage, in his spoken reminiscence to the MPA at their quarterly meeting on 21 February 1918, described him as 'a man not given to social intimacy'.[198]

Despite such comments, his manner was clearly not incompatible with an extremely successful private practice. Furthermore, no one could deny that he had a 'great mind' and was able to quote impressively from Shakespeare, Goethe *et al.* to his last years. He certainly could amuse and charm, as witness the report of the BMA meeting in 1883 that he 'set on a roar'.[199] The *BMJ* obituarist described him 'coming in and reading a case of mistaken identity from *The Times*, and commenting upon it in a way that immediately attracted the attention of the students by his originality, humour and critical insight'.[200] This was during his time as lecturer, in medical jurisprudence, at University College. In his later years he was 'rather awe-inspiring', with 'a huge head, straggling beard and piercing eyes, a low quiet voice'.[201] The same writer also described his tendency 'to suddenly fire a question at one', but had no doubt that his patients 'liked him and looked forward to his visits'. He was apparently keen to know what younger people were reading (this was when he was about 65), was fairly active for his age, and walked the two miles to the station and back 'wet or fine'. Savage supports some of this, recalling that 'he allowed his hair and beard to grow long and he had rather the aspect of an aged prophet'.[202] It is not surprising that he was respected and liked by his patients. There is a touch of the entrepreneur about Maudsley and the photograph of him reproduced in the *JMS* with his obituary is of a grave, bearded, Victorian-figure, not unlike those of Marx, or Darwin, or other learned gurus. Norman Douglas was reported to have been led 'to the great Sir Harry Maudsley' to see if his novel *Nerinda* conformed to the development of a recognizable madness. Apparently 'Sir Harry', 'after careful reading, said that he had handled to perfection "the symptoms of paramorphic insanity"'.[203] Armed with such impressive verbiage and knightly accoutrements – though of course he was definitely not knighted – it is perhaps not unreasonable to accept Maudsley's clinical presence, personal *potestas*, and money-making potential.

There seems to have been little else to distract him in the way of vices or family. We have seen how he railed at masturbation, and his views on sexual behaviour were no less pronounced. At a meeting in 1873 he gave his opinion, 'a very definite one', concerning the cause of general paralysis of the insane. This he held to be 'that quiet, steady continuance of (sexual) excess for months or years', quoting a wife who had informed him that 'during the whole period of her married life . . . he (her husband) had not refrained for a single night, except at certain periods'. (Later speakers at this debate pointed out the rarity of the disease in India, but Maudsley's reply is not recorded.)[204] Havelock Ellis quoted a line from the *Physiology of Mind* ('were man robbed of the instinct of procreation, and of all that spiritually springs therefrom, that moment would all poetry, and perhaps also his own moral sense be obliterated from his life')[205] that has a poignant ring. Was his childlessness related in some way? Psychoanalysts might suggest impotence as uniting this with his sexual prudery; degenerationists might point to hints at mental illness in Conolly's wife as necessitating prudent sterility in a son-in-law convinced of Morel's notions; his wife's age at their marriage (36) and simple bad luck might be the safest analysis. This same wife, a very 'sweet woman' whom he regarded as his 'foolometer'[206] and whose passing he greatly mourned – she died aged 81, of senile decay and heart failure on 9 February 1911 – was five years older than Maudsley but little else is known of her, apart from her being Conolly's youngest daughter. Maudsley loved cricket, 'attending Lord's cricket ground pretty regularly',[207] 'where he was bowled at by professionals'.[208] In 1903 he went to Australia 'to see the best of cricket in its best home', and used elaborate cricketing analogies in some of his later work, describing the stroke of the expert batsman as something 'he could not do if he had not diligently organised the proper mental plexuses'.[209] There is, however, no record of his ever having been a member of the MCC.

There are of course two major areas of his life that have not been covered. First, his interest and activity in forensic work, which has been discussed in some detail by Scott.[210] This author writes of 'his picture of extreme degeneracy presenting as a "precocious prodigy of all proclivities", a description which is . . . reminiscent of "poor protoplasm poorly put together", and about as useful a concept'. Scott also points to the contradictions of Maudsley's position on motivation, which though officially 'physiological', often has the look and tone of moral condemnation, as witness his views on self-abuse and his letter about Lady D—. What cannot be gainsaid, though, was his absolute condemnation of the capital punishment of lunatics in his time, and his later papers on crime and insanity consistently called for changes in the legal system.

Secondly, the act for which he is most famed, the donation of £30,000 to found the Maudsley Hospital, has also not been analysed in detail, not least because the facts are fixed in legend. He was certainly dogged in his pursuit of the LCC and described having 'secured my place among those who try to perpetuate themselves' in a letter to Vernon Briggs in January 1913.[211] But it is also clear that Mott originated the idea via a preface to the *Archives of Neurology* (1907) after visiting Kraepelin's clinic in Munich,[212] *after* which Maudsley made his financial offer, in a letter to the London County Council.[213] (At least, this is Mott's account as told in his Maudsley lecture on 7 June 1921.)[214] Given that Maudsley was by then a retired recluse, it is likely also that Mott was much more significant a figure in the subsequent complex politics of the LCC, the Asylums Board and London University. But £30,000 was a lot of money and Maudsley's epitaph was secured. Of course he had tried to raise awareness of psychological medicine in his earlier days, attending, for example, the Convocation of London University in 1865 to urge 'that students show evidence of having attended a course in clinical instruction in mental diseases'.[215] But as Alexander Walk[216] admits, 'nothing was further from Maudsley's mind than the creation or the retention of a hospital for mental disorders in London', and the credit for such a proposal is attributed to a Dr J.G. Davey.

Conclusions

Is any useful synthesis possible on Maudsley and his career, given that we have only some outline facts, his multifarious opinions, and an accepted version of influential and worthwhile achievement? Certainly he was much quoted by contemporary British authors of psychiatric textbooks.[217] Fielding Blandford inscribed his work to him, referring to him also in the text on 'classification', 'asylum restraint', and 'impulsive insanity'. Bucknill and Tuke mentioned him frequently, in particular with regard to the 'insane temperament' or 'diathesis'. Sankey (1884), Mickle (1886), Savage (1891), Hyslop (1895), Bevan Lewis (1899), and Clouston (1904), all have several references to his work. After this his name starts to fade, at least from the references, and he slowly becomes the 'shadowy figure of the Victorian past' described by Aubrey Lewis in 1951. That he was notorious, though, is illustrated by Bernard Shaw in *The Sanity of Art*. Shaw wrote (of Nordau) that 'he is so utterly mad on the subject of degeneration that he finds the symptoms of it in the loftiest geniuses as plainly as in the lowest jailbirds, the exceptions being himself, Lombroso, Krafft-Ebing, Dr Maudsley, Goethe, Shakespeare and Beethoven'.[218]

But specific influences are difficult to trace, since concrete evidence may not reflect the subtler ways in which attitudes, ideas, and clinical behaviour are transmitted. There is certainly something of the cul-de-sac about Maudsley. An increasingly isolated figure, he turned to philosophy more and more as he witnessed his therapeutic attempts founder on the cruel historical facts of a limited art. Crichton-Browne recalled:

> In a moment of bitterness Maudsley once imagined a physician, who had spent his life in ministering to the mind diseased, looking back sadly on his track, recognising the fact that one half of the diseased beings he had treated had never got well, and questioning whether he had done real service to his kind in restoring the other half to reproductive work.[219]

Nor was this philosophical leaning entirely a product of later life, for the book *Survey of Opinion* concerning diplomas in public health (1868)[220] reported him as suggesting Mill's *System of Logic* as a basic text. It was part and parcel of his career, which may be seen as representative of a whole area of alienist logic. This was materialism, rooted in 'organicity', and it led to a 'pessimism' that was truly shocking to his contemporaries. Based on degenerationist notions, it viewed individuals as sliding inevitably, evolutionarily, towards personal or family extinction. Yet Maudsley was dealing with the leading members of his society, the successful and aristocratic. If such people could develop disabling psychotic illnesses, despite all the logic of Spinoza and the advances of neurology and physiology, what did this say about his world? He himself was sneered at in reviews (cf. Mercier). Isolated, childless, lonely, temperamental, and ageing, might he not have been prey to doubts, depression, even a significant depressive illness? How did degeneration theory fit with the evidence of his own temperament? Can his generous gift to psychiatry perhaps be understood as the offerings of penance, a paying of his dues to the struggling, stigmatized, laughable even, MPA as its variably competent members tried to manage the monolithic psychiatric structures of their time? He had left them, in 1890, for the prosperous hills of private practice and philosophical writing. But in 1863 he himself had written[221] that 'the supposition that definite laws of chemical combination do exist ... can afford no possible excuse for *the selfish indolence of inactive fatalism*', as if prophesying the course of his own career. In his 1876 introductory lecture to the students of University College he stated that 'if medical practice be pursued as a mere means of money-getting, assuredly it causes the deepest demoralisation of him who so uses it, as best things turned to basest ends breed the greatest corruption'.[222] While there is much to admire in his work, there is also no doubt that his legacy has flaws, flaws that still permeate areas of modern medicine. The dangers of drawing philosophy from clinical experience, the sterility of pure materialism in the face of human needs, the easy lapse into unscientific thinking, all these are part of Maudsley's heritage.

Perhaps it was no coincidence that on a voyage back from Australia in

1904 he should meet and talk with the mystic 'beast', Aleister Crowley. Describing him as 'one of the three greatest alienists in England' who went 'rather further than Spencer in the direction of mechanical automation', Crowley felt he was 'the very man I wanted'. They talked apparently of 'Dhyana' and 'Samadhi', of methods 'pharmaceutical, electrical or surgical' of inducing genius, of 'the Stone of the Wise and the Elixir of Life'. It must have been an odd conversation on that Victorian steamer in the Arabian Sea, as the monstrous bohemian Crowley pumped the dry, bearded sceptic for ideas and knowledge. To Crowley's surprise Maudsley 'agreed with all these propositions'. But it is no surprise that he should also record that Maudsley, despite his lauded past and later eponymous fame, 'could not suggest any plausible line of research'.[223]

Table 6:1 *Books published by Henry Maudsley (English editions)*

Year	*Title*	*Publisher*
1867	*The Physiology and Pathology of Mind*	Macmillan (2nd edition, 1868)
1870	*Body and Mind: An Inquiry into their Connection and Mutual Influence*	Macmillan
1874	*Responsibility in Mental Disease*	King
1876	*The Physiology of Mind*	A revised and enlarged 3rd edition of the 1867 work (Macmillan)
1879	*The Pathology of Mind*	
1883	*Body and Will: In its Metaphysical, Physiological and Pathological Aspects*	Kegan Paul
1886	*Natural Causes and Supernatural Seemings*	Kegan Paul
1902	*Life in Mind and Conduct: Studies of Organic in Human Nature*	Macmillan
1908	*Heredity, Variation and Genius, with Essay on Shakespeare and Address on Medicine*	John Bale, Sons & Danielsson
1916	*Organic to Human: Psychological and Sociological*	Macmillan
1918	*Religion and Realities*	John Bale, Sons &

Notes

1 Henry Maudsley (1918) *Religion and Realities*, London: John Bale, Sons & Danielsson.

2 (1870–1) *Journal of Mental Science* (hereafter *JMS*), 16: 454–8.

3 (1863) *JMS* 9: 427.
4 See (1868–9) *JMS* 14: 574–87.
5 (1870–1) *JMS* 16: 152 He had also been elected an Hon. Member of the Society for the Promotion of Psychiatric and Forensic Psychology of Vienna.
6 The marriage certificate is dated 30 January 1866; Conolly died on 5 March 1866; (1866) *JMS* 12: 146.
7 Autobiography dated 1912. This unpublished manuscript some 4,000 words in length is in the Aubrey Lewis File in the archives of Bethlem Royal Hospital (hereafter ALF). It was used by Aubrey Lewis extensively for the 25th Maudsley lecture – (1951) 'Henry Maudsley: his work and influence', *JMS* 97: 259–77. See also (1918) *JMS* 64: 229.
8 Henry Maudsley (1867) *The Physiology and Pathology of Mind*, London: Macmillan; see also Lewis, 'Henry Maudsley: his work and influence', 269.
9 (1867) *JMS* 13: 383 quoting the *British Medical Journal* of 18 May 1867.
10 (1870–1) *JMS* 16: 454–6.
11 (March 1875) *Popular Science Monthly* VI: 612.
12 Bryan Donkin (22 October 1910) 'Some aspects of heredity in relation to mind', *Lancet*: 1187–93.
13 See the review of *Religion and Realities* in (1918) *JMS* 64: 306–8.
14 Lewis, 'Henry Maudsley: his work and influence', 259.
15 Peter Scott (March–April 1956) 'Henry Maudsley 1835–1918', *Journal of Criminal Law, Criminology, and Police Science* 46, 6: reproduced in S. Mannheim (ed.) (1972) *Pioneers in Criminology*, Montclair, N.J.: Patterson Smith.
16 In the ALF. A modern one is in preparation.
17 See (1862) *JMS* 8 for the report of the annual general meeting of 3 July 1862 where 'there was the largest attendance of members that has ever met'.
18 I have used those from Dr Denis Leigh's private collection, the Bethlem Royal Hospital Archives, the Autograph letter Series (ALS) of the Wellcome Institute Library, and the case books of the Ticehurst Asylum in the Wellcome Library.
19 See (1918) *JMS* 64: 227–30; (2 February 1918) *Lancet*: 193–4; (2 February 1918) *British Medical Journal*: 161–2; (1918) *Journal of Nervous and Mental Diseases* 48: 95–6; George Savage (1918) 'Henry Maudsley MD', *JMS* 64: 117–23.
20 Sir James Crichton-Browne (1920) 'The first Maudsley Lecture', *JMS* 66: 199–225; Sir Frederick Mott (1921) 'The second Maudsley Lecture', *JMS* 67: 319–37.
21 For example, his meeting with Aleister Crowley (see note 223), or the comments made on Norman Douglas's 'Nerinda' (note 203), or an apparent visit to Sweden mentioned in the Aubrey Lewis File (ALF).
22 Minutes of Evidence taken before the Select Committee on Lunacy Law (24 April 1877): 176–81 and (5 June 1877): 320–7 (London: HMSO).
23 Report of the Manchester Royal Lunatic Asylum 25 June 1858 to 24 June 1859; 25 June 1859 to 24 June 1860; 25 June 1860 to 24 June 1861 (Manchester: Sowler & Sons, 1859, 1860, 1861).
24 Elaine Showalter (1985) *The Female Malady: Madness and English Culture 1830–1980*, New York: Pantheon Books. See especially chapter 4, 'On the borderland', pp. 101–20.
25 The report of this London County Council Committee was fiercely criticized

by the Medico-Psychological Association (MPA). See D. Yellowlees (1890) 'Presidential address', *JMS* 36: 473–89 and further discussion at the annual meeting: 583–7.
26 Andrew Scull (1979) *Museums of Madness*, London: Allen Lane.
27 Ernest Jones (1954) 'The early history of psycho-analysis', *JMS* 100: 198–210.
28 Report of the committee of the Medico-Psychological Association on the status of British psychiatry and of medical officers of asylums (July 1914) London: Adland & Son. See also (12 September 1914) *British Medical Journal* 475 for the discussion of this report at the MPA's annual meeting.
29 See (22 February 1908) *British Medical Journal*: 457, (24 April 1909) *British Medical Journal*: 1020–1.
30 (1 June 1918) *British Medical Journal*: reports £60,318 net. He also left £2,000 to the MPA; (8 June 1918) *British Medical Journal*: 660.
31 Maudsley, 'Autobiography'.
32 (1887) *JMS* 32–3: 467–8.
33 Crichton-Browne, 'The first Maudsley lecture', 200.
34 Eugen Bleuler (1950) *Dementia Praecox or the Group of Schizophrenias*, trans. Joseph Zinkin, New York: International University Press.
35 (1912) *JMS* 58: 380.
36 Maudsley, 'Autobiography'.
37 Henry Maudsley (1917) 'Materialism and spiritualism', *JMS* 63: 494–506.
38 Maudsley, *The Physiology and Pathology of Mind.*
39 Maudsley, 'Autobiography'. In fact he states he is 72 in this piece, which places its composition as 1907.
40 Crichton-Browne, 'The first Maudsley lecture'.
41 Savage, 'Henry Maudsley MD'.
42 (1858) *JMS* 4: 156.
43 ibid., 57.
44 Maudsley, 'Autobiography'.
45 Lewis, 'Henry Maudsley: his work and influence'.
46 Maudsley, 'Autobiography'.
47 Extracts from the minutes of the Committee of Management of the Manchester Royal Lunatic Asylum at Cheadle Royal. Maudsley resigned in January 1862, and actually left in March 1862.
48 Reports of the Manchester Royal Lunatic Asylum 1858–1861 (see note 23).
49 Henry Maudsley (1860) 'The correlation of mental and physical forces; or man a part of nature', *JMS* 6: 50–78.
50 (22 July 1865) *Lancet*: 97.
51 (1865) *JMS* 11: 441–2.
52 Alexander Walk (1976) 'Medico-psychologists, Maudsley and the Maudsley', *British Journal of Psychiatry* 128: 19–30.
53 (1862) *JMS* 8: 310.
54 (1918) *JMS* 64: 229.
55 Crichton-Browne, 'The first Maudsley lecture'.
56 See (1932) *JMS* 78: 243–5, and Walk, 'Medico-psychologists . . . the Maudsley', footnote p. 19.
57 As recorded in the relevant volumes of the *JMS* and his obituaries (note 19).
58 See, for example, (1870–1) *JMS* 16: 454–5, where Maudsley speaks at the annual meeting, saying 'it is not desirable for us to commit suicide', and wins the motion by 13 to 8.

59 Walk, 'Medico-psychologists ... the Maudsley'.
60 See note 35.
61 (1912) *JMS* 58: 702–3.
62 (1862) *JMS* 8: 343.
63 (1865) *JMS* 11: 424.
64 (1868–9) *JMS* 14: 406–16.
65 Henry Maudsley (1863) 'Delusions', *JMS* 9: 1–24.
66 Henry Maudsley (1871–2) 'Presidential address – insanity and its treatment', *JMS* 17: 311–34.
67 ibid., 463.
68 (1874–5) *JMS* 20: 478.
69 See note 1.
70 (1918) *JMS* 64: 307.
71 Almost every article in the 1860s and 1870s is laden with such references.
72 Henry Maudsley (1860) 'Edgar Allan Poe', *JMS* 6: 328–69.
73 Maudsley, 'Autobiography'.
74 Crichton-Browne, 'The first Maudsley lecture', 14.
75 See note 53.
76 Maudsley, 'Autobiography'.
77 Henry Maudsley (1866) 'Memoir of the late John Conolly', *JMS* 12: 151–74. See especially p. 173.
78 Maudsley, 'Autobiography'.
79 (1862) *JMS* 8: 464.
80 Henry Maudsley (1862) 'Middle-class hospitals', *JMS* 8: 356–63.
81 There is a copy of this letter in the archives of the Royal College of Psychiatrists.
82 J. Stevenson Bushnan (1862) 'On the practical use of mental science', *JMS* 8: 132–52, and (1862) 'On the principles and method of a practical science of mind, in reply to Dr Thomas Laycock, Professor of Medicine in the University of Edinburgh', *JMS* 8: 235–49.
83 (1862) *JMS* 8: 451–2.
84 ibid., 444–57 and 464.
85 ibid., 327–8.
86 See Kenneth Dewhurst (1982) *Hughlings Jackson on Psychiatry*, Oxford: Sandford Publications.
87 Maudsley, 'Delusions'; Henry Maudsley (1864) 'Classification of the sciences', *JMS* 10: 242–53; Henry Maudsley (1866) 'On some of the causes of insanity', *JMS* 12: 488–502; Henry Maudsley (1864) 'Syphilitic diseases of the brain' (review), *JMS* 10: 82–96; Henry Maudsley (1865) 'Recent metaphysics', *JMS* 11: 533–56.
88 (1863) *JMS* 9: 426–7.
89 Letter to Bastian (22 November 1865) from the Autograph Letter Series of the Wellcome Institute Library.
90 (1866) *JMS* 12: 150.
91 See note by C.L.R. in (1862) *JMS* 8: 461–4; also Lewis, 'Henry Maudsley: his work and influence'.
92 (1868–9) *JMS* 14: 86.
93 (1872–3) *JMS* 18: 457.
94 Henry Maudsley (1867) *The Physiology and Pathology of Mind*, London: Macmillan; (1870) *Body and Mind: An Inquiry into their Connection and*

Mutual Influence, London: Macmillan; (1874) *Responsibility in Mental Disease*, London: Henry S. King & Co.

95 (1867–8) *JMS* 13: 403–5.

96 See (1874–5) *JMS* 20: 471–84 for the 1874 annual meeting. See ibid., 663 for his attendance at the first congress of the Società Freniatrica Italiana, at Imola in Italy, where he and Robertson were given honorary membership.

97 Letter to Bastian (22 November 1865), Wellcome Institute Library.

98 (1873–4) *JMS* 19: 469–85 (especially 472, 476).

99 (1876–7) *JMS* 23: 428–33.

100 Crichton-Browne, 'The first Maudsley Lecture', p. 199.

101 Walk, 'Medico-psychologists . . . the Maudsley'.

102 See, for example, Maudsley, 'The correlation of mental and physical force'; also his reviews of *Psychological Enquiries* by Sir Benjamin Brodie (1862) *JMS* 8: 211–34, and of *Limits of a Philosophical Enquiry* (1869–70) *JMS* 15: 269–86.

103 (1888) *JMS* 33–4: 496–7.

104 Henry Maudsley (1888) 'Remarks on crime and criminals', *JMS* 33–4: 159–67.

105 (1888) *JMS* 33–4: 311.

106 Henry Maudsley (1883) *Body and Will: In its Metaphysical, Physiological and Pathological Aspects*, London: Kegan Paul. See (1884) *JMS* 29–30: 280–4 for the review.

107 Henry Maudsley (1895) 'Criminal responsibility in relation to insanity', *JMS* 41: 657–65, and 665–74 for the discussion that ensued. Read at a BMA meeting (Psychological Section) on 1 August 1895; the chairman stated his pleasure at having 'drawn our learned friend from his privacy'.

108 Henry Maudsley (1900) 'The new psychology', *JMS* 46: 411–26 *et seq.*

109 (1887) *JMS* 32–3: 467–8.

110 See Scull, *Museums of Madness*, and chapter 9, by David Cochrane, in this volume.

111 For example, see (April 1890) 'The cerebral cortex and its work', *Mind*, and see Savage, 'Henry Maudsley MD'.

112 Clark Bell (March 1910) *Medico-Legal Journal of New York* 27, 4.

113 See, for example, (1871–2) 'Presidential address; insanity and its treatment', *JMS* 17: 311–34; also (1884–5) *JMS* 30: 466, where he is quoted: 'Sedatives . . . are seldom useful and sometimes positively mischievous.' For self-abuse, contrast the measured remarks in (1895) *The Pathology of Mind: A Study of its Distempers, Deformities and Disorders*, London: Macmillan, later reprinted (1979) with an introduction by Sir Aubrey Lewis (London: Julian Friedmann), pp. 399–414, with those of (1868) 'Illustrations of a variety of insanity', *JMS* 14: 149–62.

114 (28 September 1895) *British Medical Journal*: 772.

115 Maudsley, 'Edgar Allan Poe'.

116 Maudsley, 'The correlation of mental and physical forces' especially 70 and 62.

117 (1859–60) *JMS* 6: 79.

118 Maudsley, 'Edgar Allan Poe'; see especially 336, 337, 340, 341, 348, 354, 359, 364 and 368 for the passages quoted below.

119 See his letter on 'Man and the Monkeys' (30 March 1861) *British Medical Journal*: 346–7.

120 Maudsley, 'Delusions'; see especially 1–3, 13, 15–17 and 19.

121 Maudsley, 'Illustrations of a variety of insanity'; see especially 155–6 and 160–2.

122 David Skae (1863–4) 'A rational and practical classification of insanity', *JMS* 9: 309–19. This was a presidential address and includes an exposition of his category of 'mania of masturbation'.
123 See, for example, (20 October 1883) *British Medical Journal*: 788, where addressing a large audience of the Medical Society of University College 'Dr. Maudsley was ever wont to delight with those flashes of merriment that set his audience "on a roar" and never fails also to supply matter for serious thought'.
124 Havelock Ellis (1926) *Studies in the Psychology of Sex*, 3rd edn, Philadelphia: F.A. Davis Co., vol. 1, note, p. 254.
125 Henry Maudsley (1863) 'Consideration with regard to hereditary influence (continued)', *JMS* 9: 506–30. The quote is from 508.
126 See, for example, Charles Darwin [1872] (1978) *The Expression of the Emotions in Man and Animals*, reprint of 1872 ed, ed. S.J. Rachman, London: Julian Friedmann.
127 See Lewis, 'Henry Maudsley: his work and influence'.
128 Henry Maudsley (1876) *The Physiology of Mind*, London: Macmillan, and (1879) *The Pathology of Mind*, London: Macmillan, were a revised, enlarged 3rd edition of the 1867 volume (see note 8).
129 (1867–8) *JMS* 13: 255–60.
130 See David Duncan (1908) *Life and Letters of Herbert Spencer*, New York: Appleton & Co., vol. 1 pp. 184–5. Spencer himself complained (p. 189) that Maudsley had adopted 'the cardinal conception of the Principles of Psychology, without at all indicating whence that conception was derived' so that 'I got all the kicks and others the halfpence'; and wrote also of 'doctrines which he [Maudsley] appropriates from me' (letter to John Tyndall, 11 May 1868).
131 See Maudsley, *Physiology and Pathology of Mind*, p. 194, and Henry Maudsley (1869–70) 'Emanuel Swedenborg', *JMS* 15: 169–96 and 417–36.
132 Henry Maudsley (1916) *Organic to Human: Psychological and Sociological*, London: Macmillan.
133 (1 September 1917) *Lancet*: 349–50.
134 (1917) *JMS* 63: 103.
135 Letter from A.H. Stoddart (6 January 1948) to Aubrey Lewis (ALF). See also Lewis, 'Henry Maudsley: his life and influence'.
136 (1868–9) *JMS* 14: 87.
137 Maudsley, *Physiology and Pathology of Mind*. See especially pp. 253, 258 and 422–4.
138 See note 23.
139 See note 22.
140 See note 113.
141 See note 94.
142 (1874–5) *JMS* 20: 446–51.
143 For example, 'Heredity and disease', reported (20 October 1883) in *British Medical Journal*: 788, and 'Heredity in health and disease' (May 1886) *Fortnightly Review* 45 OS: 648–59 (1876–7) 'The alleged increase of insanity', *JMS* 23: 45–54; (September 1878) 'Hallucinations of the senses', *Fortnightly Review* 30 OS: 370–86; and the 'Introductory lecture' delivered at University College (to the freshmen of the year), (7 October 1876) *Lancet*: 490–5.
144 Maudsley, *Body and Will*, and Maudsley, *Organic to Human*. Henry Maudsley (1886) *Natural Causes and Supernatural Seemings*, London: Kegan Paul, and Henry Maudsley (1902) *Life in Mind and Conduct: Studies of Organic in Human Nature*, London: Macmillan.

145 I have culled this quotation from a selection of comments appended on p. 101 of Maudsley, *Religion and Realities*, as an advertisement for *Organic to Human*.
146 Havelock Ellis (1890) 'The criminal', *JMS* 36: 5–6.
147 Max Nordau (1895) *Degeneration*, London: William Heinemann; translated from the 2nd German edition.
148 (28 September 1895) *British Medical Journal*: 769–73: see especially 771.
149 Henry Maudsley (1908) *Heredity, Variation and Genius*, London: John Bale, Sons, & Danielsson; see (1909) *JMS* 55: 110–12 for review.
150 (1917) *JMS* 63: 102–4.
151 These letters are in the private collection of Dr D. Leigh, to whose kind generosity I owe the chance to read through them. See also Lewis, 'Henry Maudsley: his work and influence'.
152 (1879) *JMS* 25: 230–8 and 538–47.
153 ibid., 587.
154 (1885) *JMS* 30–1: 597–603.
155 (1884) *Brain* 6: 531–8.
156 Henry Maudsley (28 November 1868 and 5 December 1868) 'Concerning aphasia', *Lancet*: 690–2 and 721–3.
157 (1896) *JMS* 42: 186–90.
158 Maudsley, 'The new psychology'; see (1900) *JMS* 46: 426–7 for the discussion.
159 Henry Maudsley (29 July 1905) 'Address in medicine', *British Medical Journal*: 227–31.
160 See note 27.
161 He had attended Galton's lectures to the Sociological Society in 1904, according to C.P. Blacker (1952) *Eugenics: Galton and After*, London: Duckworth & Co., p. 113.
162 Showalter, *The Female Malady*.
163 Maudsley, *Physiology and Pathology of Mind*; see his Introduction.
164 Maudsley, *The Physiology of Mind*, p. 401.
165 Maudsley, *Responsibility in Mental Disease*, p. 33 and, for the following quote, p. 304.
166 (1 September 1917) *Lancet*: 349.
167 Henry Maudsley (1913) 'Mental organisation', *JMS* 59: 1–14.
168 Henry Maudsley (1917) 'Materialism and spiritualism', *JMS* 63: 494–506.
169 Henry Maudsley (1919) 'War psychology: English and German', *JMS* 65: 65–86; it has a brief introduction also.
170 This seems to be hinted at in a letter from his nephew in the ALF but the evidence is anecdotal.
171 See (1932) *JMS* 78: 243–5.
172 (1918) *JMS* 64: 118; see also note 19.
173 Maudsley, *Religion and Realities*.
174 The letters quoted are in the Historical Collection of the Library of the Institute of Psychiatry, folded into several editions of Maudsley's books. This one is dated 10 March 1915.
175 Maudsley, *Physiology and Pathology of Mind*, pp. 8–9.
176 Maudsley, 'Memoir of the late John Conolly'.
177 From his obituary (2 February 1918) *Lancet*: 193.
178 See note 30: and add £30,000 given to the LCC to found a hospital!
179 Sir James Clark (1869) *A Memoir of John Conolly*, London: John Murray; and see also Maudsley, 'Autobiography'.

180 See Charlotte MacKenzie (1985) 'Social factors in the admission, discharge and continuing stay of patients at Ticehurst Asylum, 1845–1917' in W.F. Bynum, R. Porter and M. Shepherd (eds), *The Anatomy of Madness*, London: Tavistock, vol. II, pp. 147–74. See also Scull, *Museums of Madness.*
181 See note 61.
182 ALF at Bethlem Archives. This one was written to Aubrey Lewis, dated 16 June 1948 in response to Lewis requesting information for his impending Maudsley lecture.
183 Crichton-Browne, 'The first Maudsley Lecture', 200.
184 See note 22; he gives a few details of his involvement with Lawn House in his preliminary answers to the 1877 Select Committee on Lunacy Law.
185 See note 9.
186 (1918) *JMS* 64: 118.
187 Crichton-Browne, 'The first Maudsley lecture', 200.
188 T.S. Eliot (1940) *The Cocktail Party*, London: Faber. An unidentified guest turns out to be a leading psychiatrist, Sir Henry Harcourt-Reilly.
189 ALF, Bethlem Archives.
190 Quoted from Stilwell's letter (see note 182).
191 Letters to H.H. Newington dated 24 March 1886 and 21 June 1886, from the Ticehurst Asylum case book no. 30 in the Wellcome Library.
192 ALF; see note 135.
193 See note 22, p. 322.
194 (1932) *JMS* 78: 244.
195 See note 20, p. 200.
196 See note 19.
197 ibid.; especially (2 February 1918) *Lancet*: 194, and *British Medical Journal*: 162.
198 (1918) *American Journal of Insanity* 75: 303; see note 19, and (1918) *JMS* 64: 228.
199 See note 123.
200 See note 19.
201 Stilwell's letter in the ALF (see note 182).
202 Savage, 'Henry Maudsley MD'.
203 Nancy Cunard (1954) *Grand Man: Memories of Norman Douglas*, London: Secker & Warburg, p. 288.
204 (1873–4) *JMS* 19: 164–5.
205 Havelock Ellis (1927) *Studies in the Psychology of Sex*, Philadelphia: F.A. Davis Co., vol. 6, p. 140.
206 See note 197 for *Lancet* obituary, 194.
207 See note 197.
208 Savage, 'Henry Maudsley MD'.
209 (1913) *JMS* 59: 7.
210 See note 15.
211 (1932) *JMS* 78: 245.
212 Preface (1907) *Archives of Neurology*, ed. F.W. Mott vol. 3, pp. iii–vii.
213 (22 February 1908) *British Medical Journal*: 457.
214 See note 19; Mott, 'The second Maudsley lecture', especially 319–20.
215 (1865) *JMS* 11: 453.
216 Walk, 'Medico-psychologists ... the Maudsley', 25.
217 G. Fielding Blandford (1871) *Insanity and its Treatment*, Edinburgh: Oliver &

Boyd; J. Bucknill and D.H. Tuke (1879) *Manual of Psychological Medicine*, 4th edn, London: Churchill; W.H.O. Sankey (1884) *Lectures on Mental Disease*, 2nd edn, London: H.K. Lewis; J. Mickle (1886) *General Paralysis of the Insane*, 2nd edn, London: H.K. Lewis; G.H. Savage (1891) *Insanity and Allied Neuroses*, 3rd edn, London: Cassell; T.B. Hyslop (1895) *Mental Physiology*, London: J. & A. Churchill; W. Bevan Lewis (1899) *Textbook of Mental Diseases*, London: H.K. Lewis; T.S. Clouston (1904) *Clinical Lectures on Mental Diseases*, 6th edn, London: Churchill.

218 Bernard Shaw (1908) *The Sanity of Art: An Exposure of the Current Nonsense about Artists being Degenerate*, London: New Age Press.

219 Crichton-Browne, 'The first Maudsley lecture', 224. He may have been quoting the last paragraph of *The Pathology of Mind.*

220 See D.E. Watkins (1984) 'The English revolution in social medicine, 1889–1911', University of London PhD thesis, pp. 108–9.

221 (1863) *JMS* 9: 530 (see note 125).

222 See note 143.

223 Aleister Crowley (1969) *The Confessions of Aleister Crowley*, London: Jonathan Cape, pp. 385–6. This is a reprint of the 1929 edition, edited by J. Symonds and K. Gruet.

CHAPTER SEVEN

The great restraint controversy: a comparative perspective on Anglo-American psychiatry in the nineteenth century

Nancy Tomes

'The great stumbling-block of the American superintendents is their most unfortunate and unhappy resistance to the abolition of mechanical restraint.'[1] So pronounced John Charles Bucknill, the influential English alienist and former asylum superintendent, in 1876. Bucknill's judgement on his American brethren formed part of a lengthy, critical commentary on American asylums, which first appeared in a series of *Lancet* editorials and was later republished as his *Notes on Asylums for the Insane in America.*[2] His criticism provoked an angry exchange between English and American psychiatrists over the propriety of using mechanical restraint – as they termed straitjackets, leather wristlets, gloves, and the like – in treating the insane. Lasting almost a decade, the great restraint controversy pitted two groups of respected psychiatrists against one another in a highly publicized, often acrimonious debate.

After the rise of the English non-restraint movement in the late 1830s, the two specialties had evolved very different therapeutic responses to patient violence. In England, the mid-nineteenth-century profession committed itself to reducing mechanical restraint to an absolute minimum, substituting in its place primarily seclusion and manual restraint by attendants. While instrumental restraint was never totally abolished in English public asylums, its use became infrequent and stigmatized. In contrast, American asylum doctors retained a strong belief in the therapeutic value of mechanical restraint, and used it much more freely than their English colleagues. Arguing that the peculiar character of American insanity made their patients more violent, they emphatically rejected the ideal of non-restraint for American institutions.

By the 1870s, these therapeutic differences had became a painful source of contention between the two specialties. While English alienists regarded the non-restraint system as one of their greatest contributions to medical progress, their professional near relations, the American asylum doctors, denied its worth vociferously.[3] Contesting one another's claims to scientific and humanitarian superiority, they carried on an exceedingly complex and increasingly contentious debate over non-restraint that spilled over from the pages of their specialty journals into the general medical literature of the day.

The restraint controversy proved all the more painful because the two specialties had so much else in common. As an English doctor wrote of the Americans in 1876, at the height of the controversy: 'We are constrained to regard them, not as offshoots or branches from our parent stem, but as part and parcel of ourselves.'[4] English and American psychiatrists shared a common medical culture, characterized chiefly by its pragmatic, empirical bent; their asylums and their medical specialties had been formed around a similar conception of moral treatment, inspired chiefly by the York Retreat. Beyond the restraint issue, the mid-nineteenth-century specialties found much common ground: they respectfully followed each other's medical literature, made common cause against such reforms as the cottage system and separate institutions for the chronic insane, and exchanged good wishes and honorary titles between their professional associations.[5]

Precisely because of the many points of similarity between English and American asylum doctors, historians have found the great restraint controversy a puzzling and obscure episode in the history of nineteenth-century psychiatry. Without denying its importance to contemporaries, scholars have given the issue scant historical attention.[6] Not only is the debate itself a complex and confusing welter of charge and countercharge, which discourages any quick insight; but also the differences between the English and American positions on restraint do not loom so large from a modern perspective. One is more inclined to be impressed by how little restraint even its most enthusiastic defenders used in this pre-thorazine age, than to enter into the fine points of their therapeutic arguments. Thus medical historians have been tempted to dismiss the episode as an example of medical 'false consciousness', resulting from excessive self-righteousness and nationalistic fervour. Given the many other, serious issues that faced Anglo-American asylum doctors in this period, issues such as overcrowding, therapeutic impotence, and declining professional autonomy, the restraint controversy seems in retrospect an unproductive diversion of their professional energies.

Yet no debate that raged so long or so violently could possibly have been peripheral to the practice of nineteenth-century asylum medicine. To be sure, the argument was fuelled by misunderstandings, deliberate and otherwise; moreover, the real extent of difference in clinical practice was unclear then and remains so now. Still, however obscure the terms of debate, the restraint controversy undoubtedly involved a problem of enormous import to nineteenth-century asylum doctors: how to fulfil the asylum's promise to provide a superior form of controlling patient violence. That the English and American asylum specialties, both devoted to the same principles of moral treatment, disagreed so violently over the proper therapeutic response to patient violence was a serious matter indeed. More than any other issue, restraint defined the therapeutic boundaries between Anglo-American psychiatrists in the mid-nineteenth century.[7]

By placing the great restraint controversy in a broad professional context, this chapter attempts to reclaim it as a significant episode in the development of Anglo-American psychiatry. In studying the non-restraint controversy, I have sought answers to three central questions: why the two specialties developed such different therapeutic perspectives on restraint; how the restraint issue shaped both practice and politics within each profession; and finally, why the Anglo-American differences exploded with such force in the mid-1870s. In answering these questions, I hope to show how the interplay between *internal* factionalism and *international* rivalries lent the great restraint controversy its peculiar intensity; and to relate this therapeutic issue to the deeper differences in the degree of centralization and class segregation that characterized the two asylum systems.

Asylum reform and the origins of the non-restraint movement

In both England and the United States, powerful reform movements advocating a new approach to the treatment of the insane emerged in the early 1800s. The embodiment of this approach, and a rallying point for change, was the York Retreat, a small Quaker institution that achieved remarkable results with a technique that came to be known as 'moral treatment'. Arguing that insanity might be cured by a more humane regimen, combining a gentle system of rewards and punishments, varied amusements, and a kind, firm discipline, Anglo-American reformers successfully crusaded for the expansion of asylum facilities, especially for the poor. Between 1810 and 1870, the asylum systems in both countries expanded rapidly, and became the locus for the new specialty of asylum medicine. But while similar in many respects, the Anglo-American experience of asylum reform and expansion differed in significant ways that directly contributed to the non-restraint controversy.[8]

In England, the non-restraint movement followed over fifty years of agitation aimed at improving an already extensive system of private profit-making madhouses and non-profit voluntary hospitals founded in the eighteenth century. Unlike their American counterparts, English reformers had to do battle on two fronts: to introduce moral treatment into these older institutions, and to finance new 'progressive' county asylums for the poor. Between 1815 and 1844, a series of parliamentary investigations and legislative proposals pitted reformers against madhouse proprietors and hospital boards with a vested interest in the asylum status quo. Ultimately the reformers triumphed in the passage of the 1845 Lunacy Acts, which mandated the construction of county asylums and set up a national Lunacy

Commission to regulate the operation of all asylums, private as well as public.[9]

The hard course of asylum reform had several important consequences for the new specialty of asylum medicine. In the first place, the complicity of many physicians in the unsavoury conditions revealed by the reform agitation gave the English asylum movement a decidedly anti-medical tone. Having faced so many physician-defenders of the old asylum system, evangelicals such as Lord Shaftesbury never quite lost their mistrust of medical intentions, and continued to regard the superintendents' claims of scientific expertise in treating the insane with scepticism. As a result, the new asylum doctors had to play an entrepreneurial role in advancing their claims to be the best practitioners of psychological medicine. At a theoretical level, this divided legacy was manifested in the much greater sense of opposition between medical and moral approaches to insanity that existed in English asylum medicine.[10]

In addition to the tension between lay and medical elements in asylum reform, the English specialty also faced factionalism within its own ranks, reflecting the strongly class-differentiated nature of asylum development. The early and strong emergence of the private madhouse trade, which came to cater almost exclusively to the middle and upper classes, was followed by the rapid growth of state care for the pauper insane, creating a highly stratified asylum system. This in turn did little to foster a cohesive sense of community among English alienists. Although they certainly made common cause on some issues, the identity of interest between the public and private men remained weak in this period. Their specialty organization, the Association of Medical Officers of Asylums and Hospitals for the Insane, which was founded in 1841, suffered as a result; in its early years, meetings were brief and poorly attended, and the association did not play a very ambitious or effective role in advancing the specialty's interests, in Parliament or elsewhere. Factionalism was even reflected in the specialty literature, with the *Journal of Psychological Medicine*, founded in 1848, and the *Asylum Journal of Mental Science*, founded in 1853, respectively championing the causes of private and public asylum medicine, often in an openly antagonistic way.[11]

Within this broader context, of a specialty highly vulnerable to moral issues and factionalized along private/public lines, the non-restraint movement allowed public asylum doctors to reclaim the moral high ground within the asylum movement. Indeed, the non-restraint system was a uniquely medical contribution to the reform effort. Prior to its inception in the late 1830s, the focus of lay reformers had been simply to moderate, not eliminate, the use of mechanical restraint. To be sure, the restraint issue had figured prominently in the asylum reform movement; one of the evangelicals' chief indictments of the old system of asylum management was its excessive and often cruel use of physical restraint, as in the celebrated confinement of James (often called William) Norris in London's Bethlem Hospital.[12] But however intent they were on reducing the physical abuse of the insane, the original exponents of moral treatment never envisioned the complete abolition of mechanical restraint. At the early York Retreat, for example, the lay-directed regimen of moral treatment did not preclude the use of physical restraint, including straitwaistcoats, restraining chairs, straps, and covered bedsteads.[13] Even allowing for the non-restraint advocates' tendency to exaggerate the terrible conditions they found before the system was introduced, it seems evident that mechanical restraint was still widely used in English asylums during the 1830s. On his tour of institutions in 1839 before taking the Hanwell post, John Conolly found straitjackets, hand and leg cuffs, and 'various coarse devices of leather and iron' employed extensively in all but one asylum.[14]

The contradiction between reliance on such devices and the ideals of moral treatment, particularly its commitment to teaching patients self-control, was not lost on some asylum doctors. Moreover, they may have sensed in this issue an opportunity to seize the moral initiative from the lay reformers. By subduing the violent insane without recourse to physical restraint, physicians might give dramatic proof of their superior powers of governing the insane. The mystique of non-restraint asserted that only the physician, with his scientific authority and moral influence, might manage the violent insane solely with what John Bucknill and D. Hack Tuke once described as 'that fascinating, biologizing power . . . which enables men to domineer for good purposes over the minds of others'.[15]

Significantly, it was the medical superintendents of the county asylums who developed this powerful scenario of the doctor controlling the madman without recourse to physical coercion. Although the non-restraint movement later found converts among the private asylum proprietors, it was uniquely the product of the new county asylums: first, the small Lincoln Asylum, where Dr E.P. Charlesworth and his successor, Dr Robert Gardiner Hill, gradually reduced their use of mechanical restraint, until by 1838 Hill dispensed with it altogether; and then, the much larger Hanwell Asylum, where John Conolly implemented non-restraint in 1839, and won international fame for the reform.[16]

Thus with the crusade for non-restraint, the medical superintendents of the county asylums reasserted their moral and medical leadership within the asylum movement. Although the reform encountered considerable resistance, especially from the medical profession, it won the influential support of the editors of the *Lancet* and *The Times* and, perhaps most importantly, Anthony Ashley Cooper, soon to be Lord Shaftesbury, the head of the asylum reform party in Parliament.[17] As a radical new system of moral control, non-restraint not only enhanced the specialty's humanitarian credentials but also lent moral treatment a new medical imprimatur.

In contrast, the course of asylum expansion and reform in the United States created a far different climate for professional development in general and the reception of non-restraint in particular.[18] From its beginnings, the American reform movement faced no entrenched asylum establishment as an obstacle to change. Only a handful of voluntary hospitals catering to the insane had been founded prior to the rise of moral treatment in the early 1800s, and these adopted its premisses with little opposition. Instead, American asylum reformers concentrated their efforts on conditions in almshouses, gaols, and private households; in other words, it was the abuse of the insane *outside* the bounds of medical authority that most concerned them. This focus on *non-medical* institutions created a very different relationship between lay and medical interests in asylum reform. American doctors had no legacy of unsavoury associations with asylum abuse to overcome; on the contrary, they could and did cite the exemplary role of medical men such as Benjamin Rush in fostering asylum reform. For their part, the lay reformers never manifested the suspicion of medical men so common among the English evangelicals. For example, quite unlike Lord Shaftesbury, Dorothea Dix, the most influential American lay reformer, maintained extremely close and respectful ties with the asylum doctors.[19]

The harmony between lay and medical interests in American asylum reform carried over into the conception of moral treatment itself. Of the early asylums in the United States, only one, the Friends' Asylum outside Philadelphia, which was directly patterned on the York Retreat, manifested a lack of faith in medical therapeutics. Perhaps because of Rush's lingering influence, American moral treatment had a robustly medical cast from its inception. In promoting the new concept of asylum treatment, American physicians did not have to overcome the same divided legacy that plagued their English counterparts. Far more easily and comfortably, physicians in the United States integrated medical and moral treatment as complementary parts of a unified system.[20]

The greater unity of the American specialty stemmed not only from the more favourable place of physicians within the asylum reform movement; it also reflected the indistinct boundaries between public and private institutions, which fostered more cohesion among the asylum doctors themselves. American asylums simply did not develop along the same clear-cut class lines that characterized English institutional development. In the first place, the private, profit-making madhouse trade never flourished in the United States; rather corporate or non-profit hospitals, such as the McLean Asylum and the Pennsylvania Hospital for the Insane, captured the patronage of the middle and upper classes. Although private institutions, they retained a charitable image and continued to treat some pauper patients. Secondly, these corporate institutions served as the direct models for the state hospitals built after the 1820s. In its early years, the American specialty consciously tried to minimize the differences between the two types of asylums; not only did they believe that state hospitals should be constructed and managed along the same lines as the corporate asylums, but also that they should have a 'mixed' class clientele of both paying and poor patients.[21]

Having charge of more similar institutions, the identity of interest among public and private asylum doctors in the United States was much greater than in England, which in turn gave them a much stronger and more cohesive professional identity. Although factionalism certainly existed among the American asylum superintendents, it did not follow the same clear-cut private/public lines found in the English specialty. Moreover, their differences tended to be more easily subordinated to a larger desire to present a strong and united front to the public. The Association of Medical Superintendents of American Institutions for the Insane, founded in 1844, reflected the cohesion of the early specialty; far more so than its English counterpart, it was a major force in building professional consensus, as well as an active political lobby for the specialty's interests. And, despite chronic dissatisfaction with its editorial policy, the *American Journal of Insanity*, also founded in 1844, served as the chief vehicle for the specialty's medical and institutional views.[22]

In sum, the circumstances that made restraint such a vital issue in England simply did not exist in the United States. American institutions were shaped more quickly and more completely to reform specifications, and their use of restraint apparently was never as extensive as in English asylums prior to the non-restraint movement.[23] More importantly, having no ambivalent legacy of asylum abuse to overcome, the American specialty had no need to prove its humanitarian credentials; in their practice, the moral and medical aspects of asylum treatment were more comfortably fused. From its inception, then, the non-restraint cause had little appeal to American asylum doctors.

Thus, due to fundamental differences in the course of institutional expansion and asylum reform in England and the United States, the two specialties were already set on divergent therapeutic courses by the 1840s. Over the next three decades, their dissimilarities continued to widen and deepen, as restraint came to play a very different role in shaping the professional identity of English and American asylum doctors.

English non-restraint: practice and politics

From the 1840s to the 1880s, the non-restraint philosophy was a powerful force shaping English asylum practice. To be sure, its implementation was neither complete nor consistent: even at the height of enthusiasm for the system, most superintendents did not endorse the concept of total abolition, and restraint continued to be employed occasionally in public asylums; among the private asylums, restraint practices were even less uniform and more extensive.[24] But the fact remains that, for all its inconsistencies, the non-restraint movement did mould English public hospitals in noteworthy ways: they not only used less mechanical restraint but also had a different, more open style of asylum management than their American counterparts.

Both the Lunacy Commission's statistics and travellers' accounts confirm the claims made by English alienists that by the 1850s their public hospitals used remarkably little restraint or seclusion. Of course, the reliability of such sources has to be treated with some scepticism, given the obvious incentives to underreport usage. But even allowing for a large 'dark figure' of clandestine use, the public hospitals still seem to have dramatically reduced the incidence of restraint and seclusion from its 1830s level. The 1870 Lunacy Commission report showed that 8 per cent of the public hospitals used neither restraint nor seclusion; 61 per cent used seclusion only; and 31 per cent used mechanical restraint. In those institutions employing restraint, the percentage of patients confined was rarely more than 1 per cent. Visitors to English asylums, with the exception of some Americans hostile to the non-restraint movement, repeatedly confirmed the same observation; English public asylums used restraint only in exceptional cases.[25]

While the medical profession certainly played an important role in fostering this policy, the single most powerful force for reducing restraint was the Lunacy Commission. Although initially ambivalent about the non-restraint system, the board, under the direction of Lord Shaftesbury, made its implementation a major administrative goal. Using its new powers of inspection and regulation, it constantly pressured asylum superintendents, as well as the madhouse proprietors, to use the least amount of physical coercion possible. Requiring that each asylum keep a register of all cases of restraint and seclusion, the visiting commissioners 'inquired minutely' into their use on tours of inspection. Despite the limitations on their power to remove recalcitrant superintendents, the board could and did make the situations of uncooperative individuals uncomfortable.[26]

In this fashion, the Lunacy Commission narrowed the range of permissible uses of mechanical restraint in English asylums; yet unlike the Americans' stereotype of it as a rigid body that harshly punished the slightest deviation from the non-restraint ideal, in actuality the commissioners neither sought nor required absolute uniformity in opinion and practice on the issue. On the whole, the non-restraint movement was never as monolithic as its critics – or, for that matter, some of its admirers – often assumed. Thus to comprehend the complexity of the therapeutic debate, both within the profession and with the Americans, it is necessary to map out the dominant tendencies in the philosophy and practice of non-restraint during the 1850s and 1860s.

The premisses of English non-restraint might be summed up as follows: first, that a proper system of asylum management could dramatically reduce the instances of patient violence; and second, that when patient violence did occur, it should be managed with the least physical coercion possible. Thus the development of non-restraint methods proceeded along two different but complementary lines: the management of the asylum milieu, and the therapeutic response to violence.

The starting-point of successful asylum management was, of course, the elimination of mechanical restraint to the fullest extent compatible with the patient's well-being. As John Conolly wrote in his first Hanwell report in 1839, mechanical restraint itself was 'creative of many of the outrages and disorders, to repress which its application was commonly deemed indispensable'.[27] But simply eliminating mechanical restraint was not sufficient; to do without it, the fundamental priorities of asylum treatment itself had to be changed. Again, in Conolly's words, 'the mere abolition of fetters and restraints constitutes only a part of what is properly called the non-restraint system. Accepted in its true and full sense, it is a complete system of management of insane patients.' The two most important elements in its success were the recruitment of a large body of co-operative attendants, who would supervise the patients closely, in lieu of restraint; and an extensive programme of employments, which would reduce the inmates' disorderly propensities. In the 1850s and 1860s, reformers experimented also with eliminating the repressive features of the asylum building itself, arguing that the constant awareness of grated windows, locked doors, and high fences undermined the good moral effect of abolishing restraint.[28]

The second tendency within the non-restraint movement was the development of less coercive measures to treat those patients who remained violent, even under the 'rule of kindness'. To control patient violence, the non-restraint system relied first and foremost upon manual restraint and temporary seclusion. When patients became violent, attendants held them temporarily and conducted them to a safe room or padded cell, where they remained until the rage had passed. If the violence persisted, various other measures might be employed: the shower-bath, often accompanied by a powerful emetic; the 'wet pack', which consisted of wrapping the patient in a wet sheet; and sedation or 'chemical restraint'.[29]

Non-restraint advocates preferred such measures to restraint, on both moral and medical grounds. First, they believed patients found it less degrading to be held by attendants and put in isolation than to be trussed up in a straitjacket. Second, they believed that restraint only worsened the diseased state of the nervous system, by its propensity to 'irritate, and heat, and disorder the body'. Seclusion was a far better therapeutic remedy for violence, because it allowed 'a simple exclusion from the irritable brain of all external causes of additional irritation'.[30]

While preferring such measures to mechanical restraint, non-restraint doctors recognized that each posed its own disadvantages. While no one could prove that manual restraint led to more protracted and violent conflicts between attendants and patients, rib-fractures and other patient injuries resulting from such struggles were in fact common and often quite serious. The practice of seclusion also gave rise to neglect, if not carefully monitored. The Lunacy Commission was particularly concerned about this problem, and discouraged superintendents from using seclusion as much as possible. Likewise, the shower-bath easily acquired a punitive meaning; after the celebrated Snape case, in which an elderly patient died after a prolonged shower-bath and a large dose of tartarized emetic, it was generally abandoned in favour of the wet pack. That method, too, had its critics, who objected to the confinement of the limbs, and the wet pack had to be reported as a form of restraint. But in spite of all these problems, the majority of superintendents still believed that these alternative methods posed far fewer problems than did instrumental restraint. As Conolly observed, 'All the substitutes for restraint are, like restraint itself, liable to be abused, but none can be made such an instrument of cruelty by abuse.'[31]

With this repertoire of admittedly imperfect alternatives, the majority of non-restraint superintendents, as well as the Lunacy Commission, acknowledged the need occasionally to use mechanical restraint to protect the patient's safety. In fact, there were firm adherents of total abolition who insisted, as did Hugh Diamond of the Surrey Asylum in 1854, that 'any person who would now use personal restraint or coercion is unfit to have the superintendence of an asylum'. But those taking such a radical position were in fact the minority, even in the early, most enthusiastic years of the reform; in the responses to the Lunacy Commission's 1854 circular on restraint, for example, the advocates for a qualified use of mechanical restraint outnumbered the advocates of total abolition by over two to one.[32]

Thus for all the play hostile observers gave extreme sentiments such as Diamond's statement, neither the Lunacy Commission nor the majority of non-restraint superintendents condemned all uses of mechanical restraint as illegimate. The views expressed by Sir James Clark in his 1869 memorial of John Conolly were far more representative of English practice: 'that mechanical restraint should never be resorted to unless there be a clear necessity, and that the existence of the clear necessity should not be too readily accepted'.[33] The real problem arose, not surprisingly, over what the superintendents construed as 'clear necessity'. While some uses of mechanical restraint – such as in force-feeding to prevent death by self-starvation, and the application of 'surgical' restraint to prevent a patient from removing stitches or otherwise aggravating a physical injury – aroused little controversy, other usages, as in the case of chronic destructiveness, provoked much more debate within the specialty.[34]

The majority opinion, as represented by the Lunacy Commission, the editorial policy of the *Journal of Mental Science*, and the 'moderate' non-restraint faction, held that mechanical restraint was rarely needed simply to control patient violence. If a doctor tried hard enough using other measures – and this was the critical point – he could manage all but a handful of cases without resorting to instrumental restraint. The determination of a physician's allegiance to non-restraint clearly depended on complex and subjective measures of good intent. Two doctors might both apply a camisole, one after several hours of trying other means to calm the patient, the other after several weeks; the former doctor might be rebuked by the Lunacy Commission, the latter be regarded as a model of non-restraint principle. The proof of the physician's non-restraint convictions rested, then, on the diligence and sincerity with which he exhausted all other means of calming a difficult patient before taking the final, drastic step of employing restraint.

From this perspective, any attempt to integrate mechanical restraint into the therapeutic regimen as a positive good was suspect. If doctors valued instrumental control too highly, it would lose its status as a therapeutic tool of last resort; they would gradually use it more and more, until the whole system of asylum treatment based on non-restraint would be destroyed. In a frequently quoted passage, Conolly warned against allowing restraint to assume too secure a place in the therapeutic armamentarium: 'No fallacy can be greater than that of imagining what is called a moderate use of mechanical restraint to be consistent with a general plan of treatment in all other respects complete, unobjectionable, and humane.'[35]

It was precisely on this issue – the legitimacy of mechanical restraint as a *therapeutic* measure – that controversy centred, both within the English specialty and, as we shall see, in the debate with the Americans as well. Those superintendents within the English system who earned a reputation for being 'unsound' on mechanical restraint did so because they believed it should be resorted to more quickly and less self-critically in cases of extreme and prolonged violence. Weighing the advantages and disadvantages of the various measures available to control patients, the 'dissidents' argued that the non-restraint faction had exaggerated the dangers of mechanical restraint, and that more humane asylum practice dictated its less sparing use.

The minority position was concisely put by Edgar Sheppard, superintendent of the Male Department of Colney Hatch, in his 1869 *Lectures on Madness*, when he wrote of the non-restraint system that 'much evil has resulted from its too rigid adoption'. The allegiance to non-restraint kept superintendents from utilizing restraint when it was truly needed. 'In cases of persistent suicidal and homicidal impulses, valuable lives are frequently preserved by the temporary adoption of what is termed "instrumental coercion"'. He concluded: 'That treatment, I repeat, cannot in the largest sense be called humane which does not make the most effective provision against these aggressive outbreaks.'[36]

The number of British superintendents openly espousing such views was small. In the 1850s and 1860s, superintendents Samuel Hill at the North and East Ridings Asylum and James Huxley at Kent earned reputations for being unsound on restraint. In the late 1860s and early 1870s, two superintendents of provincial asylums, David Yellowlees in Wales, and W. Lauder Lindsay in Scotland, joined Sheppard of the Colney Hatch Asylum in the ranks of critics. While few in number, the dissenters gained considerable renown because of the hostile scrutiny they encountered from the Lunacy Commission and the *Journal of Mental Science*. Their views provoked a strong reaction because they combined a contrary view about non-restraint with a challenge to the Lunacy Commission's regulatory authority.[37]

The case of James Huxley is particularly revealing in this regard. Unlike his contemporary, Samuel Hill, who openly argued that mechanical restraint be used to control violent patients, the 'peculiarity' of Huxley's views lay in his argument that restraint might occasionally have a remedial use. Complaining that in the non-restraint movement, 'the ground of dispute has been narrowed to the single proposition, "All or none"', he insisted that the doctor's *motivation* in using restraint had to be considered in judging its appropriateness. If mechanical restraint was used not to *punish* but to *treat* the patient, it was legitimate. 'We are inclined to place it in the list of indispensable adjuvants to treatment, whilst we believe it to exert sometimes a direct remedial agency of its own of considerable value,' he wrote in his *Annual Report* for 1853. Huxley further strayed from the path of right belief by questioning the Lunacy Commission's authority to interfere with the exercise of medical judgement. Lacking 'practical experience' in the care of the insane, they should defer more to medical opinion on matters such as restraint, he argued.[38]

Not surprisingly, given these views, Huxley soon ran foul of the Lunacy Commission. After preliminary skirmishes over the care of incontinent patients, the commission strongly reprimanded him in 1861 for leaving one patient in restraint and seclusion for four months, and another without clothes for twelve months. 'The Board consider that such cases, which they believe to be without parallel in any similar institutions in the country, are discreditable to the management of, and ought not to be found in, a County Asylum.' Huxley's local board of visitors defended him, and he remained in office. But again, in 1863, the commission complained about conditions at his asylum, particularly the excessive number of patients in 'strong dresses' (restrictive canvas garments). That same year, Huxley resigned and was replaced by John Kirkman, a staunch non-restraint man.[39]

Edgar Sheppard also had his problems with the Lunacy Commission, yet managed to maintain his post in spite of his deviant views on restraint. In 1866, the board took Sheppard to task for his unorthodox treatment of patients suffering from general paresis who had an uncontrollable impulse to remove and destroy their clothing. Arguing that their skin was galled by the clothing, Sheppard proposed to put them in warm padded cells without clothing or bedding. Notwithstanding his therapeutic rationale for this plan of action, the board took grave exception to it, as did the editors of the *Journal of Mental Science*. Yet Sheppard survived the controversy and remained a visible figure in the specialty.[40]

While the *Journal of Mental Science* and the *Lancet* took up the cudgels against the dissenters on non-restraint, they found a sympathetic hearing in the *JMS*'s rival publication, the *Journal of Psychological Medicine*. Until his death and the journal's demise in 1863, the editor Forbes B. Winslow, who was a private madhouse proprietor himself, espoused the causes of private asylum doctors in general and mechanical restraint in particular. Winslow's journal provided a continuous critique of the non-restraint party and commended those superintendents, such as Hill and Huxley, who defied its allegedly fanatical excesses. In disputing non-restraint, the *JPM* not only attacked the extremists in the specialty, but also questioned the Lunacy Commission's judgement in pressing their ideals too vigorously.[41]

In reality, then, English opinion on non-restraint was far from uniform.

Among the county asylum superintendents, significant differences of opinion existed and often became the focus of bitter public debate. Perhaps more importantly, the non-restraint issue became closely linked to a larger debate over the Lunacy Commission's authority to regulate medical practice. As we shall see, precisely because the American specialty criticized centralized authority in much the same way, its practice threatened the weakest point in the English consensus on non-restraint.[42]

The 'American system' of restraint

The restraint issue also played a prominent role in shaping the professional identity of American asylum doctors, albeit in a different fashion. While the English specialty viewed non-restraint as their greatest contribution to medical progress, the Americans found their professional satisfaction in *resisting* that same system. For the first generation of American psychiatrists, the critique of English practice helped to define their own distinctive style of asylum medicine, a style that championed not only the therapeutic value of mechanical restraint, but also the physician's right to prescribe it without external interference.

By the early 1840s, influential American asylum doctors such as Samuel Woodward and Isaac Ray had already enunciated the two therapeutic principles that would guide American practice for the next three decades: that while it was desirable to reduce its use, total abolition of mechanical restraint was not warranted, because of its exceptional value in some cases; and that the peculiar character of American society and American madness meant that more frequent use of restraint was required in the New World than in the Old. With remarkable agreement, the specialty endorsed these principles in 1844, when at the first meeting of their association, they passed a resolution 'that it is the unanimous sense of this convention that the attempt to abandon entirely the use of all means of personal restraint is not sanctioned by the true interests of the insane'. But while American physicians were quick to reject it, the English reform none the less continued to influence them in contradictory ways: at the same time as it encouraged individual superintendents to reduce the amount of restraint they employed, it also made rejection of non-restraint in principle the primary article of therapeutic faith among American alienists.[43]

As followers of moral treatment, American asylum doctors certainly believed that enlightened practice required the least amount of restraint compatible with the patient's safety; where they differed with their non-restraint colleagues was in refusing to endorse the concept of total abolition as a desirable goal. To a much greater degree than their English counterparts, American superintendents believed that restraint was an essential part of asylum treatment. As Isaac Ray wrote in the Butler Hospital annual report in 1863; 'In some shape or other, restriction is an essential element in all hospital management of insanity.' Given their premiss that 'coercion is a powerful adjuvant, in itself a moral instrument', American doctors were far more comfortable with the repressive functions of the asylum building and regimen; they thought patients needed to feel physically safe and protected from the consequences of their mental disease as the first step towards regaining their self-control.[44]

American resistance to non-restraint also stemmed from a dislike of the alternative forms of controlling violence upon which the English system depended. Comparing the advantages and disadvantages of mechanical restraint with the means favoured by the non-restraint school, the Americans did not find the latter so decidedly superior. In their minds, the moral and physical ill-effects of prolonged struggles with attendants or long stays in a padded cell equalled, if not surpassed, the dangers of mechanical restraint. Many American superintendents agreed with their Canadian colleague, Joseph Workman, who, after returning from a tour of non-restraint hospitals, declared their means of controlling patients were 'much more annoying, and must be more hurtful, both bodily and mentally'.[45]

Besides these general therapeutic objections, superintendents frequently invoked a form of therapeutic nationalism to explain why non-restraint would not work in their institutions. In the first place, they believed that in the United States mental illness was more likely to manifest itself in violence; their patients came to the asylum in a more excited state and stayed that way, regardless of how they were treated. The supposedly greater intensity of American mental disease was compounded by the social customs of a democratic nation, which made patients more impatient of authority. American superintendents were fond of contrasting their boisterous, freedom-loving inmates with the passive, beaten-down masses of the English public asylum. They argued that the free use of alcohol and tobacco, grinding poverty, and a rigid class system made the average Englishman a more manageable inmate than his Yankee cousin. As John Butler of the Hartford Retreat put it crudely in 1855: 'The great secret of non-restraint [is] the stupidity of their patients.' The 'mixed' character of American asylums also made non-restraint hard to implement in American hospitals, because with paying patients in public asylums, it was difficult to develop employment programmes that might make inmates more tractable; those who paid board refused to work, and those who did not pay board imitated them.[46]

Rather than slavishly following the non-restraint system, American superintendents felt that they had developed a style of practice much better suited to their patients and their institutions; the 'true humanity of the American system' allowed for 'the use of mild forms of restraint *pro re nata*', in the words of one doctor. Resisting the excesses of *ultra* reform, they had retained in their medical armamentarium an invaluable aid, foolishly abandoned by their English brethren. Charles Nichols summed up their credo at the 1859 AMSAII meeting in these words: 'I take pride in the belief that we have an American practice in the use of restraint, which is at once benevolent, enlightened, and practicable. It is, therefore, catholic and not subject to those revulsions which lead to ambitious antagonisms in sentiment, and dangerous extremes and substitutions in practice.'[47]

Perhaps the greatest virtue of the American system in the superintendents' estimation was the freedom it allowed the physician to choose the proper course of treatment. They frequently contrasted their independence from outside interference with what they perceived to be the 'servile' position of the English superintendents *vis à vis* the Lunacy Commission. As determined critics of all forms of centralized asylum regulation, most American asylum doctors attributed the follies of the non-restraint system to the excessive interference of the Lunacy Commission; they firmly believed that the majority of English superintendents wanted to use more mechanical restraint, but dared not because of the commission's excessive power over them. Having to answer to no such oppressive body, the Americans believed that they had arrived at a more scientific and humane position on the restraint issue.[48]

Prior to the 1870s, the specialty displayed a remarkable professional consensus around the central premisses of the 'American system', that is, the therapeutic value of restraint in certain cases, and its absolute necessity for treatment of American patients. But these general principles still allowed considerable scope for determining the proper use of mechanical restraint; moreover, without any centralized body to encourage conformity, there was no external pressure to narrow the range of acceptable opinions on the issue. As a result, the actual practice of restraint varied widely in the United States, 'many of its advocates scarcely resorting to it at all, and others resting upon it as a frequent and potent aid', as the *British and Foreign Medical-Chirurgical Review* quite accurately observed in 1876.[49]

With no state boards to collect even imperfect statistics before the 1880s, estimates of American practice are even more unreliable than the English figures. Not until the 1880 census was there any large-scale effort to gather information on the use of restraint and seclusion. Yet piecing together the superintendents' own observations about their practice, travellers' accounts, and the 1880 census data, one is led to the same general conclusion: that American asylums not only used more restraint than their English counterparts, but also that their practice was far less uniform. The *least* amount of mechanical restraint used in the United States corresponded with the *most* amount used in England, and the highest estimates of American usage were ten to fifteen times the English average.[50]

Although the 1880 census returns were flawed in certain respects – the census agent who collected them, Frederick Wines, himself stated that the statistics on seclusion were not reliable – they still provide the clearest sense of national practice at a time when the restraint controversy was at its height. Summarizing reports from some 139 public and private asylums, Wines put the ratio of patients under restraint at the time of the census at 1 in 21, or almost 5 per cent, a statistic that confirms the characterization of general American practice as quite 'robust', compared to the English. The

1880 census returns also demonstrated the great *variance* in institutional experience with restraint. The figures for individual hospitals given in table 29 revealed at one extreme a few hospitals using no restraint; a larger minority having between 1 per cent and 2 per cent in restraint; a middle group ranging from 3 to 5 per cent in restraint; and at the far extreme, reputable state asylums with 8 per cent, 11 per cent, and even a remarkable 21 per cent in restraint. The variance showed no apparent relationship to region or institutional type; hospitals at either end of the restraint-use spectrum could be found in every region of the country, even within the same state hospital system. While the corporate hospitals tended to use less restraint than the 5 per cent average, their practice varied, too, from the 0.5 per cent at the Pennsylvania Hospital for the Insane to the 5.5 per cent at the much smaller Hartford Retreat.[51]

This lack of uniformity in American practice was a major factor complicating the debate with the English specialty. Supporters of the 'American system' often pointed to the superintendents who used mechanical restraint so sparingly as to approximate the 'exceptional use' school in England, and concluded that the actual differences in Anglo-American practice were not so great as the English claimed.[52] Yet the 'minimalists', as I term them, by no means represented the whole specialty; equally strong was the tendency towards a much more 'robust' use of restraint. While these differences were not openly acknowledged by the superintendents themselves, they were none the less very real.

Although they rejected total abolition of restraint, a considerable number of American asylum doctors were inspired by English example to reduce their use of mechanical restraint to the mildest forms – that is, wristlets, mittens, and the bedstrap – and to use even those means quite sparingly. In the place of restraint, they substituted close supervision, strong dresses, and temporary seclusion, exactly as did the English (although they never shared the latter's enthusiasm for hydrotherapy). Had they practised in England, the minimalists would not have been regarded as exceptional in their usage of restraint. Where they chiefly disagreed with the English movement was in their refusal to endorse total abolition as the proper goal of enlightened practice.[53]

The best-known representative of this faction among the American superintendents was Thomas Story Kirkbride of the Pennsylvania Hospital for the Insane. In his *Notes*, Bucknill described him as a non-restraint man who simply refused to call himself by that name. Indeed, until the end of his long career, when the *Lancet* controversy lent a sharper tone to his pronouncements on the subject, Kirkbride's statements on restraint had much in common with the moderate faction of the English non-restraint party. He characterized the frequent resort to mechanical restraint as 'a great evil', claiming always to feel a sense of regret when forced to employ it. Kirkbride also believed that his institution had benefited enormously from lessening its reliance on instrumental restraint. Yet he refused to endorse total abolition as a desirable aim of asylum practice. In a small number of cases, usually less than 1 per cent in his practice, he found it to be an invaluable, sometimes life-saving remedy. So long as the doctor retained strict control over its use, he should be able to employ it without adverse results. In a frequently cited passage from his 1852 annual report, Kirkbride argued: 'A proper discipline and a judicious use of apparatus may make it like many other remedies, valuable or injurious, according to the wisdom exhibited in their use.'[54]

Supporters of the 'American system' frequently invoked Kirkbride's practice as its exemplar, yet in point of fact the 'robust' tendency in American practice was apparently more common. 'Robust' practitioners not only prescribed restraint more frequently, but also relied on its more restrictive forms, such as the straitjacket and the protection bed. The best-known representative of this school was John Gray, the superintendent of the Utica asylum from 1854 to 1882. In his own practice, Gray gained particular notoriety for his extensive employment of the crib bed; in the early 1880s, he had some fifty of them in use. Whereas Kirkbride always referred to mechanical restraint as a treatment of last resort, to be avoided if at all possible, Gray presented it as a more routine and benign form of therapeutic intervention. 'We look upon restraint and seclusion, directed and controlled by a conscientious and intelligent medical man, as among the valuable alleviating and remedial agents in the care and cure of the insane,' he wrote in 1861. As editor of the *American Journal of Insanity*, Gray wielded his considerable influence to champion the therapeutic uses of mechanical restraint. Besides frequently airing his own pro-restraint views in the *Journal*, he also reprinted articles by English critics of non-restraint such as W. Lauder Lindsay.[55]

To advocates of total abolition, the differences between Kirkbride's and Gray's practice may not have seemed so important, yet within the American specialty, they represented a significant, albeit unacknowledged, faultline in therapeutic belief. Whereas a minimalist might try seclusion or a canvas strong dress to control destructive behaviour or self-abuse, a more robust-minded physician would immediately apply restraint. Likewise, the minimalist tended to justify restraint only in cases of extreme and life-threatening violence, while the robust practitioner advocated its use for far less serious behaviours such as disrobing or destruction of clothing. Perhaps the contrast between the two tendencies is best indicated by the surgical analogies their exponents used to discuss the place of mechanical restraint in the therapeutic armamentarium: the minimalist Richard Gundry likened it to amputation, while the robust practitioner Eugene Grissom compared it to a crutch or a cane.[56]

Thus a careful reading of the American superintendents' views suggests that despite their public agreement about the premisses of the 'American system', they none the less had some significant differences of opinion over the proper use of mechanical restraint. Yet in striking contrast to Great Britain, where much less marked disagreements prompted bitter debate, in the United States the differences within the specialty were rarely acknowledged, much less debated. With their strong sense of professional cohesion, the 'brethren' chose rather to submerge their differences and present a united front to the outside world. Kirkbride's professional leadership – or rather lack of it – on the restraint issue is a case in point. Although his own practice won him the title of 'the American Conolly', he played no role similar to the English reformer within the larger profession. The need to stand firm with men such as Gray on other issues, such as the defence of the 'mixed' class asylum, outweighed any impulse Kirkbride might have had to force the restraint issue.[57]

The precipitant for a more open and hostile debate of restraint originated primarily *outside* the main ranks of the American specialty, within a small group of lay reformers, private practitioners, neurologists, and 'dissident' superintendents who launched a determined attack on the asylum association in the two decades after the Civil War. The restraint issue was but one aspect of these post-bellum reformers' critique of the specialty. Comparing American mental hospitals with their European counterparts, they found them lacking on many counts. Architecturally, American asylums were too grand and too monotonous; therapeutically, their regimen was unnecessarily restrictive and offered patients too little useful employment; administratively, they imposed so many duties on the superintendent that he had no time to be a real physician. Worst of all, men such as Kirkbride countenanced no deviation from the ideal of small 'mixed' state asylums, serving both paying and poor, acute and chronic patients; by refusing to approve cheaper facilities for the chronically ill, the asylum association condemned the poor insane to languish in almshouses and gaols.[58]

The asylum critics regarded the American specialty's hostility to the non-restraint movement as but one more sign of its backwardness. Yet prior to the mid-1870s, restraint remained a relatively muted element in the reformers' overall attack; the debate over separate institutions for the chronic insane and the need for more employment programmes occupied their energies much more closely. Restraint usually came up in the context of other debates as, for example, in the critique of the repressive lines of Kirkbride-style hospitals, or in the arguments for more extensive employment of patients as a means to reduce asylum disorder.[59] In other words, as the battle lines between the 'old guard' and the 'young Turks' began to form in the 1860s, restraint did not immediately surface as a leading point of contention. But as we shall see, once English alienists began to attack the 'American system', the internal debate over restraint became much more heated.

The great restraint controversy

Thus by the early 1870s, significant differences in both the philosophy and practice of restraint existed in English and American asylum medicine. From the 1840s on, the English specialty was guided by a conviction that mechanical restraint had such grave moral and physical disadvantages that its use should be at least severely curtailed, at best eliminated entirely. Through the concerted efforts of the Lunacy Commission and a powerful non-restraint lobby within the specialty, the range of acceptable opinion and practice of restraint in public asylums was greatly narrowed between the mid-1840s and the 1870s. In striking contrast, the American specialty retained a strong faith in the therapeutic properties of restraint. Perhaps as a lingering influence of 'heroic' medicine, they perceived American patients as in particular need of physical control. Stressing physician autonomy rather than therapeutic conformity as a guide to practice, the American leadership did not make the reduction of restraint an important professional goal. Although significant differences of opinion about its use certainly existed among American asylum doctors, they suppressed those disagreements for the sake of professional solidarity.

As we have seen, these Anglo-American therapeutic differences over restraint were quite well established by the 1850s, yet they did not become the focus of open conflict between the two specialties until the 1870s. To be sure, the Americans had been criticizing non-restraint since its inception; they quite self-consciously moulded their practice in opposition to English precedent. But prior to the 1870s, English asylum doctors had never bothered to reply directly to their American critics; in defending the cause of non-restraint, they concentrated instead on *continental*, chiefly German and French, arguments against the English reform.[60] When the Americans were mentioned in discussions of the international progress of non-restraint, they were as often as not portrayed in a favourable light; for example, in 1864, the *Journal of Mental Science* referred to the United States as a place 'where the principle of non-restraint has been so well-received and generally acted upon'.[61]

But in the late 1860s and 1870s, English commentaries on American practice became much more hostile. It was this greater determination to criticize and improve American practice that precipitated the bitter Anglo-American debates of the 1870s. The content and timing of the English specialty's critique suggests a connection between its own internal dynamics and the new imperative to discredit the Americans. Thus we must look for the proximate cause of the great restraint controversy in the English asylum politics of the early 1870s.

These were in fact years of discouragement for the English specialty; by the early 1870s, the fate of moral treatment in the public asylums seemed to many quite uncertain. A steadily falling cure rate, the accumulation of chronic cases, and the growing size of county institutions made any form of therapeutic care exceedingly difficult. The sense of crisis in the asylum system gave rise to the *Lancet* Commission, headed by J. Mortimer Granville, which investigated conditions in the metropolitan asylums during the mid-1870s. Criticizing the mechanical, impersonal quality of care they found there, the Commission concluded in its 1877 report that the public asylum system had hardly improved since its inception in 1845, and in some respects had regressed.[62]

Amidst this general climate of concern about the state of asylum affairs, the debate over non-restraint within the English specialty became even more pointed and personal. By the early 1870s, many observers sensed a waning of commitment to non-restraint ideals; both the Lunacy Commission and the specialty as a whole seemed to be moving away from the goal of total non-restraint towards a more relaxed acceptance of its exceptional use in cases of extreme violence. In retrospect, the Lunacy Commission's statistics for 1880 show that this perception of a 'reaction' against total non-restraint was correct: while the percentage of patients so confined remained quite low, the percentage of asylums using some mechanical restraint rose from 31 per cent to 47 per cent.[63]

The majority of English superintendents seem to have welcomed a more open acceptance of the occasional use of mechanical restraint. But for those with strong views, either for or against the system, the alleged 'reaction' in restraint could not pass unnoticed. The total abolition faction was alarmed at the increasingly public advocacy of mechanical restraint by superintendents such as Sheppard and Yellowlees, and lamented the Lunacy Commission's failure to discipline them severely enough. Warning against the dangers of 'moderation' on this issue, Conolly's son-in-law, the eminent alienist Henry Maudsley, stated ominously in 1870 that 'the principle of the non-restraint system will admit of no compromise'. The critics of non-restraint responded in kind, using their annual reports and letters to the editor to challenge the extremist tendency within the non-restraint movement. 'Unnecessary restraint cannot be too strongly condemned,' Yellowlees wrote to the editor of the *Lancet* in 1872, 'but to reject its use when necessary for the patient's welfare is to sacrifice the patient to a sentiment, and to degrade "non-restraint" from the expression of a great principle into the tyranny of a mere name.'[64]

Nowhere was the new stridency in the non-restraint debate more evident than in the writings of W. Lauder Lindsay of the Murray Royal Institution for the Insane. First classed as one of the 'traitors in the camp, who would undermine the great structure of non-restraint' in the late 1860s, because of his advocacy of the protection bed, Lauder Lindsay wrote an article in the *Edinburgh Medical Journal* in 1870, innocently titled, 'Mollities ossium in relation to rib-fracture among the insane', which concluded with a stinging attack on the non-restraint system. '*Rib-fracture* may legitimately be regarded as one of the many fruits of the *non-use of mechanical restraint* in cases where it is really required,' he wrote. The excesses of the 'Conollyites,' and the misguided public opinion they had created on the subject, had created a new form of restraint, according to Lauder Lindsay: the 'terrorism' fostered by the Lunacy Commission, which 'restrained' the English superintendents from exercising their own medical judgement.[65]

Significantly, in making his argument against the 'tyranny' of non-restraint sentiment, Lauder Lindsay contrasted English servility with the 'manly independence that exists on the same subject, as regards both action and opinion in America!' Indeed, not only Lauder Lindsay, but other English critics of non-restraint drew strength from the American specialty's philosophy of restraint. In England, their dissident views might warrant public censure, but in the United States men such as Lauder Lindsay and Sheppard were hailed as practical, scientific, even courageous men. The *American Journal of Insanity* reprinted Lauder Lindsay's articles criticizing the non-restraint system; Sheppard was warmly received on a visit to the United States in the early 1870s. Not surprisingly, in their struggle against the Lunacy Commission's authority, these 'deviant' superintendents found kindred souls in the Americans, who so vehemently argued for physician autonomy, and were only too glad to pillory the Lunacy Commission for the excesses of non-restraint.[66]

Herein lies the critical link between the English specialty's internal debate over non-restraint and the growing antagonism towards American practice. The more English critics of non-restraint invoked practices across the Atlantic to support their call for moderation, the more threatening that foreign precedent became to the advocates of asylum reform. What was particularly dangerous about the 'American system' was not so much its therapeutic argument against non-restraint – the Germans and French had been making similar arguments for decades – but rather its *celebration of physician autonomy*. The American critique of centralization too closely paralleled the dissidents' resentments against the Lunacy Commission. Thus the critical sights of the non-restraint party settled on the Americans.

In the political climate of the 1870s, attacking American asylum practice had several useful functions for English reformers: by comparing their achievements with American conditions, they sustained the impression that whatever the faults of English asylums, they were still far more humane than their Yankee counterparts. Second, by discrediting American practice, the reformers also aimed at disarming the internal critics of non-restraint, such as Lauder Lindsay and Sheppard, who appealed to American precedent as proof for their own convictions. Once exposed as inhumane and unscientific, the American practice of 'moderate' restraint would serve as a warning to all who proposed a freer use of mechanical restraint in English asylums, and reaffirmed the value of centralized regulation.

The tensions between the two specialties over the restraint issue exploded in the mid-1870s. The first skirmish came in 1874, at the AMSAII meeting in Nashville. Mark Ranney of the Iowa asylum presented a critical paper on the non-restraint system, which ended with the observation that English practice was becoming more like the American, citing Sheppard, Yellowlees, Lauder Lindsay and others in support. In the discussion that followed, the president of the association, Clement Walker, observed that on a recent trip to the British Isles, he had found four-fifths of the superintendents favoured mechanical restraint and would use it more, if the Lunacy Commission would only allow it, adding, 'They say the Superintendents are emulous, one of another, to report the smallest number of restraints during the year.'[67]

The AMSAII discussion distressed John C. Bucknill, then Lord Chancellor's Medical Visitor of Lunatics, because it clearly revealed how little the Americans understood the non-restraint system. In a letter to Kirkbride, he attributed Walker's supposedly misinformed views on the English situation to Edgar Sheppard, a man with 'no reputation' who had been blackballed by the College of Physicians. The following year, Bucknill took a leave of absence from his post to visit the United States, where he inspected ten asylums and attended the AMSAII meeting in May 1875; while he avoided the restraint issue to avoid offending his hosts, he made a brief speech, after being elected an honorary member of the Association, in which he challenged English and American specialists to provide one another with 'a friendly competition, and an appreciative audience outside of their own country, so that their opinions may be sifted and their practice criticized, not by entire strangers and foreigners but by an audience, to a certain extent, generic'.[68]

The competition that ensued was far from friendly, however, due to an editorial excoriating the American superintendents that appeared soon after in the *Lancet* of 13 November 1875. Significantly, the author was J. Mortimer Granville, the physician heading the *Lancet* Commission, and a keen asylum reformer; his dual role as critic of English asylums and scourge of the American specialty suggests the connection between the internal and international politics of reform. Identifying three stages in the care of the insane – the barbaric, the humane, and the remedial – Granville claimed that the Americans had barely emerged from barbarism. Suggesting that slavery had coarsened their moral fibre, he characterized American alienists as both unscientific and inhumane for their continued use of mechanical restraint. 'If the medical superintendents of American asylums resort to the old system, they do so in the face of patent facts, and their practice has no claim to be classed as medical, hardly can it be called humane.' Questioning whether they had really mastered the principles of moral treatment, Granville concluded: 'They adhere to the old terrorism tempered by petty tyranny.'[69]

The *Lancet* editorial infuriated the American superintendents, who besieged their colleague Bucknill with angry letters; he dutifully came to their defence in a letter to the *Lancet*, alluding to his own observations of American institutions. When the journal responded by asking him 'to make known what I had seen in America', as he later wrote, Bucknill saw an opportunity to chide his American friends for their wayward views on non-restraint. In a series of *Lancet* articles, later revised and republished as his *Notes on Asylums in America*, he provided his own critique, which was in every way more potent than Granville's caricature of American asylum practice.[70]

Bucknill denied that the use of restraints in the United States was part of 'a system of negligence and inhumanity', characterizing American asylums as on the whole well managed. The best American precedent, as that of Kirkbride, was quite acceptable by English standards; but the worst American practice, as at the Philadelphia and New York City asylums, was very bad indeed, and far worse than any conditions in his own country. 'They are men, as I most willingly testify,' he wrote of the American superintendents, 'animated by the highest motives of humanity, but ignorant and mistaken in their appreciation of means to the furtherance of that great end to which we all press forward, namely, to the care and cure of the insane, with the least amount of suffering.' Referring particularly to the argument that the distinctive forms of American mental illness necessitated more restraint, he replied that this 'spread-eagle apology for the bonds of freeman is the most feeble, futile, and fallacious which could possibly be imagined'.[71]

Thus, while seeking to defend the American specialty against Granville's indiscriminate condemnation, Bucknill attempted 'to distinguish the good from the evil' in their practice and so prod his American brethren to take a more aggressive stance against mechanical restraint. Far more than Granville's exaggerated claims, Bucknill's criticisms identified the real fault-lines in American practice: the extreme variance in their usages of restraint, and the curious unwillingness of the specialty to confront and discuss its own differences on the subject. In his private correspondence, he made clear that Kirkbride's unwillingness to take a stand on the issue puzzled and disturbed him; by so directly challenging the specialty's leadership, he hoped to provoke a franker discussion of the subject.[72]

Unfortunately for Bucknill's good intentions, his attempts to provoke self-reflection came at a time when the American specialty was little inclined to listen sympathetically to English criticism. By the mid-1870s, the older generation of asylum superintendents felt themselves under siege by internal critics who, in their mounting frustration with the 'iron rule' of AMSAII, turned increasingly to English precedent to support their proposals for change. As the English dissidents Sheppard and Lauder Lindsay took solace in American views, so, too, the American dissenters looked across the Atlantic for moral support. In the United States as in England, internal factions and international debates coincided to make restraint an explosive issue.

The same year that Bucknill took to the pages of the *Lancet* to criticize American asylum practice, a young physician named Hervey B. Wilbur prepared a report for the New York State Board of Charities comparing the state of English and American mental institutions. Concerned with declining cure rates and growing costs, the board hired Wilbur, the superintendent of the state idiot asylum, to tour English public asylums and gather ideas for improving the state hospitals under their supervision. On his return, Wilbur published *The Management of the Insane in Great Britain*, a report that lavishly praised the English at the American specialty's expense. Wilbur wrote approvingly of the good order and extensive employment schemes in the public asylums, crediting the latter with the extremely rare use of restraint and seclusion in English asylum practice. In response to those American superintendents who claimed non-restraint caused more patient injuries, he included statistical data that suggested American accident and suicide rates were far higher than those in England. Wilbur concluded that if American asylums were to catch up with their

English counterparts, they needed to be brought more completely under the discipline of state boards of inspection.[73]

Wilbur was but one of a number of determined asylum reformers who tried to use English precedent to discredit the specialty's conservative leadership.[74] Thus in the United States, the restraint issue became closely tied up with the larger conflict between the asylum superintendents and the state boards of charities over asylum design and management. The older doctors such as Kirkbride and Gray saw the non-restraint agitation as but one more aspect of the plot to turn the 'mixed' asylums of the United States into pauperized institutions; by resisting it, they were defending their peculiar concept of the state hospital. In the context of their own factional strife, the timing of Bucknill's criticism could not have been worse for the American leadership. The well-meaning criticisms of Bucknill, a trusted colleague whom they might expect to defend the cause of high asylum standards, must have seemed like a bitter betrayal to Kirkbride and his colleagues. Unintentionally, the English alienist appeared bent on furnishing additional ammunition to their enemies among the neurologists and state boards of charities.[75]

As a result, Bucknill's efforts at constructive criticism had quite the opposite effect from his intentions. In the first place, far from endorsing the English alienist's criticisms and calling for reform, the minimalists such as Kirkbride, whom Bucknill looked to for leadership on the restraint issue, emphatically closed ranks with their more robust-minded brethren. For example, in his 1877 annual report, Kirkbride denied the criticisms from both home and abroad that American hospitals were not as progressive as their European counterparts. Likewise he disputed the argument that a centralized authority should oversee the proper use of restraint, writing that 'no outside commission nor any non-professional board is competent for such a duty'. Clearly, in Kirkbride's mind, the issues of professional solidarity and physician autonomy overrode any concern that some American superintendents might be using more restraint than they need be.[76]

Among the more 'robust' supporters of restraint, Bucknill's comments had an equally unproductive effect. The criticism from abroad only strengthened their commitment to defend the therapeutic value of non-restraint. At the 1877 association meeting, Eugene Grissom of the North Carolina state asylum took to the floor to deliver a paper entitled 'Mechanical protection for the violent insane', which presented an exhaustive, often emotional defence of American practice, summarizing arguments against non-restraint that had been developed and refined over three decades: that the moderate use of mechanical restraint was therapeutically and morally sound; that it was required by the peculiar violence of American insanity; and that it prevented tragic accidents and injuries. For good measure, Grissom threw in statistics purporting to show a higher mortality rate in British asylums, and a reference to poor conditions in Irish asylums; then concluded with a proverb suggesting that his English brethren attend to their own failings before judging anyone else.[77]

But while in the short run, the *Lancet*-Bucknill controversy intensified the older superintendents' defence of mechanical restraint, it contributed to a more positive view towards non-restraint among the younger asylum doctors entering practice in the 1870s. Among those who chafed at the conservative leadership in the specialty, advocacy of non-restraint became the mark of a new, more scientific approach to psychiatry. As an editorial in the *Medical Record* proclaimed in 1876: 'So long as it is the ambition of alienists to be considered scientific physicians, and not mere jailors, this idea [of non-restraint] will be kept in view, and all the hindering circumstances to its fulfillment will be patiently and strenuously combated.'[78]

One manifestation of this new 'scientific' approach to restraint was the attempt to compare systematically Anglo-American therapeutic practices. Responding to the frequently heard argument among the American superintendents, that the English only did without restraint by overdrugging their patients, Hervey Wilbur decided to collect more information on the restraint issue, and in 1881, published an article entitled, '"Chemical restraint" in the management of the insane', in the *Archives of Medicine*. Using comparative statistical data, Wilbur professed to show that not only did English asylums use less mechanical restraint, less seclusion, and fewer drugs, but also that they had lower rates of accident and suicide. Thus, in this widely cited article, he challenged the superiority of American practice on every count.[79]

The new association of non-restraint with 'scientific psychiatry' encouraged some superintendents to implement the system in their own institutions. In the late 1870s and 1880s, the English system finally found some genuine advocates among American asylum doctors, including Peter Bryce, who introduced it at the Alabama State Hospital in the late 1870s; John C. Shaw at the asylum in Kings County, New York, who introduced it in the early 1880s; and Alice Bennett, who introduced it in the women's department of the Norristown, Pennsylvania, state hospital in the late 1880s. Their successes posed a serious challenge to the old therapeutic nationalism by demonstrating that the supposedly more violent, ungovernable 'Yankee' patients could indeed be managed by the milder system. In describing his methods, Bryce explicitly attacked the notion of a peculiar violence among American patients in his 1876 annual report, concluding, 'Men are too nearly the same in every civilized country to warrant such an assumption.' His experience seemed to prove the argument, made frequently by the English, that the non-restraint system had not previously succeeded in the United States only because it had never been given a fair trial.[80]

Conclusion

In retrospect, the great restraint controversy of the 1870s can perhaps best be understood as a reflection of two fundamental differences in the Anglo-American asylum systems: their varying degrees of centralization and levels of class differentiation. For all their many points of commonality, English and American superintendents practised within asylum settings that varied significantly in governance and clientele. The non-restraint movement grew out of a more centralized system of institutions designed primarily for pauper patients. In contrast, American state hospitals, at least until the 1870s, enjoyed far greater autonomy and catered to a more 'mixed' class clientele. In debating their therapeutic philosophies concerning restraint, English and American doctors returned to these two themes again and again.

Within the English specialty, the non-restraint issue was closely bound up with perceptions of the Lunacy Commission's role in asylum practice. For those who accepted the premiss of state control, the reduction of restraint in English asylums served as proof of the commission's usefulness; it had been a powerful (if occasionally not quite zealous enough) ally in enforcing orthodoxy on the restraint issue. The board's role in producing a more uniform, self-critical practice was exactly the point of contention among the English critics of non-restraint, who resented its encroachments on the physician's therapeutic autonomy. By challenging the wisdom of non-restraint, they were also challenging the larger process of centralization and its effects on medical practice.

Not surprisingly, in resisting the 'terrorism' of the Lunacy Commission, the English dissidents made common cause with the Americans, whose 'American system' of restraint celebrated the principle of physician autonomy above all else. But as their asylums also deteriorated over the course of the mid-nineteenth century, American asylum doctors faced their own group of 'young Turks', who believed that more centralized authority was the only means to improve asylum conditions. For the post-bellum asylum reformers, the extensive and divergent use of mechanical restraint in the United States was proof that the system needed external regulation; in envisioning a new asylum order, they looked to England and the achievements of state supervision for inspiration.

Thus the central tendencies in the two specialties were exactly opposite: in England, centralization of asylum policy, with a minority resisting and drawing strength from the American emphasis on autonomy; in the United States, a strong and independent asylum specialty gradually being brought under more state supervision, aided by dissidents who admired the English system. As reverse images each of the other, the internal divisions within the two specialties intersected to produce a painful international confrontation.

Beneath the rhetoric about the nature of their patient populations, there was another point of difference involved in the Anglo-American controversy: the class differentiation in their respective public asylums. This issue of clientele is perhaps most clearly revealed in the discussions of acceptable *risk* in asylum practice. As the English superintendents themselves admitted, the non-restraint system worked upon the principle that it was preferable to take some chance with patient safety than to risk the moral dangers of mechanical restraint. As an editorial in the *Journal of Mental Science* said in 1858: 'It is better to submit to defeat from the unmanageable exceptions than to break the rule of kindness.' Criticizing what he perceived to be the excessive caution of the American superintendents, an English alienist wrote to Charles Folsom, 'It seems to me that the only way we are ahead of you is this: we run risks, you endeavour not to do so.'[81]

Without implying deliberate callousness on their part, it is worth noting that in dealing chiefly with a pauper clientele, English public asylum superintendents did not have to worry excessively about the impact of suicides and rib-breakings on their institutional livelihoods. Of course, cases of flagrant abuse could cause them grave difficulties with the Lunacy Commission or the press; but on a daily basis, having an assured clientele of poor patients whose board was guaranteed by the state, they were not so vulnerable to the adverse publicity surrounding patient mishaps. From this perspective, the fact that the private asylums consistently used more restraint than their public counterparts makes sense: the more 'valuable' the patient, the less willing the asylum doctor was to run unnecessary risks.

That the Americans placed a higher premium upon safety was surely a reflection of their greater dependence on certain kinds of public patronage. Although American state hospitals certainly had a guaranteed population of chronic pauper patients, whose board was paid by local and state authorities, they also attracted and prized a paying clientele of more affluent and acutely ill patients. While often few in number, these paying patients contributed not only to the economic viability of the mixed state asylums, but also to the superintendents' interest and satisfaction in institutional work. Compared to their English counterparts, the American state hospital doctors were far more concerned with the cultivation of a paying clientele.[82]

As a result, the American conception of 'acceptable' risk was apparently far more conservative than the English. Wanting to preserve their more respectable patrons, American asylum doctors naturally wished to avoid charges of neglect; suicides and accidents posed a serious 'public relations' problem in terms of the paying patients and their families. A strict asylum regimen including the use of mechanical restraint helped to guarantee asylum patrons that their relatives would be safer and more secure in an institution than at home. Unfortunately, in gaining popular confidence, the American asylum doctors suffered certain disadvantages as a result of their greater autonomy; precisely because they lacked centralized regulation, they had no authority, other than their own boards of trustees, to defend them against charges of abuse and neglect. While both specialties endured their share of public clamour in this period, the American superintendents seem to have been far more nervous about their public image. To them, the benefits of non-restraint simply did not balance the potential for adverse publicity from patient accidents. As Kirkbride stated their position in a discussion of open hospitals, 'No slight advantage can compensate the loss of a single life, for the destruction of property or the hundred kinds of mischief that may be perpetuated by insane thus given their freedom.'[83]

After peaking in the late 1870s, the great restraint controversy continued into the 1880s, but gradually lost its force as the older asylum superintendents passed from the scene, and the younger doctors taking their place confronted new institutional realities with different professional ideals. As the asylum system in both countries aged, such issues of centralization and clientele became progressively less important. State regulation of asylum practice became a fact of life even American superintendents had to accept in the late nineteenth century. On both sides of the Atlantic, institutional psychiatry became synonymous with the loss of medical autonomy. For the Americans, issues of patronage and clientele grew steadily less important as state hospitals assumed a more custodial identification with the chronic pauper class.

Last but not least, the lessening concern with mechanical restraint reflected the abandonment of moral treatment as the guiding principle of Anglo-American asylum medicine. To use or not to use restraint was an important therapeutic choice only so long as moral influences were conceived of as important factors in the cure of insanity. As somatic approaches and therapeutic pessimism gained ascendance in the late nineteenth century, restraint became much more simply an issue of efficient patient management.

In the 1880s and 1890s, opinion in the English and American specialties about the use of restraint converged more closely around a similar set of principles. English asylum doctors ceased to worry about the moral dangers of its occasional use, allowing it a legitimate, albeit circumscribed, role in treatment; the Americans endorsed the general principles of non-restraint as consistent with 'scientific psychiatry'. In both countries, mechanical restraint became but one element in an expanded repertoire of responses to manage patient violence, including improved forms of sedation, hydrotherapy, and occupational therapy.[84]

For all its greater acceptance in theory, non-restraint proved no less utopian an ideal in subsequent years. Even as they held up the reduction of restraint as a desirable goal, Anglo-American psychiatrists and hospital administrators declared that the exigencies of asylum economics made it increasingly difficult to practise in the late nineteenth century. As Conolly observed at its inception, the philosophy of non-restraint required an extremely labour-intensive style of asylum management; without ample resources to provide co-operative attendants, occupational programmes, and the like, restraint had to remain an integral aspect of treatment. By the 1890s, even the most optimistic asylum reformers knew that such resources were not likely to be forthcoming. Thus in the long run, the fervour of non-restraint became but one more casualty of the increasingly limited institutional horizons of late-nineteenth-century psychiatry.

Notes

I would like to thank the members of the history of medicine seminar at the Wellcome Institute for the History of Medicine, London, who commented on an early draft of this paper, especially W.F. Bynum and Charlotte MacKenzie; and Gerald Grob, who shared his own research on the topic with me.

1 John C. Bucknill (18 March 1876) 'Notes on asylums for the insane in America', *Lancet*: 418.

2 Bucknill's articles on American asylums appeared in the following numbers of the *Lancet* for 1876: (12 February): 263–4; (18 March): 418–19; (25 March): 455–7; (8 April): 529–30; (22 April): 595–6; (13 May): 701–3; (3 June): 810–12; (24 June): 918–21. They were republished (1876) as *Notes on Asylums for the Insane in America*, London: Churchill.

3 See W.F. Bynum (1983) 'Themes in British psychiatry, J.C. Prichard (1786–1848) to Henry Maudsley (1835–1918)', in M. Ruse (ed.), *Nature Animated*, Dordrecht, Holland: D. Reidel, esp. pp. 226–9, on the importance of non-restraint to the mid-nineteenth-century specialty.

4 [Anonymous] (1876) 'Lunacy in the United States', *British Foreign Medical-Chirurgical Review* 58: 74.

5 For a more extended discussion of the similarities and differences between the two specialties, see Nancy Tomes (forthcoming) 'The Anglo-American asylum in historical perspective', in J. Giggs and C. Smith (eds), *Location and Stigma: Emerging Themes in the Study of Mental Health and Mental Illness*, London: Unwin Hyman.

6 There is surprisingly little written on the non-restraint movement. Useful accounts can be found in Albert Deutsch (1949) *The Mentally Ill in America*, 2nd edn, New York: Columbia University Press, pp. 213–28; Gerald Grob (1973) *Mental Institutions in America*, New York: Free Press, pp. 206–10; and Kathleen Jones (1972) *A History of the Mental Health Services*, London: Routledge & Kegan Paul, pp. 14–21. Andrew Scull presents an extremely useful account of the non-restraint movement's most famous publicist in (1985) 'A Victorian alienist: John Conolly, FRCP, DCL (1794–1866)', in W.F. Bynum, R. Porter, and M. Shepherd (eds), *The Anatomy of Madness* 2 vols, London: Tavistock, vol. I, pp. 103–50.

7 John Warner (1986) *The Therapeutic Perspective*, Cambridge, Mass.: Harvard University Press, reminds us how important therapeutics were to the construction of medical identity in the nineteenth century, and this was no less true in psychiatry. Warner's analysis suggests some valuable insights into the non-restraint controversy, which I plan to explore in a second article focusing more closely on the therapeutic arguments between English and American psychiatrists.

8 The summary that follows draws heavily on my 'Anglo-American asylum in historical perspective'.

9 For general accounts of English asylum reform, see Jones, *A History of the Mental Health Services*, esp. pp. 1–149; and Andrew Scull (1979) *Museums of Madness*, London: Allen Lane, esp. pp. 50–119.

10 On this 'divided legacy' in English asylum practice, see W.F. Bynum (1974) 'Rationales for therapy in British psychiatry, 1780–1835', *Medical History* 18:

317–34; Nicholas Hervey (1985) 'A slavish bowing-down: the lunacy commission and the psychiatric profession', in Bynum, Porter, and Shepherd (eds), *The Anatomy of Madness*, vol. II, pp. 98–131; and Scull, *Museums of Madness*, pp. 129–85.

11 Bynum, 'Themes', pp. 229–30 discusses the feebleness of the early English asylum association. Scull, *Museums of Madness*, pp. 164–5, 204–5, discusses class segregation and factionalism within the specialty. Contemporary observers often noted that the American association seemed much more active than its English counterpart. See, for example, (1854–5) 'Proceedings of the 9th annual meeting of the Association of Medical Superintendents of American Institutions for the Insane [hereafter AMSAII]', *Journal of Mental Science* (hereafter *JMS*) 1: 130–3.

12 See, for example, the references to restraint Jones mentions in her survey of early asylum reform, *A History of the Mental Health Services*, pp. 64–107.

13 Ann Digby (1985) *Madness, Morality and Medicine: A Study of the York Retreat, 1796–1914*, Cambridge: Cambridge University Press, pp. 78–82.

14 John Conolly (1854–5) 'Inauguration of the statue of the late Dr Charlesworth', *JMS* 1: 105. Accounts of the non-restraint movement abound with gruesome descriptions of the 'bad old days' before restraint was abolished. See, for example, the remarkable list of restraining devices in use at the Lancaster Asylum in 1840 given in D. Hack Tuke (1882) *Chapters in the History of the Insane in the British Isles*, London: Kegan Paul, pp. 268–9.

15 J.C. Bucknill and D.H. Tuke (1858) *A Manual of Psychological Medicine*, 1st edn, London: Churchill, p. 509. Bynum, 'Themes', pp. 228–9, argues that Conolly's medically oriented version of non-restraint appealed to the specialty more than Gardiner Hill's humanistic conception of the reform.

16 There was a bitter controversy over who should get credit for 'inventing' non-restraint. The followers of Charlesworth and Gardiner Hill fought one another bitterly; Gardiner Hill also resented Conolly's subsequent fame as the champion of non-restraint. See Jones, *A History of the Mental Health Services*, pp. 117–19; and Scull, 'A Victorian alienist', pp. 124–5, for brief accounts of the controversy.

17 Scull, 'A Victorian alienist', pp. 122–3.

18 The following points are elaborated in my 'Anglo-American asylum'.

19 One need only examine Dix's extensive correspondence with the 'brethren' to get a sense of how much more harmonious was the relationship between lay reformers and medical superintendents in the United States. The Dix papers are in the Houghton Library, Harvard University.

20 On the Friends Retreat, see Norman Dain and Eric Carlson (1960) 'Milieu therapy in the nineteenth century', *Journal of Nervous and Mental Diseases* (hereafter *JNMD*) 131: 277–90. On the theoretical basis of American asylum medicine, see Nancy Tomes (1984) *A Generous Confidence: Thomas Story Kirkbride and the Art of Asylum-Keeping, 1840–1883*, Cambridge: Cambridge University Press, pp. 75–85.

21 Tomes, *A Generous Confidence*, esp. pp. 264–301.

22 See Grob, *Mental Institutions*, pp. 132–50; and Constance McGovern (1985) *Masters of Madness*, London: University Press of New England, for an overview of the founding of AMSAII and its early activities.

23 American asylum doctors insisted that prior to the 1840s, their asylums used far less mechanical restraint than their English counterparts. See, for example,

Luther Bell's remarks (1855–6) 'AMSAII proceedings', *American Journal of Insanity* (hereafter *AJI*) 12: 86–7.

24 The whole problem of restraint in the private asylums is one I simply had to exclude from consideration here, due to limitations of time and space. Based on my reading of the English sources, I think it is safe to characterize the non-restraint movement as primarily a product of the public hospital system; despite the Lunacy Commission's efforts to reduce its use, private asylums continued to employ more restraint.

25 I derived these statistics from Commissioners in Lunacy (hereafter CL) 24th *Annual Report* (hereafter *AR*) (1870), pp. 115–226. I realize my remarks here finesse many difficult issues concerning the actual extent of restraint use. But I am convinced, after reading widely in the published sources, that English asylums did indeed use far less restraint than their American counterparts, and that is the central point I am trying to make here. I base my conclusions on the commission's yearly reports on individual asylums and the numerous travellers' accounts describing English asylums. Even Americans hostile to the non-restraint system did not contest the claim that English asylums used less restraint, but rather argued that they did not practise total abolition. See, for example, A.O. Kellogg (1868–9) 'Notes of a visit', *AJI* 25: 281–304.

26 CL (1854) 8th *AR*: 40–3, has a nice discussion of the board's methods in this regard. The published appendices in each annual report give ample testimony of their continued efforts to eliminate excessive and undesirable forms of restraint. The 1844 *Report of the Metropolitan Commissioners* was ambivalent on the non-restraint system, but the new national board set up under the 1845 Lunacy Act gradually 'converted' to the cause, according to John Conolly (1856) *The Treatment of the Insane Without Mechanical Restraint*, London: Smith, Elder, & Co., p. 300.

27 Quoted in James Clark (1869) *A Memoir of John Conolly*, London: John Murray, p. 21.

28 Conolly, *Treatment of the Insane*, p. 35. This book remains the single best statement of the non-restraint philosophy. Conolly devoted special attention to the attendant question on pp. 97–104. The 'open hospital' movement was associated first with the Lincoln and Rainhill asylums, later with the Fife and Kinross asylum in Scotland. For two admiring American accounts of these institutions, see Edward Jarvis to Samuel G. Howe, 1 June 1869, Howe Papers, Houghton Library, Harvard University; and (1875–6) 'A Scotch insane asylum', *AJI* 32: 252–4. (This article was first published in the *Boston Medical and Surgical Journal*, and reprinted in the *AJI* with a critical comment from the editor.)

29 Conolly, *Treatment of the Insane*, esp. pp. 40–2, covers the basic techniques of manual restraint and seclusion. For a good overview of therapeutic responses to violence, see Bucknill and Tuke, *Manual*, 1st edn, pp. 511–28. On bathing, see Harrington Tuke (1858) 'On warm and cold baths in the treatment of insanity', *JMS* 4: 532–52. On the wet pack, see C. Lockhart Robertson (1861) 'On the sedative action of the cold wet sheet', *JMS* 7: 265–77.

30 Conolly, *Treatment of the Insane*, pp. 256, 231.

31 Conolly (1840) Hanwell Asylum 2nd *Annual Report*, quoted in his *Treatment of the Insane*, p. 207. The superintendents themselves were extraordinarily reluctant to link patient injuries to attendant violence, but any perusal of the

Lunacy Commission reports certainly suggested a connection, which the Americans were only too glad to make. See, for example, Isaac Ray to Edward Jarvis, 21 November 1863, Jarvis Papers, Countway Library, Harvard Medical School (hereafter C. Lib.).

For debates over seclusion, see, for example, CL (1854) 8th *AR*, pp. 42–3; CL (1859) 13th *AR*, pp. 67–8; J.C. Bucknill (1854–5) 'On the employment of seclusion in the treatment of the insane', *JMS* 1: 180–9. On the Snape incident, see CL (1857) 11th *AR*, pp. 32–9; and [Editorial] (1856–7) 'Mr. Snape', *JMS* 2: 282–3. For a criticism of the wet pack, see Bucknill and Tuke (1879) *Manual of Psychological Medicine*, 4th edn, London: Churchill, pp. 744–5.

32 CL (1854) *AR*, p. 140. Appendix G of that report, pp. 123–209, gives the individual responses to the circular on restraint.

33 Clark, *A Memoir*, p. 158.

34 John Conolly (1854–5) 'Second notice of the 8th report', *JMS* 1: 145, allowed that temporary restraint for the purpose of force-feeding was acceptable under the non-restraint system. Likewise, Robert Gardiner Hill (1854–5) 'On the non-restraint system', *JMS* 1: 154, stated that surgical restraint was also exempted from censure. The appendices to the Lunacy Commission's annual reports give an idea of the type of cases that fell under the rubric of surgical restraint.

35 Conolly, *Treatment of the Insane*, p. 31.

36 Edgar Sheppard (1873) *Lectures on Madness in its Medical, Legal, and Social Aspects*, London: J. & A. Churchill, pp. 181, 183.

37 The *JMS* was edited by a long line of staunch non-restraint men, including John C. Bucknill, C. Lockhart Robertson, and Henry Maudsley. For examples of its hostile commentary on the dissidents, see (1854–5) 'The restraint system, as practised at the North and East Ridings Asylum ...' *JMS* 1: 81–3 [Hill]; John Conolly, 'Second notice of the 8th report', 147–8 [Hill and Huxley]; (1856–7) 'Annual reports of the county lunatic asylums', *JMS* 2: 267 [Huxley]. Yellowlees was taken to task in the *Lancet* (4 May 1872): 626. Lauder Lindsay is discussed later in this chapter.

38 (1857) 'Annual reports of county asylums, 1856', *JMS* 3: 482; (1854) 'Letter to the editor', *JMS* 1: 174; (1853) 'British institutions for the insane', *Journal of Psychological Medicine* (hereafter *JPM*) 6: 16. Huxley wrote an article critical of the Lunacy Commission (1858) entitled 'On the existing relation between the Lunacy Commission and medical superintendents of public asylums', *JMS* 5: 95–100. See Hervey, 'A slavish bowing down', pp. 109–11, for more on Huxley's resistance to the Lunacy Commission.

39 CL (1861) 16th *AR*, p. 187. See pp. 187–200 for a long discussion of the whole case. See also CL (1863) 17th *AR*, pp. 74–8; and CL (1864) 18th *AR*, pp. 13–4. The (1858) *JMS* 4: 118–27 mentions Huxley's first problem with the board over the 'wet and dirty' patients.

40 Edgar Sheppard (1867–8) 'On the treatment of a certain class of destructive patients', *JMS* 13: 65–75; (1869–70) 'Correspondence', *JMS* 15: 658–9; and CL (1867) 21st *AR*, pp. 40–2, convey the gist of Sheppard's problems.

41 Winslow's lengthy critique (1854) of the CL 8th *AR*, 'On non-mechanical restraint in the treatment of the insane', *JPM* 7: 541–72, nicely conveys the journal's hostile tone towards non-restraint. Compare also the treatment of Hill's views in (1851) 'British lunatic asylums', *JPM* 4: 557, with the *JMS*

articles cited in note 37. Bynum, 'Themes', pp. 229–30, provides background on Winslow and his journal. Note also that the *JPM* reported favourably on the American views of non-restraint. See, for example (1853) *JPM* 6: 605–7.

42 Hervey, 'A slavish bowing down', provides an excellent exposition of the tensions over centralization.

43 The AMSAII resolution is quoted in John Curwen (ed.) (1875) *History of the Association of Medical Superintendents of American Asylums for the Insane*, privately printed, p. 7. Significantly, it was deleted from the transcript of the proceedings published in the *AJI* in 1844. See Samuel Woodward (1840–1) *Worcester State Hospital, 8th Annual Report*, pp. 79–80; and Isaac Ray (1844) *Maine Hospital for the Insane, Annual Report for 1844*, pp. 30–40, for two early American responses to non-restraint.

44 Ray was quoted in (1863–4) 'Reports of American asylums', *AJI* 20: 488. 'Lunacy in the United States', p. 69, referred to the Americans' conception of restraint as a moral instrument.

45 Joseph Workman to Edward Jarvis, 17 September 1868, C. Lib.

46 Butler's remarks appear in (1855–6) 'AMSAII proceedings', *AJI* 12: 90. The most eloquent explication of this point of view is Isaac Ray's remarks in (1862–3) 'AMSAII proceedings', *AJI* 19: 58–61. The link between arguments against non-restraint and problems in getting patients to work are evident in the discussion following Edward Jarvis's paper on patient employment (1862) 'AMSAII proceedings', *AJI* 19: 57–71. As Warner notes in *The Therapeutic Perspective*, the concept of therapeutic specificity was central to mid-nineteenth-century American medicine.

47 Joshua Worthington (1855–6) 'AMSAII proceedings', *AJI* 12: 90; Charles Nichols (1859–60) 'AMSAII proceedings', *AJI* 16: 61.

48 See D. Tilden Brown (1863–4) 'Meeting of the British Association ... ', *AJI* 20: 270–84, for a good example of the 'servility' argument about the English specialty. The majority of American asylum superintendents opposed the principle of a lunacy commission, passing a resolution to that effect in their 1864 meeting. See (1864–5) 'AMSAII proceeding', *AJI* 21: 152. See also Grob, *Mental Institutions*, pp. 294–7.

49 'Lunacy in the United States', p. 69.

50 Again, I base these conclusions on a wide reading in the superintendents' correspondence, published debates on restraint, and travellers' accounts of American asylums, as well as the 1880 census returns (see note 51). I will cite here only one of the most important sources. Frederick Manning (1868) *Report on Lunatic Asylums*, Sydney, Australia: Richards, has the best claim to be an unprejudiced observer of both English and American hospitals. An Australian physician, he was sent by his government on a grand tour of European and American hospitals in the mid-1860s. Manning stated unequivocally that the Americans used the most mechanical restraint, more even than the continental alienists (p. 120). He also claimed that he saw no restraint in use during his tour of English asylums (p. 116).

51 Frederick Wines (1888) *Report on the Defective, Dependent, and Delinquent Classes of the Population of the United States*, Washington, DC: Government Printing Office, pp. xlii, 145–57.

52 Edward Jarvis made this argument to Sir James Clark in a lengthy letter reviewing American practice, 25 June 1868, Jarvis Letterpress, 1867–9, C. Lib.

53 Other superintendents I would class as 'minimalists' include William Chipley of

the Eastern Lunatic Asylum in Kentucky, Richard Gundry of the Athens, Ohio, asylum; and Joshua Worthington of the Friends Asylum. See Chipley to Jarvis, 4 April 1868, and Worthington to Jarvis, 22 April 1868, C. Lib., for good expositions of the minimalist approach. D. Hack Tuke (1885) *The Insane in the United States and Canada*, London: H.K. Lewis, pp. 58–9, commented on the fact that the American asylum doctors used neither the shower bath nor the wet pack.

54 Thomas Story Kirkbride, *Pennsylvania Hospital for the Insane, Annual Report 1852*, pp. 37, 38. This report contained a full explication of his views on pp. 33–9, passages that were frequently cited as typical of American attitudes towards restraint. See also Tomes, *A Generous Confidence*, pp. 197–8. Bucknill, 'Notes', 4–6, discusses Kirkbride's practice.

55 John Gray (1861) *Utica Lunatic Asylum, 18th Annual Report*, p. 25. On Gray's extensive use of restraint and the protection bed, see Tuke, *The Insane in the United States*, pp. 55, 118. Other practitioners I would describe as 'robust' in their outlook are Pliny Earle and Eugene Grissom.

56 Richard Gundry's remarks (1877) 'AMSAII proceedings', *AJI* 31: 223; Eugene Grissom (1877–8) 'Mechanical protection for the violent insane', *AJI* 34: 31.

57 Edward Jarvis to Sir James Clark, 25 June 1868, C. Lib., cites Kirkbride as the closest representative of Conolly's ideals in the United States. For a larger sense of the asylum politics involved here, see Tomes, *A Generous Confidence*, pp. 264–310.

58 ibid., pp. 281–8; Grob, *Mental Institutions*, pp. 303–42.

59 See, for example, the criticisms in John Galt (1855) 'The farm of St Anne', *AJI* 11: 352–7.

60 Conolly, *Treatment of the Insane*, pp. 343–68, reviews the arguments against non-restraint without once mentioning the United States; his main concern is clearly with the French and German critics.

61 (1864) 'Report on the progress of psychological medicine', *JMS* 10: 574.

62 J. Mortimer Granville (1877) *The Care and Cure of the Insane*, 2 vols, London: Hadwicke & Bogue, reported the *Lancet* Commission findings. On the general sense of demoralization in the specialty, see Bynum, 'Themes', pp. 239–40; and Scull, *Museums of Madness*, pp. 186–220.

63 CL (1880) 34th *AR*, pp. 172–346. On the 'reaction' against non-restraint, see, for example, Thomas L. Rogers (1874) 'The president's address', *JMS* 20: 328–37.

64 Henry Maudsley (1870) 'The treatment of the insane without mechanical restraints', *Practitioner* 5: 197; David Yellowlees (22 June 1872) 'Mechanical restraint in cases of insanity', *Lancet*: 881. Yellowlees's letter was but one of several written in defence of a more flexible interpretation of non-restraint. See 25 May 1872 [J. Murray Lindsay] and 8 June 1872 [W.C. Hills]. Rogers, 'President's address', presents the 'reaction' in a favourable light, as does 'Lunacy in the United States', pp. 69–70.

65 C. Lockhart Robertson (26 December 1868) 'Dr Lauder Lindsay's protection bed . . . ', *Lancet*: 826; W. Lauder Lindsay (1870–1) 'Mollities ossium in relation to rib-fracture among the insane', *AJI* 27: 320, 321 (reprinted from *Edinburgh Medical Journal*, hereafter *EMJ*).

66 Lauder Lindsay, 'Mollities ossium', p. 322. Edgar Sheppard to Isaac Ray, 3 January 1877, Ray Papers, Butler Hospital, refers to his pleasant visit to the US. For the rest of Lauder Lindsay's critical opus, see (1878–9) 'The theory and

practice of non-restraint in the treatment of the insane', *AJI* 35: 272–306 (reprinted from *EMJ*, 1878); (1878–9) 'Mechanical restraint in English Asylums', *AJI* 35: 543–55; and (1879–80) 'The protection bed and its uses', *AJI* 36: 404–21 (reprinted from *EMJ*, 1880).

67 Clement Walker's remarks (1874–5) 'AMSAII proceeding', *AJI* 31: 182. See 160–6 for the abstract of Mark Ranney's paper. Note particularly how he incorporates the arguments of the English dissidents into his defence of American practice on p. 166.

68 J.C. Bucknill to T.S. Kirkbride, 30 March 1879, Institute of the Pennsylvania Hospital Archives (hereafter IPHA); Bucknill's remarks (1875–6) 'AMSAII proceedings', *AJI* 32: 269. J. Bucknill to E. Jarvis, 31 October 1875, C. Lib., refers to his feeling that non-restraint was 'dangerous ground' for discussion during his visit.

69 [J. Mortimer Granville] (13 November 1875) *Lancet*: 706, 707. In a subsequent issue (16 September 1876) the editor printed a retraction of sorts. See Bucknill, 'Notes', vii.

70 John Bucknill (1876) 'Speech ... ', *AJI* 33: 327. Bucknill defended the Americans in this speech to the Medico-Psychological Association, referring indignantly to subsequent attacks in the *Lancet* on Charles Nichols, the beleaguered superintendent of the Government Asylum. The association passed a resolution expressing sympathy with physicians who were innocent victims of partisan politics, but explicitly withheld approval of American medical practice. Bucknill's original letter defending the Americans, 'American lunatic asylums', appeared (12 February 1876) in the *Lancet*: 263.

71 Bucknill, 'American lunatic asylums', p. 263; (25 March 1876) 'Notes on asylums for the insane', *Lancet*: 457.

72 Bucknill, 'Speech', p. 327. J. Bucknill to T. Kirkbride, 30 March 1879, IPHA, conveys his sense of puzzlement about Kirkbride's lack of professional leadership on restraint.

73 Hervey Wilbur (1877) *The Management of the Insane in Great Britain*, Albany, NY: Weed, Parsons & Co.; his study first appeared in 1876 as part of the State Board of Charities report. That same year, Wilbur wrote another controversial paper (1876) 'Governmental supervision of the insane', *Conference of Charities Proceedings* 3: 82–90.

74 For other examples of how the asylum critics used English precedent, see [Charles Folsom] (13 April 1876) 'The treatment of insanity', *BMSJ* 94: 435–7; and [Editorial] (2 September 1876) *The Medical Record (N.Y.)*: 575–6.

75 (1877) 'AMSAII proceedings', *AJI* 31: 217–37 suggests the range of reactions to Bucknill's comments.

76 Thomas Story Kirkbride (1877) *Pennsylvania Hospital for the Insane Annual Report*, p. 35. Although he mentions no names, pp. 29–52 of this report can be read as an extended critique of Wilbur, Folsom, and Bucknill.

77 Grissom, 'Mechanical protection', 58.

78 (2 September 1876) *The Medical Record (N.Y.)* 575.

79 Hervey B. Wilbur (1881) '"Chemical restraint" in the management of the insane', *Archives of Medicine* 6: 271–92. For a similar study that reaches similar conclusions, see J.M. Bannister and H.N. Moyer (1882) 'Non-restraint and seclusion in American institutions for the insane', *JMND* 9: 457–78.

80 Peter Bryce (1876) *Alabama Insane Hospital Annual Report* 16: 25. For accounts of these early non-restraint asylums in the US, see Peter Bryce (1890–

1) 'Mechanical restraint of the insane', *Medico-Legal Journal* 8: 311–13; John C. Shaw (1880) 'The practicability and value of non-restraint in treating the insane', *Conference of Charities and Corrections Proceedings* 7: 137–42; Alice Bennett (1884) 'Mechanical restraint in the treatment of the insane', *Medico-Legal Journal* 1: 285–96.

81 (1858–9) *JMS* 191; [Folsom], 'Treatment of insanity', 228. Folsom was quoting a letter he had received from an English alienist (unidentified).

82 See Tomes, *A Generous Confidence*, esp. p. 269.

83 Kirkbride's remarks (1875–6) 'AMSAII proceedings', *AJI* 32: 338–9. Bucknill related the Americans' timidity on restraint to their 'painful sensibility to public opinion' in his article (18 March 1876) *Lancet*: 418.

84 For a sense of the convergence of attitudes, see A.M. Shew (1879) 'Mechanical restraint', *AJI* 35: 556–62. I have not yet done enough work in the 1880s and 1890s to assess how far this convergence really went. I suspect that American practice stayed less uniform well into the early twentieth century.

CHAPTER EIGHT

Hysteria, hypnosis, and the lure of the invisible: the rise of neo-mesmerism in *fin-de-siècle* French psychiatry

Anne Harrington

> Some of the most advanced practitioners in Paris are being led back to processes and theories strangely like Mesmer's own, but even more transcendental.[1]

Historians of medicine (unless they are explicitly concerned with popular culture) generally regard the history of mesmerism and the history of hypnosis more or less as a seamless entity, with the 'modern science of hypnosis' rising, phoenix-like, from the ashes of Anton Mesmer's animal magnetism. Although these historians differ in their chronological emphasis and the orientation of their analysis, consensus is pretty broad that it was some time in the nineteenth century that medical thinking passed from its so-called 'pre-scientific' era (dominated by speculation about 'fluids' or occult forces flowing between operator and subject), to its 'scientific' era (oriented towards experimentation and positivist description). The story of how this alleged cognitive shift took place boasts a number of heroes; and historians differ again in their assessment as to which of these should be given pride of place. One man, however, always figures high on the list: the charismatic, somewhat forbidding figure of Jean-Martin Charcot (1825–93), France's pre-eminent clinical neurologist in the late nineteenth century.

Indeed, the historical record is quite clear on certain basic facts. In the late 1870s, Charcot first began to turn his attention to the study of hypnosis, finally reading a report of his findings before the French Académie des Sciences in 1882. This was the same learned body that had harshly condemned hypnosis twice in the past century under the name of animal magnetism. Charcot, however, was a man whose reputation was such that he could not be denied a hearing, and the academy listened to what he had to say – soberly and respectfully. In his 1882 paper, the great neurologist sternly eschewed any reference to invisible fluids or occult forces. Instead he described hypnosis as an artificially induced modification of the nervous system that could be produced only in hysterical patients. It manifested itself in three distinct phases: catalepsy, lethargy, and somnambulism. Each of these was induced by strictly physical means, and could be identified by special physiological signs: waxy rigidity, neuro-muscular hyper-excitability, somnambulistic contractures, etc.[2] By transforming hypnosis into a type of artificially induced pathology that followed physiologically explicable laws, Charcot managed, in one fell swoop, both to give an aura of medical respectability to a formerly shunned and suspect subject, and simultaneously to stake a clear claim to the medical profession's exclusive competency to deal with this subject. It was, as Janet[3] would later put it, a true *tour de force* of persuasion that opened the door to a 'golden age' in France of hypnosis and hysteria research and theory.

All this is true enough as far as it goes, but the picture it conveys is all the same misleading in its selectivity. A wider perspective on research activities within the great hospitals and asylums of nineteenth-century France shows that Charcot's views on hypnotizable hysterics did *not* spell the death toll of Anton Mesmer's animal magnetism. Quite the contrary: the work of the Charcot school on hypnosis and hysteria was conceptually linked to – and actually helped inspire – a reawakening of interest in the fundamental ideas of biomagnetism as taught by the old mesmerists. Both for the fresh angle it offers on France's intellectual love affair with hypnosis and for the broader questions it raises about the social and institutional context of this affair, French 'neo-mesmerism' is a subject that is ripe for serious historical scrutiny.[4]

Metalloscopy and the birth of 'grand hypnotisme'

Mesmerism walked into the wards of Charcot's Salpêtrière – incognito – in 1876. The bearer was a French doctor whose name deserves to be better known in the history of psychiatry: Victor Jean-Marie Burq (1822–84).[5] In August 1876, Burq wrote a letter to Claude Bernard, the illustrious president of the no less illustrious Paris Société de Biologie. Here he explained how over the past twenty-five years he had been curing women suffering from hysterical anaesthesia by applying metallic plates to the afflicted parts of their bodies. This system of treatment, christened by Burq 'metallotherapy', had been scorned or ignored by the official medical community for decades (in spite of the fact that Burq presented the French academies of science and medicine with no fewer than twenty-two reports of his findings between 1847 and 1853 alone!). In a more or less desperate final attempt to gain recognition, Burq now asked Bernard if the Société de Biologie would be willing to investigate and pass judgement on the validity of all his life's labour.

Bernard, with commendable courtesy and open-mindedness, agreed. Not only that, but he took Burq seriously enough to appoint what surely struck contemporaries as a first-rate commission to investigate the old man's work: Jean-Martin Charcot, chief physician at la Salpêtrière hospital and vice-president of the Société de Biologie since 1860; Amédée Dumontpallier (1827–99), a neuropathologist at la Pitié hospital and former favoured student of Claude Bernard himself; and Jules Bernard Luys (1828–96), a neuroanatomist and physician at la Salpêtrière, and soon to be appointed chief physician at la Charité hospital.

Burq was invited to Charcot's Salpêtrière, where a series of experiments and clinical trials was carried out between 1876 and 1877, focusing chiefly on a select group of female patients suffering from hysterical hemi-anaesthesia (anaesthesia affecting one lateral half of the body only). And when the commission reported back to the Société de Biologie one year later, it was thoroughly enthusiastic.[6] It is true that there were some doubts about the long-term therapeutic value of Burq's method; and it was for this reason that the commission dropped the term 'metallotherapy' and limited its discussion in this report to *metalloscopy* – the 'immediate phenomena determined ... by the action of metals on the cutaneous surface', but without curative intent. At the same time, the genuineness of the metallic effects on hysterical insensibility was resoundingly affirmed, and it was reported that other agents – notably magnets, static electricity, and electric currents – had also been found effective (all these agents would eventually be subsumed under the umbrella heading 'aesthesiogens'). In addition to confirming Burq's essential claims about the effects of metals on hysterical anaesthesia, the commission reported that successful trials had also been carried out on cases of hysterical paralysis, amblyopia (blindness), achromatopsia (colour-blindness), deafness, and even – in a few carefully observed instances – hemiparalysis of known organic or toxic origin. Keenly aware of the startling nature of its claims, the commission then proceeded to air a variety of sober-sounding electrical, electrochemical, and physical theories intended to bring the whole enterprise safely back into the uncompromising framework of nineteenth-century science.[7]

Finally, the Société de Biologie was told how a wholly new discovery – unsuspected even by Burq – had been made in the course of investigation. It seemed that when sensation was restored to a region on one half of the body of a hemi-anaesthetic patient, a symmetrical region on the normally healthy or sensitive side of the body *lost* its normal cutaneous sensibility – or motor capacity, vision, auditory capacity, etc. As Charcot put it at the time: 'It appears with these hysterics, that the nervous fluid, if one will pardon the expression, does not transport itself to one side until after it has in part abandoned the other.'[8] It was Dumontpallier who – inspired by a morning visit to the bank – had proposed to christen this most striking and novel finding the 'law of transfer'.[9]

The discovery of transfer occupies an important place in our story, for the idea of transfer (much extended beyond its original metalloscopic roots) would go on to play an important role in later neo-mesmeric practice and theory. Before all that could happen, however, another critical event in French medicine had to occur: Charcot had to discover hypnosis.

Now there is no denying that Charcot probably became interested in hypnosis for a number of reasons.[10] Nevertheless, the historical record is also quite clear that Burq's metalloscopy was critical to Charcot's decision in the late 1870s to involve himself and his entourage in a full-scale investigation of artificial catalepsy, lethargy, and somnambulism.

To understand how this might have been, it is now necessary to explain that the treatment of hysterics using metals had been tangled up with mesmerism from its earliest beginnings under Burq. A believer since the 1840s in the virtues of Anton Mesmer's animal magnetism, Burq's interest in the therapeutic value of metals took its starting-point from his early interest in the phenomenon of mesmeric insensibility or anaesthesia in the trance state. In 1847, he made the fateful discovery that *copper* tended at once to restore the sensibility of subjects with a strong mesmeric aptitude *and* to dissolve the mesmeric state (or, alternatively, to make such a state impossible to induce). That is to say, this metal was at one and the same time an anti-anaesthetic and an anti-mesmeric agent. Why should this be? Burq's answer was that there was something special about insensibility in mesmerism; it was not simply one of the signs, but the actual groundwork of mesmerism – in Burq's words, 'an essential condition of magnetic sleep'. No anaesthesia, no magnetic sleep. Copper's capacity to restore sensibility and dissolve a mesmeric trance were simply two sides of the same coin.[11]

Now, that there was some sort of unclear affinity between the mesmeric state and the hysterical condition had long been recognized by Burq, as indeed by many of the early magnetizers in general.[12] Burq's copper experiments, however, now predisposed him to focus particularly on the fact that both conditions were typically characterized by anaesthesia. It occurred to him that perhaps loss of sensibility in hysteria was, just like in mesmeric sleep, the essential phenomenon, the precondition for producing all the other symptoms. If this were so, then conceivably a metal like copper – which could stop a mesmeric trance dead in its tracks – could equally cure patients suffering from hysteria. Trials were made (with copper and soon with a variety of other metals as well), and proved successful, at least to Burq's satisfaction. Metallotherapy was born.

It is true that when Burq wrote to Claude Bernard in 1876, he prudently made no reference to the pivotal role played by mesmerism in the development of his metallic therapy. Nevertheless, there is good reason to believe that his interest in the relationship between hysteria and magnetic sleep did not escape the notice of the 1876 Société de Biologie Commission. Admittedly, the commission's 1877 report on Burq limited itself to the data gathered on hysteria and made no reference to hypnosis (let alone mesmerism with its postulated fluids). Nevertheless, by the time that report was presented, the first investigations into hypnosis had already begun, and not a few of these explicitly focused on the effective role of aesthesiogenic agents in artificial catalepsy, lethargy, and somnambulism.

Some of the new studies, like the work carried out by Dumontpallier and his assistant Paul Magnin, essentially confirmed Burq's view of the stimulating, anti-hypnotic nature of such agents as metals.[13] Other studies, however, seemed to suggest that at least some aesthesiogenic agents, notably the magnet, could also *cause* hypnosis.[14] This idea, that one and the same agent could have a diametrically opposite physiological effect, is not simply a flagrant contradiction in the literature which somehow was overlooked. The key to understanding it is to be found in one aspect of the commission's metalloscopy research not yet mentioned. This was the discovery – following the discovery of transfer and closely linked to it conceptually – that the same agents which *restored* sensibility on the anaesthetic side of the body could, when applied to the sensitive or healthy side, cause *loss* of sensibility.[15] Charcot called this phenomenon 'provoked anaesthesia' or 'metallic anaesthesia', and he came to believe that it could serve as a powerful diagnostic tool in cases where a patient might seem to be cured, but in fact still possessed latent hysterical tendencies.[16]

Now, if aesthesiogenic agents could both inhibit and provoke a state of hysteria, and if Burq were right in arguing for a close physiological relationship between hysteria and mesmerism, then the conclusion followed that such agents might equally be able to provoke or inhibit a trance state in an appropriately sensitive (hysterical) subject. What happened next, it seems, is that this basic idea became increasingly generalized and dissociated from its original metalloscopic roots.[17] Finally, by 1882 or so, when Charcot presented his hypnosis paper to the Académie des Sciences, it had been transformed into the Salpêtrière doctrine that hypnosis could be induced and broken using a wide range of physical agents acting on the nervous system of the hysterical patient via the sensibility (including the special senses). And the curious property of such agents to both provoke and inhibit hypnotic phenomena would soon be generalized by Dumontpallier into the paradoxical 'law' of hypnosis: '*la chose qui fait, défait*'.[18]

Two points must now be made. First, even if it is true that the rise of hypnosis research in Paris owed much to the influence of an old mesmerist named Burq, it is also clear that Charcot himself can in no sense be called a mesmerist, since he rejected the notion of a biomagnetic fluid. At the same time (and this takes us to our second point), Charcot's entry into hypnosis via metalloscopy meant that he did end up acknowledging important chunks of the same phenomenological reality as the old magnetizers, who had long associated metallic and magnetic therapies with animal magnetism. This is significant because it implies that some form of biomagnetism was always one of his cognitive options (though doubtless his most dangerous one). Consequently, even if he and his followers at the Salpêtrière chose to empty mesmerism of its fluidistic soul and call it 'hypnosis', that does not mean that all his colleagues in other institutions – seeking to make sense of more or less the same phenomenological reality as he – would necessarily toe the line with the Salpêtrière workers on that decision.

The rise of neo-mesmerism: basic issues and themes

Sure enough, the primary literature attests to the continuing viability of the biomagnetic alternative in orthodox French medicine during the last two decades of the nineteenth century. The story which can be pieced together from this literature is rich with colourful personalities and dramatic confrontations, and in a longer work would certainly deserve to be told in full. For the purposes of this chapter, however, I must be content with a brief descriptive overview of the key themes running through French neo-mesmerism as it evolved – and declined – during the period from *c.* 1880 into the first years of the new century. By focusing first on the intellectual parameters of neo-mesmerism, I will then be in a position, in the concluding section of this chapter, to suggest some ways in which the movement might begin to be understood within the larger institutional and social context of *fin-de-siècle* French psychiatry.

The 'radiating neurique force'

Neo-mesmerism began the process of defining itself by taking the old biomagnetic fluid of Mesmer and the old magnetizers, and recasting it in terms of the professional concerns and technical vocabulary of late-nineteenth-century French psychiatry. In its new form, Mesmer's animal magnetism was to be viewed as a problem for neurology; a force that would ultimately be demystified through increased understanding of the physics and physiology of human nervous activity. It was the French physician, A. Barety, who coined the term, soon to be widely adopted, 'radiating neurique force' (*'force neurique rayonnante'*), in the course of calling for a scientific rehabilitation of fluidism before the Société de Biologie in 1881.

Barety had a great deal to say about both the physics and physiology of his neurique force, but it will suffice here simply to note his belief – based, as he stressed, on careful clinical and experimental observation – that this force 'radiated' from the nervous system through three principal ports: the eyes (or optic nerves), the fingers (or palmar and dorsal collateral digital nerves), and the mouth via the breath (or pneumogastric nerves). These three types of radiating neurique force (optic, digital, pneumatic) produced distinct physiological effects on predisposed or sensitive subjects: variously causing hyperaesthesia, anaesthesia, muscular contractions and decontractions, somnambulism, etc. Barety's findings on this point cast considerable new light, he believed, on the odd (indeed, rather unseemly) methods traditionally used by mesmerists to manipulate their subjects (the 'passes' up and down the length of the body, the mutual locking of gazes, the intimate mingling of breath, etc.). Barety called attention as well to the conceptual continuity between his own work and the recent metalloscopy and hypnosis studies, pointing out that all the physiological modifications produced by the neurique force were 'strongly analogous to those produced by electricity, and more particularly the magnet, from whence the name *animal magnetism* created by Mesmer'.[19] The Société de Biologie – which had by now become rather accustomed to bearing witness to the domestication of the extraordinary – could hardly but agree that the notion of a human biomagnetic force was, at least in principle, scarcely more remarkable than metallic and magnetic therapies and the provoking of bizarre artificial neurological states. Dumontpallier, for example, declared that the idea of a neurique force was the only means of accounting for the singular way hysterics react under the impression of the hypnotist's fingers, gaze, and breath. Over the next several months, he would publish a number of papers analysing the potential of the neurique fluid as a new approach to cerebral localization – before finally recanting in a major 1882 paper before the Académie des Sciences, and more or less aligning his school of hypnosis at la Pitié hospital with that being developed by Charcot at la Salpêtrière.[20] Ultimately (as will be seen shortly) it would fall to the third member of the 1876 Société de Biologie Commission – Jules Bernard Luys and his school of hypnosis at la Charité – to carry the case for human biomagnetism into ever more transcendent realms.

Action of medicines 'at a distance'

Luys' entry into the history of neo-mesmerism is inextricably bound up with the rise of the next key theme on our roster: the so-called action of medicines 'at a distance'. The basic idea here was that, under certain circumstances, the peculiarly sensitive nervous system of the hysterical patient was capable of responding to the action of medicines and toxic substances sealed in glass containers and placed at a distance from the subject. The phenomenon had been discovered accidentally at the École de médecine navale at Rochefort by the physicians Henri Bourru and Ferdinand Burot, in the course of performing some metalloscopy experiments on their highly talented (male) hysterical patient, Louis Vivé. The discovery some months later of a second appropriately sensitive subject, Victorine M., permitted the two doctors to confirm their ever more intriguing results, and to present a report of their findings to the 1885 congress of the Association française pour l'Avancement des Sciences in Grenoble. There they explained how potassium set on a table some feet away caused patients to sneeze and yawn compulsively; how opium applied to the head brought on a state of deep sleep; and how valerian had the particularly striking effect of causing patients to drop to all fours and behave like cats.[21] Although reluctant to commit themselves prematurely to any one theory, the two doctors tentatively sought an explanation for all these data in 'radiations'.[22] Others were less prudent. A. Berjon's book-length 1886 analysis of the case of Louis Vivé argued strongly for a link between the action of medicines at a distance and Barety's radiating neurique fluid, and Eugene Alliot that same year made the Rochefort findings the centrepiece of his lyrical microcosmic/macrocosmic analysis of the universe as an infinitely huge battery.[23]

While attempts were made in hospitals all over Paris and the provinces to reproduce Bourru and Burot's results, it was Luys – newly appointed chief physician at la Charité hospital – who would really make this subject his own. In August 1887, he presented the Académie de Médecine with a résumé of his extensive researches into the 'experimental solicitation of emotions' in hypnotized hysterics through the action of medicines at a distance. Startled by his claims (which, as the secretary wryly observed, were reminiscent of tales 'aux temps fabuleux'), the Académie took the unprecedented step of appointing a commission to investigate the research claims of one of its own members. The commission's report, presented to the Académie in 1888, was highly critical. Yet – ironically enough – this censuring, far from squelching the nascent neo-mesmeric movement, would actually play a pivotal role in its further consolidation. After 1888, Luys and the other neo-mesmerists would increasingly close ranks, seek fresh allies from other, less orthodox corners, and turn to publishing in journals founded explicitly for the purposes of championing the new biomagnetic ideas.[24]

The discovery of human polarity

Matters took a new turn with the announced discovery by the French physicians, L.-Th. Chazarain and Ch. Dècle, in 1886 (coinciding with the first rush of studies on medicines acting 'at a distance') that the human biomagnetic force was *polarized*, just like the electro-magnetic force of the physicists. This was an important development from a metaphysical perspective, since it brought to the foreground the idea that there were essential links of continuity flowing between the human and the cosmic realms of action. It was also important, however, because it enabled the neo-mesmerists to draw sweeping conclusions about the biomagnetic 'laws' operating in metalloscopy, transfer, and hypnosis. By purporting to reveal the dynamic pattern of currents and polarized forces operating beneath the flux of experimental phenomena, the neo-mesmerists put themselves in a position to achieve two significant ends. First and foremost, they could disarm those outright critics of the metalloscopy, transfer, and hypnosis experiments, who – favouring one or another psychological explanation of these studies – pointed to the apparently equivocal, conflicting nature of the results. Second, they could claim a conceptual victory over their colleagues in the field who had chosen to follow the Charcot school in its physiological but *non-fluidist* approach to the phenomena of metalloscopy and hypnosis. In contrast to the neo-mesmerists, it was clear that non-fluidists like Charcot were in no position to offer science any all-embracing framework capable of synthesizing all the hypnosis and hysteria data gathered over the past decade.[25]

For Luys and his workers at la Charité hospital, the discovery of human polarity would also serve as a source of inspiration for a variety of new directions in biomagnetic research. In the last years of the 1880s, this school established to its satisfaction that magnets and certain metals were capable of polarizing the opposing emotional states associated with the positive and negative sides of the biomagnetic force. These opposing emotional states could then be localized in the two lateral halves of a hypnotized subject's body (while a line of artificially induced emotional 'indifference' would spontaneously manifest itself in the middle). The Charité also extensively documented the contrasting psychological and physiological effects induced by bringing hypnotized patients in near proximity to the two opposing poles of a mineral magnet. In general, the north (positive) pole brought on a feeling of well-being and pleasure, the south (negative) pole a sense of repulsion and fear.[26]

New biomagnetic directions in 'transfer' research

Since the late 1870s, research into the phenomena of transfer had been proceeding at a brisk pace. In 1885, two of Charcot's most able students, Alfred Binet and Charles Féré, announced in the pages of Théodule Ribot's distinguished journal *Revue philosophique* that they had been able to use a magnet to transfer from one half of the body to the other, not only sensory-motor symptoms, but psychological phenomena as well – unilateral voluntary actions, hallucinations and certain forms of intellectual activity (especially verbal tasks which could exploit the fact that language is a unilateral cerebral function, normally controlled by the left side of the brain). Binet and Féré called this phenomenon 'psychic transfer'.

A second report published by the authors shortly afterwards went one step further, arguing that 'the idea of transfer is too narrow to embrace the totality of phenomena which the magnet is capable of provoking in the organism, within a certain category of subjects at least'. A new interpretive framework was now volunteered, under the name of 'psychic polarization'. This referred to the alleged capacity of the magnet to turn a sensation, perception, and even emotional state into its corresponding opposite. Working mostly with the Salpêtrière's star hysteric, Blanche Wittmann, Féré and Binet explained how they had been able to transform a hallucination of red into its polar opposite, green; to make a subject successively 'recall' and 'forget' a particular memory; to turn laughter into depression, anger into love.[27]

More startling still was the announced discovery in 1886 by another of Charcot's most gifted students, Joseph Babinski, that the magnet could be used to transfer hysterical disorders, not just between different halves of the body, but between different *patients*. Speaking before the Paris Société de Psychologie Physiologique, Babinski described how one hemi-anaesthetic patient, A., had been made to take up the half-sensibility of another hemi-anaesthetic patient, B., making A. fully sensitive and B. fully anaesthetic. The transfer had then reversed itself, B. taking back both her own sensibility and that of A., leaving the latter anaesthetic on both sides of her body.[28]

Now, it is true that these new transfer researches were not explicitly interpreted by Charcot's students from a fluidist or biomagnetic perspective, but that in the end hardly mattered. For any observer with fluidist leanings, the data reported by these representatives of Charcot's camp spoke for themselves. Consequently, in 1891 Jules Bernard Luys and his young colleague Gérard Encausse (soon to become renowned in occult circles as 'Papus') were pleased to cite the precedent of Babinski when they announced before the Société de Biologie that an iron crown placed on the head of a patient was capable of absorbing and artificially preserving the pathological biomagnetic effluvia underlying his or her neuropathic states, hallucinations, and delusions. These disorders could then be transferred to a second patient by placing the same crown on his or her head. In outlining the details of their findings, Luys and Encausse also spoke hopefully about their therapeutic implications – if *pathological* nervous states could be artificially absorbed, stored, and transferred, then perhaps *healthy* ones could as well.[29]

Luys had in fact at this time already developed the idea of transfer into a powerful therapeutic technique, but without the use of iron crowns. In his 'laboratoire d'hypnologie' at la Charité (overseen since 1889 by Gérard Encausse) a trained hypnotized subject would be seated facing the patient targeted for treatment. The two would clasp hands, and Luys would then pass a magnet over the body of the patient in order to draw out his diseased 'effluvia' and pull them into the body of the subject. At each such pass, the subject would experience an involuntary convulsion as magnetic absorption was supposedly effected. At length the subject would have acquired the symptoms of whatever disorder the patient was suffering from (and generally his personality as well), while the patient himself would normally feel much better. The subject would then be rid of her acquired disease through the force of 'imperative suggestion'.[30]

The exteriorization of the sensibility

Early in the 1890s, the Charité also began to report that certain highly sensitive hysterics had proved themselves capable of *seeing* the magnetic effluvia radiating from the bodies of living beings (notably the doctors themselves), as well as from such non-living sources as mineral magnets and electrical currents. Resembling a flickering flame, the effluvia were a brilliant and beautiful blue colour when emanating from the positive (attractive) pole of a magnet and the left side of a human being, and a rather hellish, frightening red when emanating from the negative (repulsive) pole of a magnet and the right side of a human being.[31] It was clear to the Charité workers that, among other things, they had stumbled here on to an important confirmation of the essential truth of human polarity.[32]

But matters were quickly to grow more complex. The leading French occultist, Colonel Albert de Rochas, who – like Encausse – had come to the Charité hospital at Luys' invitation to carry out biomagnetic research, was working during this period with a certain hysterical subject, Albert L. This young man not only had a highly developed ability to perceive the biomagnetic effluvia, but was a trained draughtsman and amateur artist as well. He was therefore able, through sketches and paintings, to clarify for his doctors exactly what this radiating fluid looked like. And out of this doctor/patient collaboration, a number of new facts became clear. The most important of these was that the biomagnetic force manifested itself in two forms. In its first, *dynamic* incarnation, it radiated outwards from key points such as the eyes, nostrils, mouth, etc., much as Barety had said. In its second, *static* form, however, it also surrounded the entire surface of the human body in a sort of blanket of luminous colour (blue on one side, red on the other).

It was then discovered that these 'enveloping layers' of biomagnetic fluid could serve as an external point of reference for the sensibility of the individual. If de Rochas plunged a needle into the floating sensible zones of an appropriately sensitive subject, he or she felt a prick in a corresponding portion of his or her body. If a child's doll was allowed to absorb some of the fluid from these zones and then covertly pricked, the subject felt a pain in a region that corresponded to the abused portion of the doll's body. If a glass of water was 'sensitized' by being placed in the subject's hand, then taken away and partially emptied, the subject experienced an overwhelming sense of suffocation until she was allowed to drink from the glass herself. De Rochas' work on the 'exteriorization of the sensibility' attracted considerable, mostly negative attention from the medical community, even as it was rapidly incorporated into the popular culture of the occult. As late as 1909, the leading popular magnetizer Hector Durville would still turn to this work as the point of departure for his own studies on the spiritist phenomenon of 'phantom formation'.[33]

Objectifying the invisible

The final stage of neo-mesmerism's (increasingly unsuccessful) effort to define and justify itself within the framework of orthodox medicine and natural science manifested itself in a series of attempts to make the radiating biomagnetic force objectively tangible to sceptical colleagues. For some neo-mesmerists concerned with this task, the technology of photography seemed to beckon like a promise. Thus the well-known Parisian physician Hippolyte Baraduc described in his works on the 'iconography of the invisible fluidic' how an impression from the luminous vibration of the soul could be captured on a sensitive photographic plate. 'Today the photographic plate permits each of us to catch a glimpse of these hidden forces, and thus subjects the marvellous to an unimpeachable control in making it enter the natural domain of experimental physics.' Similarly, Luys and a colleague David told the Société de Biologie and the Académie des Sciences how the biomagnetic effluvia emanating from the human body had proved itself susceptible to 'photographic registration' through new techniques developed at la Charité. Through photography, the doctors affirmed, the fluid of the old magnetizers would find its final 'certificate of scientific reality'.[34]

The photographic plate, however, was not the only means employed to make the emperor show his clothes. Others sought scientific certification through the construction of special instruments designed to register and measure the action of the biomagnetic force. Professor Paul Joire's 'sthénomètre' – a needle suspended inside a hermetically sealed glass globe – was at the time probably the best known of these, coming as it did from such an impeccably respectable source. As a human hand approached the instrument, the needle inside was said to move. Technology thus served witness to the fact – whatever narrow-minded critics might say – that there existed in nature (in Joire's words) '*a special force, which transmits itself at a distance, emanating from the living organism, and seeming to be particularly dependent on the nervous system*'.[35]

Neo-mesmerism in *fin-de-siècle* medicine: towards a framework for interpretation

The rise, consolidation, and ultimate decline of a neo-mesmeric movement within the great hospitals and asylums of France raises questions far too numerous and complex to receive anything approaching adequate treatment in a brief chapter such as this. My goal in this final section is therefore not so much to place neo-mesmerism in its larger intellectual, social, and institutional context myself, as to signpost at least some of the issues which I believe any adequate contextual analysis would have to address.

The intellectual context

One could begin then with some questions about the plausibility of the biomagnetic thesis as a system of medical or scientific thought according to the standards of the time. It is noteworthy, for example, that there was nothing in late-nineteenth-century French neurophysiology that *a priori* ruled out the possibility that nervous energy could 'radiate' out of the body. In these years before nervous action had come to be necessarily or even normally conceived in terms of measurable impulses passing over defined nervous fibres, such leading physiologists as Charles Edouard Brown-Séquard would speak regularly in their writings about the 'nervous energy' as if this were some sort of commodity that accumulated in the nervous system and was then released along channels of least resistance – if denied one pathway, it would take another.[36] If things really functioned this way, who was in a position to say arbitrarily that nervous action might not sometimes be perpetuated down paths beyond the strict confines of the nervous system?

The world of late-nineteenth-century physics – a splendid baroque world of rarefied ethers, invisible energy fields, moving lines of force, waves and undulations – certainly did not appear to rule out this provocative possibility, any more than did the world of neurophysiology. Quite the contrary; from the beginning, the 'invisible Universe proclaimed by the new physics' (as the astronomer Camille Flammarion put it in 1886) was regarded by the neo-mesmerists themselves as one of their most important allies. Drawing on the claims and vocabulary of physics (especially electromagnetism) in much the same loose way that some parapsychologists today draw on that of quantum mechanics, these men stressed how (in the words of one of the Charité school workers):

> We are surrounded in nature by a subtle force that scientific men call ether, and which is supposed to be imponderable; it would seem possible that this ambient medium – the nature of its substance being unknown – may transmit the perturbations of nerve power.... The brain nerve cells vibrate under the influence of different causes, why should it be thought that the movement does not extend further than the cranium?[37]

The fact that the neo-mesmerists sought to locate their work squarely in the world of nineteenth-century physics and physiology is important because it forces one to focus on the fact that neo-mesmerism must in the end be judged a *materialistic* doctrine.[38] On the intellectual battlefield of late-nineteenth-century hypnosis research, it stood firmly beside Charcot's physiological school in its opposition to the 'unscientific' psychologizing associated with the Bernheim school at Nancy. This state of affairs had certain necessary repercussions on the relationship which would develop between the hypnosis workers at la Salpêtrière and those, say, at la Charité. While neo-mesmerism may have started out as a sober rival to the non-fluidist alternative of Charcot, it had evolved by the early 1890s into a slightly embarrassing eccentric relation that the Charcot workers could not easily condemn outright because such condemnation would have been seen by enemies at Nancy and elsewhere as having too many uncomfortable self-referential implications. As things stood, it was already all too easy for outside observers indiscriminately to lump the groups together. Fulgence Raymond was not saying anything particularly original when he expressed his belief before the second Congrès International de l'Hypnotisme Expérimental et Thérapeutique in 1890, that 'the quarrel which has arisen between the Salpêtrière school and the Nancy school is nothing but a renewal of that which formerly divided the fluidists and the animists' in the time of Mesmer.[39]

The social/political context

The neo-mesmeric movement in late-nineteenth-century France also raises a number of important questions about the relationship between French neuropsychiatry at this time and the wider landscape of French politics, anti-clericalism, and secularism. Jan Goldstein has argued that important aspects of French research into hysteria at this time can be understood only in the context of the anti-clericalism of the Third Republic's government and its social programme for secularization through science. She focuses on the extent to which the Charcot school's early work on hysteria was directed towards a reinterpretation of various Catholic religious categories into 'natural-pathological' ones. By denigrating the putative saints and demons of the past into nothing more than a series of undiagnosed cases of hysteria, Goldstein argues that Charcot and his workers consciously and actively collaborated with the government in its attempt to undermine the ideological foundations of the church and thus strip it of its political power.[40]

But is this the whole story? The neo-mesmeric movement – a product of the same social and political environment as the anti-clerical hysteria studies with which Goldstein is concerned – suggests that in fact French psychiatry's relationship with the supernatural under the Third Republic was as much interactive as parasitic. Certainly, some medical men might have used science to 'pathologize' the supernatural, but there was nothing in the rules that forbade others from setting the equation up the other way – and using French psychiatry's appropriation of the bizarre world of hysteria and hypnosis as a pathway back to the supernatural. The story of neo-mesmerism thus highlights an important ambivalence in the way nineteenth-century psychiatry in France (as elsewhere) tended to conceptualize the relationship between the pathological and the supernatural, and offers itself as an instructive example of how that ambivalence played itself out within a particular social and political environment.

In this case, the environment would seem to be one that, as much as it may have been conducive to anti-clericalism in science, was no less a breeding-ground for the rise of a certain disillusionment with cold, impersonal secularism. A full analysis of neo-mesmerism in French psychiatry would surely have to ask questions about how far the medical men who became involved in the movement found in their research (much like the British psychical researchers working during this same period) a means of giving voice to a type of ill-defined, unchurched or non-institutionalized religious yearning after the transcendent or miraculous.

The institutional/interpersonal context

Now, all these tensions running under the surface of the neo-mesmeric movement naturally did not exist in an institutional vacuum, but acted themselves out in the real world of doctor/patient relations. Most historical studies that focus more or less exclusively on Charcot and his immediate circle tend to emphasize the exploitative nature of the French hysteria and hypnosis research programme, in which an aggressive male doctor manipulates his passive, intimidated female patients in pursuit of some abstract scientific aim. The neo-mesmeric literature, however, reveals that a more complex interpersonal relationship may have developed in at least some French asylums. The hysterical patient was not only a degenerate wretch; he or she was also gifted with supernormal powers to see and respond to a marvellous reality beyond the perception of the doctor. We thus see here the human face of the intellectual ambivalence already noted in the nineteenth century's conception of the relationship between the pathological and the supernatural – an ambivalence that would in turn spawn another one. Yes, French asylum hypnosis and hysteria researchers exploited and manipulated their patients, but at least some of them were not a little awed by the results they were producing, and not a little susceptible to being manipulated themselves. Indeed, the Belgian medical hypnotist Crocq, looking back in 1902 at his earlier – and apparently resoundingly successful – efforts to call forth exteriorization of the sensibility, and the visibility of electric and magnetic effluvia in his hypnotized subjects, would go so far as to remark categorically: 'If you want to be duped, then experiment with hysterical patients.'[41]

In light of this, one could argue that any attempt to ground neo-mesmerism in the wider context of French asylum medicine would necessarily have to pay a certain amount of attention to the important institutional phenomenon of the 'gifted hysteric': that (usually female) individual with one foot in the world of the miraculous and the other in the backwaters of neuropathic degeneracy. And questions would inevitably have to be asked about the extent to which these specially gifted patients actively collaborated with their doctors in defining the contours of neo-mesmerism as a system of knowledge-claims.

But French neo-mesmerism did not only break apart the traditional doctor/patient power relationship; in its attempt to consolidate itself, it also broke down certain traditional social and cultural barriers. Indeed, in the final analysis, the story of neo-mesmerism in French medicine reveals itself as at least in part a story about the rise of a quite remarkable dialogue between representatives from élite culture and representatives from popular culture; between people operating from under the banner of medical orthodoxy and people speaking from the margins of science and medicine; between hospitals and scientific societies with impeccable pedigrees (la Charité, la Société de Biologie), and basement occult groups publishing journals with names like *L'Initiation, Le Voile d'Isis, La Paix Universelle, La Chaîne Magnetique*, and *Le Magicien*.

The dialogue of which I am speaking seems to have endured for about twenty years. Finally, however, as the voices of medical orthodoxy became increasingly drowned out by those of popular culture, it became too one-sided to be sustained. And it is at precisely this point of transition from *dialogue* to *monologue*, that one might say neo-mesmerism ceases to be a part of the history of French medicine, and becomes more or less exclusively part of the history of spiritualism and the occult arts in early-twentieth-century France.

Notes

1 (28 December 1892) 'The new mesmerism' (from an occasional correspondent), *The Times*: 6.

2 J.M. Charcot (1882) 'Sur les divers états nerveux determinés par l'hypnotisation chez les hystériques', *Comptes-Rendus hebdomadaires de l'Académie des Sciences* 94: 403–5.

3 P. Janet (1925) *Psychological Healing: A Historical and Clinical Study*, trans. Eden and Cedar Paul, 2 vols, London: George Allen & Unwin.

4 The present introductory overview of neo-mesmerism as a movement in French *fin-de-siècle* medicine makes no attempt to relate it to the vast history of fluidist and biomagnetic thinking in general, important though such an task would be. For an introduction to some of the key issues, see R. Amadou (1953) 'Esquisse d'une histoire philosophique du fluide', *Revue métaphysique* 21 NS: 5–33; H. Schott (ed.) (1985) *Franz Anton Mesmer und die Geschichte des Mesmerismus*, Stuttgart: Franz Steiner, with a valuable bibliography of secondary and primary sources compiled by H. Schott; E.J. Dingwall (ed.) *Abnormal Hypnotic Phenomena*, 4 vols, London: Churchill; (1967–8) H. Ellenberger (1970) *The Discovery of the Unconscious*, New York: Basic Books, esp. chapters 2 and 3; and the classic social interpretation of eighteenth-century mesmerism by R. Darnton (1968) *Mesmerism and the End of the Enlightenment in France*, Cambridge, Mass.: Harvard University Press.

5 I have described Burq's life and career in more detail in my essay 'Metals and magnets in medicine', in *Psychological Medicine* (1988) 18: 21–38. Portions of the first section of the present work necessarily summarize arguments presented in this earlier paper.

6 See A. Dumontpallier, J.-M. Charcot, and J.B. Luys (1877) 'Rapport fait à la Société de Biologie sur la métalloscopie du docteur Burq', *Comptes Rendus de la Société de Biologie (sec. mémoires)* 4, 6th series: 1–24. For the second report of the commission, which assessed the therapeutic value of Burq's work, see A. Dumontpallier, J.-M. Charcot, and J.B. Luys (1878) 'Second rapport fait à la Société de Biologie sur la métalloscopie et la métallothérapie du docteur Burq', *Gazette médicale de Paris* 7, 4th series: 419–23, 436–40, 450–2.

7 For an overview of the earliest electro-physiological explanations for the metalloscopic effects, see A. Dumontpallier *et al.* (1877) *Comptes Rendus de la Société de Biologie* 4: 1–24; L.-H. Petit (1879) *Sur la métallothérapie, ses origines et les procédés thérapeutiques qui en dérivent*, Paris: Octave Doin; and the English-language review in A.S. Adler (1880–1) 'A contribution to the doctrine of bilateral functions after experiences of metaloscopy [*sic.*]', *San Francisco Western Lancet* 9: 536–52. For some early alternative theories, see R. Vigouroux (1878) 'Sur la théorie physique de la métalloscopie', *Lancette française: Gazette des hôpitaux* 51: 780; E. Schiff (1879) 'Prof. Schiff über Metalloskopie und Metallotherapie', *Wiener Medizinische Presse* 20: 1379–82; and the psychological explanation championed by D.H. Tuke (and indignantly disputed by the French) in (1878–9) 'Metalloscopy and expectant attention', *Journal of Mental Science* 24: 598–609.

8 Cited in Ch. Féré (1902) 'L'alternance de l'activité des deux hémisphères cérébraux', *L'année psychologique* 8: 108.

9 For descriptions of the transfer phenomenon, see A. Dumontpallier *et al.* *op. cit.*: 22; R. Vigouroux (1880–1) 'Métalloscopie, métallothérapie, aesthe-

siogènes', *Archives de neurologie*, 2, 1: 414–15; P. Richer (1881) *Études cliniques sur l'hystéro-épilepsie ou grande hystérie*, Paris: Delahaye & Lecrosnier, p. 536. For some attempts to account for transfer within a variety of physical/physiological frameworks, see A. Adamkiewicz (1880) 'Über bilateralen Functionen', *Archiv für Physiologie*, Leipzig, pp. 159–62; A.S. Adler (1879) *Ein Beitrag zur Lehre von den 'bilateralen Functionen' im Anschlusse an Erfahrungen der Metalloscopie*, inaug. dissertation, Univ. Frederick-Guillaume, Berlin: Gutman, with an English-language summary in Adler, 'A contribution . . . ', 536–52; Ch.-E. Brown-Séquard (1882) *Recherches expérimentales et cliniques sur l'inhibition et la dynamogénie. Application des connaissances fournies par ces recherches aux phénomènes principaux de l'hypnotisme et du transfert*, Paris: G. Masson; [extract from the *Gazette hebdomadaire de médecine et de chirurgie*]; M. Rosenthal (1882) 'Untersuchungen und Beobachtungen über Hysterie und Transfert', *Archiv für Psychiatrie und Nervenkrankheit* 12, 1: 201–31; Ch. Féré (1902) 'L'alternance de l'activité des deux hémisphères cérébraux', *L'année psychologique* 8: 107–49.

10 See the various discussions on this issue by I. Veith (1965) *Hysteria: The History of a Disease*, Chicago and London: Chicago University Press, p. 238; H. Ellenberger (1970) *The Discovery of the Unconscious*, New York: Basic Books, p. 90; A.R.G. Owen (1971) *Hysteria, Hypnosis, and Healing: The Work of J.-M. Charcot*, London: Dennis Dobson, p. 184; Th. R. Sarbin and W.C. Coe (1979) 'Hypnosis and psychopathology: replacing old myths with fresh metaphors', *Journal of Abnormal Psychology* 88: 511.

11 For a discussion of these issues and more details about the origins of Burq's discoveries, see V. Burq (1853) *Métallothérapie, traitement des maladies nerveuses, paralysies, rhumatisme chronique, spasmes . . . par les applications métalliques. Abregé historique, théorique et pratique, extrait de vingt-deux mémoires ou notes aux deux Académies*, Paris: G. Ballière; J. Elliotson (1852–3) 'Nervous affections: metallo-therapia, or metal-cure: new properties of metals illustrated through mesmerism, by Dr Burq of Paris', *The Zoist* 10: 121–140 229–78; V. Burq (1882) *Des origines de la métallothérapie. Part qui doit être faite au magnétisme animal dans sa decouverte. Le Burquisme et le Perkinisme*, Paris: A. Delahaye & Lecrosnier.

12 See Ellenberger, *The Discovery of the Unconscious*, p. 123.

13 See A. Dumontpallier and P. Magnin (1881) 'Expériences sur la métalloscopie, l'hypnotisme et la force neurique', *Comptes Rendus de la Société de Biologie* 3, 7th series: 359–64, esp. 361. Cf. A. Dumontpallier and P. Magnin (1882) 'Étude expérimentale sur la métalloscopie, l'hypnotisme et l'action de divers agents physiques dans l'hystérie', *Comptes Rendus Hebdomadaires des Séances de l'Académie des Sciences* 94: 60–3.

14 See the examples reported by L. Landouzy, experimenting at Charcot's request, in (1879) 'Relation d'un cas de léthargie provoquée par l'application d'un aimant', *Le Progrès Médical* 7: 60–2; and in (1879) 'Effets de l'application d'un aimant chez une hystérique [with discussion]', *Gazette des hôpitaux* 1: 45–6. Interest in the hypnotic qualities of the mineral magnet would persist through the end of the century. See, for example, the well-known works by the Polish physician and philosopher, J. Ochorowicz (1884) 'Note sur un critère de la sensibilité hypnotique: I'hypnoscope, une nouvelle méthode de diagnostic', *Comptes Rendus de la Société de Biologie* 1, 8th series: 324–7, and (1884) 'Le sens du toucher et le sens du magnetisme', *Revue Scientifique* 4, 3rd series:

324–7. Cf. the similar arguments of the German worker, G. Gessmann (1886) 'Magnetismus und Hypnotismus', *Sphinx: Monatschrift für die geschichtliche und experimentale Begrundung der übersinnlichen Weltanschauung auf monistiche Grundlage* 2(1): 43–50.

15 J.-M. Charcot (1883) *Exposé des titres scientifiques du M.J.-M. Charcot*, Paris: Victor Goupy & Jourdan, pp. 146–7.

16 'One thus has in provoked anaesthesia, or more generally in the property the anaesthesiogenes have to evoke certain symptoms that [before] only existed in latent form, a *veritable touchstone of hysteria*': R. Vigouroux (1880–1) 'Métalloscopie, métallothérapie, aesthesiogènes', *Archives de Neurologie* 1: 423 (emphasis added).

17 See, for example, Charcot's 1881 report to the Société de Biologie in which it is clear that the term 'aesthesiogène' has come to mean *any* agent (heat, light, a puff of cold air, etc.) that induces hypnosis. J.-M. Charcot (1881) 'Métallothérapie [index title]', *Comptes Rendus de la Société de Biologie* 3, 7th series: 403.

18 E. Bérillon (1899) *L'oeuvre scientifique de Dumontpallier*, Paris: A. Quelquejeu. Later, Dumontpallier would also pay explicit tribute to the catalytic role played by Burq and metalloscopy in the rise of hypnosis research under Charcot. See A. Dumontpallier (1889) 'Discours de M. Dumontpallier au congrès de l'hypnotisme', *Revue de l'hypnotisme et de la psychologie physiologique* 4: 79–82.

19 For Barety's original paper to the Société de Biologie, which concentrated mostly on the physical aspects of the radiating neurique force, see A. Barety (1881) 'Des propriétés physiques d'une force particulière du corps humain (force neurique rayonnante) connue vulgairement sous le nom de magnétisme animal', *Comptes Rendus de la Société de Biologie (sec. mémoires)* 3, 7th series: 5–34. For an exhaustive analysis of the neurique force, see Barety's great tome (1887) *Le magnétisme animal etudié sous le nom de force neurique rayonnante et circulante dans ses propriétés physiques, physiologiques et thérapeutiques*, Paris: Octave Doin.

20 See Dumontpallier and Magnin, 'Expériences sur la métalloscopie, l'hypnotisme et la force neurique', 359–64; A. Dumontpallier (1881) 'Action de divers agents physiques dans l'hypnotisme [index title]', with a lively discussion session in which Charcot warns against the dangers of running after the marvellous, *Comptes Rendus de la Société de Biologie* 3, 7th series: 394–8; and Dumontpallier and Magnin, 'Étude expérimentale sur la métalloscopie, l'hypnotisme et l'action de divers agents physiques dans l'hystérie', 60–3.

21 The occultist researcher Colonel Albert de Rochas would later suggest that the singular effects of valerian at a distance cast light on the old legends of witches who turned into cats by night to suck the blood of children, and seemed to offer a new perspective generally on the prominent place of cats in the history of sorcery. See A. de Rochas (1904) *Les Frontières de la Science*, 2nd series, Paris: Librairie des Sciences Psychologiques, p. 103.

22 Bourru and Burot's report at Grenoble received special notice in the national weekly journal, *Le Temps*, and led to a repeat performance before a session of the Société de Psychologie Physiologique. For details, see H. Bourru and P. Burot (1887) *La Suggestion Mentale et l'Action à Distance des Substances Toxiques et Médicamenteuses*, Paris: J.B. Baillière et Fils.

23 See A. Berjon (1886) *La Grande Hystérie chez l'Homme*, Paris: J.B. Baillière et Fils; E. Alliot (1886) *De la Suggestion Mentale et de l'Action des Médicaments à Distance*, Paris: J.-B. Baillière et Fils.

24 For Luys' report to the Académie de Médecine, see J.B. Luys (1887) 'De la solicitation expérimentale des phénomènes emotifs chez les sujets en état d'hypnotisme', *Bulletin de l'Académie de Médecine* 18, 2nd series: 291–306 (with discussion). For the commission's report on Luys' work, see (1888) 'Rapport par MM. Hérard, Bergeron, Brouardel, Gariel, et Dujardin-Beaumetz', *Bulletin de l'Académie de Médecine* 19, 3rd series: 330–51. For Luys' defiant reply to his critics, see (1888) *Bulletin de l'Académie de Médecine* 20: 246–66, and also Luys' comments in his (1890) *Hôpital de la Charité. Leçons cliniques sur les principaux phénomènes de l'hypnotisme dans leurs rapports avec la pathologie mentale*, Paris: Georges Carré, pp. 254ff. In the wake of his censureship, Luys' demonstrations of his work in this area would grow increasingly sensational, drawing crowds from tout Paris, as ruthlessly satirized in Léon Daudet (1956) *Les Morticoles*, Paris: Bernard Gasset, pp. 164–7. Auvray-Escalard is right to point out in her thesis on Luys, that the character of Foutange in this novel – normally assumed to be modelled after Charcot – gives every indication of really being a Charcot/Luys composite. See B. Auvray-Escalard (1984) 'Un méconnu de l'hystérie: Jules Bernard Luys (1828–1897)' Université de Caen thèse pour le doctorat de médecine, 1984.

25 The key sources here are L.-Th. Chazarain and Ch. Dècle (1886) *Découverte de la Polarité Humaine*, Paris: O. Doin, which includes an 'equisse historique sur la métallo-thérapie et la magnéto-thérapie'; and the follow-up work by the same authors, portions of which were first presented to the 16th (1887) session of the Association française pour l'avancement des sciences at Toulouse, *Les Courants de la Polarité dans l'Aimant et dans le Corps Humain*, Paris: privately printed by the authors (a copy of this second work, with a flyleaf inscription by Chazarain, can be found at the Paris Bibliothèque Nationale). See also the rival theory of human polarity published at this same period by the leading (but non-medical) mesmerist Hector Durville (1886) *Lois physiques du magnétisme. Polarité humaine. Traité expérimental et thérapeutique de magnétisme. Cours professé à la Clinique du Magnétisme en 1885–86*, Paris: Librairie du Magnétisme.

26 For the studies on the lateral polarization of emotional states in the hysterical nervous system, see J.B. Luys (1890) *Hypnotisme Expérimentale. Les emotions dans l'état d'hypnotisme et l'action à distance des substances médicamenteuses ou toxiques*, Paris: J.-B. Baillière et Fils, pp. 126–31. For the studies on the attractive and repulsive effects of magnetic poles on hypnotized subjects, see J.B. Luys (1890) 'Action psychiques des aimants, des courants electromagnétique, et des courants electriques continus', published in his own journal, *Revue d'Hypnologie Théorique et Pratique*: 74–83, 107–12.

27 A. Binet and Ch. Féré (1885) 'L'hypnotisme chez les hystériques. I. Le transfert psychique', *Revue Philosophique de la France et de l'Etranger* 19: 1–25; A. Binet and Ch. Féré (1885) 'La polarisation psychique', *Revue Philosophique de la France et de l'Étranger* 19: 369–402; see also the experiments described by these authors in their (1887) *Animal Magnetism*, Int'l Science Series, London: Kegan, Paul, Trench & Co.

28 J. Babinski (1886) *Recherches servant à établir que certaines manifestations hystériques peuvent être transferées d'une sujet à un autre sous l'influence de l'aimant*, Paris: A. Delahaye & E. Lecrosnier.

29 J.B. Luys and G. Encausse (1891) *Du Transfert à Distance à l'Aide d'une Couronne de Fer Aimanté d'états nevropathiques variés, d'une sujet à l'état de*

veille sur un sujet à l'état hypnotique [extrait des *Annales de Psychiatrie et d'Hypnologie*, mai 1891], Clermont: Daix Frères.

30 I have adapted my description of Luys' transfer therapy from G.M. Robertson (1892) 'Hypnotism at Paris and Nancy. Notes of a visit', *Journal of Mental Science* 38: 523–4; but see also J.B. Luys (1890) 'Du transfert comme methode thérapeutique dans le traitement des maladies nerveuses', *Revue d'Hypnologie*: 39–48.

31 Some patients would later reverse these data, claiming to see the *left* side of the human body as red (negative, repulsive), and the *right* side as blue (positive, attractive). See A. de Rochas (1899) *L'Extériorisation de la Sensibilité. Étude expérimentale et historique*, 5th edn, Paris: Chamuel, pp. 6–7, and also de Rochas' explanation for these inconsistencies in patients' reports, p. 41.

32 J.B. Luys (1892) 'De la visibilité des effluves magnétiques & électriques chez les sujets en état hypnotique', *Annales de Psychiatrie et d'Hypnologie* 2, NS: 193–5; J.B. Luys (1892) 'De la visibilité par les sujets en état hypnotique des effluves degagés par les êtres vivants', *Annales de Psychiatrie et d'Hypnologie* 2, NS: 321–3.

33 See J.-S. de Plauzoles (1893) 'Les expériences du Dr Luys et de M. de Rochas sur l'exteriorisation de la sensibilité', *Annales de Psychiatrie et d'Hypnologie dans leurs rapports avec la psychologie et la médecine légale* 3 (1), NS: 51–7; de Rochas, *L'Extériorisation de la Sensibilité*; and also the final (6th) edition of this work (1909), augmented with new experiments by Boirac, Joire, Broquet and others (Paris: Bibliothèque Charcornac). For a harsh denunciation by medical orthodoxy of the de Rochas studies (and most of the rest of the Charité's hypnosis research in general), see E. Hart (1893) *Hypnotism, Mesmerism, and the New Witchcraft*, New York: D. Appleton & Co. For Durville's incorporation of the de Rochas studies into the world of living phantoms, see H. Durville (1909) *Les Fantômes des Vivants. Anatomie et physiologie de l'âme. Recherches expérimentales sur le dédoublement des corps de l'homme*, Paris: Librairie du Magnétisme.

34 For Baraduc's work (with photographic plates), see (1896) *L'Âme Humaine, ses mouvements, ses lumières, et l'iconographie de l'invisible fluidique*, Paris: Carré; (1904) *Les Vibrations de la vitalité humaine. Méthode biométrique appliquée aux sensitifs et aux névrosés*, Paris: Librairie J.-B. Baillière et Fils; and the provocative analysis in G. Didi-Hubermann (1982) *Invention de l'hystérie: Charcot et l'iconographie photographique de la Salpêtrière*, Paris: Macula, pp. 89–97. (The Baraduc citation in this paper is also taken from this source, p. 93.) For the Charité's work on photographing the effluvia, see J.B. Luys and David (1897) 'Note sur l'enregistrement photographique des effluves qui se dégagent des extrémités des doigts et du fond de l'oeil de l'être vivant, à l'état physiologique et à l'état pathologique', *Comptes Rendus de la Société de Biologie* 4, 10th series: 515–19; (1897) 'Fixations par la photographie des effluves qui se dégagent de l'appareil auditif. Réponse à certaines objections concernant l'émission des effluves digitaux', *Comptes Rendus de la Société de Biologie* 4, 10th series: 676–8. See also the technical doubts cast on the Charité's work by C. Martin (1897) 'De l'importance des actions physico-chimiques dans l'obtention des-preuves photographiques par le procédé de MM. Luys et David', *Comptes Rendus de la Société de Biologie* 4, 10th series: 722–3.

35 P. Joire (1908) *Traité de l'hypnotisme expérimental et thérapeutique*, Paris: Vigot Frères. Cf. the 'magnétomètre' developed a number of years earlier by the

abbé Fortin and presented to the Académie de Sciences for evaluation, as recounted in L. Moutin (1907) *Le magnétisme humain, l'hypnotisme et le spiritualisme moderne, considérés au point de vue théorique et pratique*, Paris: Perrin, pp. 185–7.

36 J.M.D. Olmsted (1946) *Charles-Edouard Brown-Séquard. A Nineteenth-Century Neurologist and Endocrinologist*, Baltimore: Johns Hopkins University Press, pp. 164–5.

37 F. de Courmelles (1891) *Hypnotism,* trans. L. Ensor, London: George Routledge & Sons, p. 48.

38 Indeed, one modern commentator, René Guenon, has spoken of fluidism in general as 'materialisme transposé'. See the thoughtful discussion on these issues in R. Amadou (1953) 'Esquisse d'une histoire philosophique du fluide', *Revue Métaphysique* 21, NS: 5–33.

39 Cited in D. Barrucand (1967) *Histoire de l'hypnose en France*, Paris; Presses Universitaires de France, p. 178.

40 J. Goldstein (1982) 'The hysteria diagnosis and the politics of anti-clericalism in late nineteenth-century France', *Journal of Modern History* 54: 209–39. I am indebted to Ruth Harris for first bringing this important essay to my attention.

41 Cited in Ellenberger, *The Discovery of the Unconscious*, p. 172. A revealing, if somewhat harsh, picture of the way in which at least some of the Charité hospital's star subjects appear actively to have manipulated their doctors can be found in Hart's *Hypnotism, Mesmerism, and the New Witchcraft*.

CHAPTER NINE

'Humane, economical, and medically wise': the LCC as administrators of Victorian lunacy policy

David Cochrane

With the passing of the 1888 Local Government Act, the new London County Council (LCC) assumed statutory responsibility for persons of unsound mind in the metropolitan parishes and unions (excluding the City of London). Before the 1888 Act, the powers and duties under statute for the capital were fragmented across the County Justices of Middlesex, Surrey, and Kent.[1] Of course Middlesex had spearheaded Victorian lunacy administration, by its pioneering development of the vast, utilitarian pauper lunatic asylums at Hanwell and Colney Hatch. By 1888 it had added a third at Banstead in Surrey, mainly for chronic cases, and embarked on the building of a fourth at Claybury in Essex. These institutions and the Claybury project were transferred to the LCC along with the Surrey Asylums at Cane Hill and, also, Wandsworth which was immediately sold to the new County of Middlesex. Kent County Council retained the one institution in which Metropolitan paupers were housed,[2] and simply began charging the LCC on a contract basis.

The LCC had a constituent population of over 4 million people and was accordingly the largest asylums authority in England and Wales. A close examination of the LCC's work is instructive particularly as it reveals a significant degree of heterogeneity and conflicting motivations in policy as well as highlighting the influence of administrative and financial relationships and expedients. This kind of detail can often become blurred in the wide sweep and thrust of some structural accounts. The temporal focus is the LCC's first twenty-five years, a period which merits attention for within it the utilitarian pauper asylum reached its zenith. Perhaps the most striking feature over the period was the inflated rate of registered lunacy in London compared to elsewhere which needs to be considered in the context of metropolitan poor law administration to elucidate how the LCC perceived its problems and the solutions it was obliged to adopt. To meet demand for places the Asylums Committee embarked on a massive asylum building programme which doubled capacity in twenty years. Each asylum project, notably the peculiar development of five large institutions on one centrally serviced site, emerges as a quintessential example of Victorian social engineering. Behind their walls we find English asylum administration typified and a brief descriptive account is therefore included. In the later years of the period under review, the LCC built the first small-scale, pauper mental hospital for acute and curable cases. The ideological foundations of this development are uncovered to support the contention that it was primarily tangential to the committee's principal policy momentum which still, at the outbreak of the Great War, implied an expanding system of mass segregation as the preferred solution to the problems posed to society by madness.

Although the LCC brought a degree of co-ordination, the management of London's insane was not unified as another authority, the Metropolitan Asylums Board (MAB), was largely unaffected by the Local Government Act. The MAB had been established in 1867 to administer relief to the capital's non-ablebodied paupers with the aim of freeing the workhouse to sanction the 'less eligible' ablebodied. Its formal remit in lunacy administration was limited to chronic cases and this it dutifully followed, building two huge barrack institutions at Leavesden and Caterham, and later adding the Darenth Training Colony in Kent, Belmont in Sutton and a further large 'asylum' principally for senile dementia cases at Tooting Bec in south-west London.[3]

The Asylums Committee was appointed in June 1889. Its powers were those of the Committee of Visitors required in statute for each county asylum,[4] and it delegated these to a separate subcommittee appointed for each of its asylums. Membership of the subcommittees was drawn from the main body thereby assuring continuity of policy and centralized control. The most important functions were the purchase of land for the purpose of asylum construction, controlling the reception of pauper lunatics, the framing of central general rules, the appointment of the senior staff for each institution, and the determination of diet.[5]

The committee's revenue and all capital expenditure exceeding £400 were subject to the sanction of the main council. The cost of the provision and repair of asylums was funded from the county's own rates. Its revenue derived from other sectors of the diverse poor law funding arrangements which had evolved in London. This elaborate financial structure was a major factor determining the high rate of lunacy in the capital compared to the rest of England and Wales. As Figure 9.1 shows, between 1890 and 1910 the total number of lunatics, idiots, and other persons of unsound mind in England and Wales continued gradually to rise as a proportion of the population from 1.87 to 3.31 per 1,000. By contrast, when the LCC came into office, the rate in London was already ahead of the national average by 23 per cent, and accelerated further until by 1910, this differential had almost tripled.

There was also a marked contrast between the respective distributions of pauper patients between the asylum and the workhouse over this period,

Figure 9:1 Comparative Lunacy Rates: London and the rest of England and Wales

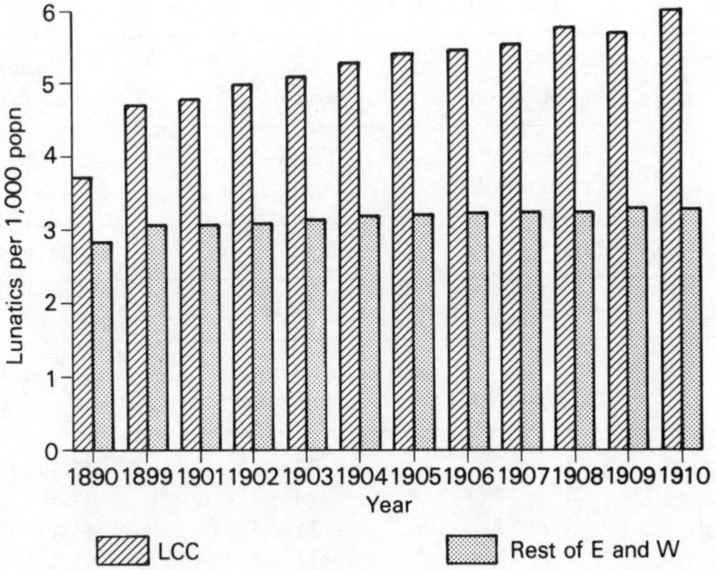

as Table 9.2 shows. In the rest of the country the proportion of pauper lunatics detained in asylums reached a plateau at 84 per cent. By the time the LCC came into office, the London asylum system already housed 96 per cent and rose to stabilize at 98 per cent. Related to this, there was also a significant if smaller divergence in the proportions of pauper patients to the total number of registered lunatics throughout the period. By the end of the nineteenth century, the proportions of paupers to the total in the country as a whole and in London had stabilized at 91 per cent and 98 per cent respectively.

In late Victorian and Edwardian London, as elsewhere, doctors and asylum authorities exercised wide discretion in certifying as insane the most economically vulnerable classes of society. But the discrepancies in the figures demonstrate the importance of financial incentives and disincentives to local unions in determining the extent of that latitude and consequent rate of incarceration. This is a factor which has received less emphasis in explanations of the national increase. However, it merits closer examination in London's case since the relative plenitude with which the capital's rates were lavished on the non-ablebodied poor, and the unique structure of its poor law administration, provided every incentive for local unions to divest themselves of their most troublesome charges.

The 1867 Metropolitan Poor Act has been heralded by Ayers as the dawn of a public hospital service delivered on criteria of need.[6] Although the argument is well supported, taken alone it misrepresents the multi-

Table 9:1 *Pauper lunatics by place of detention*

Year	Workhouses	Relatives and others	County[1] asylums
England and Wales except London			
1889	11,827–14%	6,856–8%	65,599–78%
1899	11,108–11%	7,707–8%	80,983–81%
1904	10,948–10%	6,597–6%	89,641–84%
1909	11,218–10%	6,108–5%	98,216–85%
County of London			
1891	275– 2%	285–2%	15,293–96%
1899	361– 2%	243–1%	20,465–98%
1904	311– 1%	151–1%	23,486–99%
1909	237– 1%	132–1%	25,924–98%

Derived from tables I and II in appendix A to the 64th Annual Report of the Commissioners in Lunacy, 1910, and the annual reports of the LCC Asylums Committee 1890–1909.

[1] Includes MAB asylums.

dimensional objectives of this statute which was a prime early instance of 'welfare serving many masters'. By passing the Act, Parliament acknowledged that the overriding belief of the 1834 Benthamite reformers, that the great bulk of pauperism was volitional, had been unsound. By the 1860s, experience had shown that the vast majority of those seeking indoor relief comprised the sick, the infirm, the elderly, and the mad. Indeed the 1832 Poor Law Commissioners had never intended the principle of less eligibility to be applied to the non-ablebodied.[7] The 1867 Act's objective was therefore to diversify poor relief according to stricter classification. Initially the major targets were chronic lunatics and those who contracted life-threatening infectious diseases. The first group were simply impervious to less eligibility, their detention in workhouses was objectionable on humanitarian grounds,[8] and they were difficult to manage in workhouse wards. In the case of the second, it was now recognized that crowding together the victims of lethal, communicable diseases constituted a major public health risk, as a recent spate of epidemics had highlighted.[9] Pauperism, criminality, and lunacy may have been social diseases largely restricted to the labouring classes, but cholera and typhus were evidently less discriminating.

The Act set up the Metropolitan Asylums Board which proceeded to develop a network of 'asylums'[10] for the victims of infectious diseases on London's urban fringe,[11] whilst simultaneously herding the capital's chronic lunatics into special, inexpensive institutions which had recently been proposed by the Commissioners in Lunacy. By 1860, the commissioners had begun to harmonize their own dual policy aim, to end the detention of the insane in workhouses and relieve overcrowding in county asylums, with the resistance of local ratepayers to yet more extravagance. Counties were advised to erect inexpensive, 'auxiliary asylums ... intermediate between the Union Workhouses and the principal curative asylums'.[12] The resultant Caterham and Leavesden asylums comprised standard-design barracks on a regimented layout which enforced the ultimate in batch-living on 1,500 (and later over 2,000) people.[13]

Despite pressure from humanitarian reformers, the Act stopped short of obliging unions to establish poor law infirmaries for the rest of the sick poor. Instead, the MAB was to create a network of outdoor dispensaries whilst unions were merely empowered to group together for the purpose of infirmary provision according to local discretion. The latter was a skilful political manoeuvre which was to stimulate the emergence of a hospital system none the less. Of special significance for our concerns, the Act also placed a duty on the Poor Law Board to levy a rate towards a new London-wide Common Poor Fund, administered by the MAB, to finance the new measures.

At the general level, the implementation of the new Act was a major precipitant of the immense and disproportionate growth in poor law expenditure in the capital which flattened the cost differentials between lunatic asylums and other forms of poor relief. Whereas total spending elsewhere increased by 66 per cent between 1867 and 1904, it rose nearly fourfold in London,[14] over the same period. Indeed poor relief in London expanded relatively faster than even the figures on net expenditure suggest, for the corresponding gradients of population growth were 80 per cent and only 40 per cent respectively.[15] By 1890 the maintenance charge in the LCC's lunatic asylums was no longer extravagant compared to the cost of the various other forms of indoor and outdoor relief which had developed in the metropolitan unions.[16] Averaged across all classes of pauper, expenditure per head in London had risen from £10 15*s* in 1870 to £22 9*s* in 1891, and had reached £28 16*s* by 1904. Over the same period, the average cost per inmate-year in a county lunatic asylum had remained relatively stable at between £23 and £26. This was in marked contrast to the equivalent relativities in the rest of England and Wales which continued to act as a financial disincentive to certification.

More specifically, the centrally administered Common Poor Fund not only covered the MAB's revenue budget, it also contributed to the cost of maintaining rate-aided lunatics in county asylums, registered hospitals, and licensed houses. This was to act as a powerful incentive to local unions to move lunatics from the workhouse where their maintenance costs were met entirely from the parish rates for which the guardians were directly accountable to ratepayers. In 1875, these converging inducements were reinforced when the Poor Law Board began offering a weekly grant of four shillings to all unions in England and Wales, towards the extra cost of maintaining a pauper lunatic in a county asylum. Considering the predictable effect that this 'wholly mischievous' subvention would have in fuelling the continued expansion of the asylum system over ensuing decades, it is surprising that it seems to have slipped through with minimum ceremony.[17] In London the payment was centralized through the Common Poor Fund but the inducement was no less strong. By the turn of the century, a local metropolitan union could save 60 per cent of its monetary obligation to maintain paupers if they were transferred to a county or an MAB lunatic asylum.[18]

Of course this is not to argue that the numbers of certified insane increased simply as a result of financial incentives. Rather, the inducements established fertile conditions for the contemporary, widening definitions of insanity formulated by asylum doctors. As Scull has shown, their advancing professionalization generated myriad subclassifications of insanity and idiocy and an unshakeable belief in their own humanitarianism which 'compelled them to seek out still more cases, rather than to reject any who were proffered'.[19] There was also a strong suspicion within the LCC Asylums Committee that the payment of certification fees to medical officers also had 'a tendency to increase the number certified'[20] given that some of them could supplement their salaries by £200 to £400 year through this source alone. Incessant pressure from the Lunacy Commissioners and the administrative convenience of clearing the workhouse of people who were difficult to manage could only accentuate the trends.

Explaining the acceleration in the rate of certification in London after 1890 is more problematic. To begin with, it coincided with a sharp downward turn in the economic cycle and a consequent increase in unemployment: this simply increased the pool from which lunatic paupers came.[21] But at the same time, the 1890 Lunacy Act legitimized the established practice of detaining chronic lunatics in the workhouse, though it might at first sight have been expected to have reduced referrals to asylums. Paradoxically, the impact of section 24 probably fuelled the demand for asylum places because it made detention in the house conditional upon the medical officer satisfying himself both that the person was a proper case, and that the place itself was suitable for 'his proper care and treatment'.[22] During the 1890s a number of considerations would have led medical officers to conclude that this was inappropriate, even without any personal financial gains.

First, the plight of indoor paupers became an important political issue in the wake of the surge in strength of working-class politics, and conditions began to improve markedly. The widening of the franchise certainly increased the sensitivity of all politicians to the popular perception of the workhouse as a poor law 'bastille'. This was reinforced by changes to the property qualification during the 1890s which enabled working-class representatives to stand for election to boards of guardians, bringing with them their deep-rooted hatred of the poorhouse and determination to correct its faults.[23] Secondly, prudent medical officers heeded the prevailing view of the Poor Law Board Inspectors who were responsible for the scrutiny of workhouse administration. During the 1890s, these inspectors adopted the stance long held by the Commissioners in Lunacy that the workhouse was not a suitable place for the detention of lunatics. For in the colourful though not untypical view of one of them, although the labour power of chronic lunatics and imbeciles was useful to the upkeep of the institution, boards of guardians were duty-bound to eradicate 'what may almost be characterised as the cruelty of requiring sane persons to associate, by day and night, with gibbering idiots'.[24]

A master-builder of barracks

Nowhere was the effect of these developments more strongly felt than in London. Throughout the period under review, the role of the workhouse in lunacy administration was purely as a place of reception for lunatics prior to virtually automatic transfer to an asylum. As a result, the demands placed on the LCC by local unions raced ahead of its ability to meet them, so that despite a massive and unprecedented building programme, the Asylums Committee was obliged to approve a series of expensive capital projects the suitability of which it profoundly doubted.

In concept, if not in design detail, the late-nineteenth-century pauper lunatic asylum owed much to Bentham's own proposed solution to the containment and control of the awkward and socially disruptive. The problem lunacy posed to social engineering remained one of reforming the deviant in conditions which allowed humanitarianism to be appropriately tempered by the imperatives of surveillance and security.[25] The Panopticon was a technical device to meet social need as defined in Bentham's philosophy of state intervention and as such was the social administration equivalent of the steam engine. By the 1890s, the purpose-built, 2,000-bed, barrack lunatic asylum mirrored the contemporary modern factory in its requirement for the scientific division of labour to maximize productivity and economy.[26] The essential difference between the two generations of institution lay in the transformation of the process from a moral to a medical endeavour, and the sheer scale of the enterprise in turn dictated by pressure of demand and the accumulation of hopeless cases. The project the LCC inherited from the Middlesex justices was a prime example.

When the council took office, housing London's pauper lunatics in 2,000-bed asylums was well established in precedent, albeit partly due to expedient.[27] The rising demand for large institutions of containment nurtured a specialist field within nineteenth-century architecture.[28] The designer of Claybury was George Thomas Hine, a noted and busy exponent of the trade, who was reared in his father's successful provincial practice in Nottingham. The younger Hine was to develop a formidable talent for warehousing the unwanted and emerged as an illustrious and influential figure in his field, particularly when he was appointed as a consultant architect to the Lunacy Commissioners in 1898. He secured the Claybury commission through the mechanism often used for these appointments, a nation-wide competition. Hine enjoyed such good fortune in these events, that the professional press began publicly to suspect that some of the judging was partial.[29]

Although the image of the late-nineteenth-century lunatic asylum as a monolithic warehouse is apposite as a general characterization, a sharper focus reveals a significant degree of heterogeneity. The Claybury design fulfilled three related but distinct functions. It was a hospital for curable 'acute' patients, a place of containment for the disruptive and unmanageable, and a repository for the socially inadequate, the feeble-minded, and chronic lunatics. As the Lunacy Commissioners were later to recommend, doubtless on Hine's advice:

> There is much to be said in favour of a plan which provides – (1) a more or less separate hospital for the treatment of acute cases . . . in which the hospital idea is primary and fundamental, and carries with it the full equipment necessary for its practical realization. The existence and administration of such a hospital would, no doubt, tend largely to keep alive the medical spirit and promote the clinical investigation which are so important to the well being of every Asylum . . . (2) a central establishment of much cheaper and simpler construction, in which can be maintained the rank and file of mental and physical decrepitude, interspersed with the subjects of troublesome propensities; and (3) a series of simple cottage residences in which the quiet and harmless, the industrious and the convalescing may live under conditions more approximating to those of their previous normal lives.[30]

Claybury was just such a mixed asylum whose design achieved separation of wards on clinical criteria and also minimized running costs. The acute wards flanked the administration block within easy access of the offices of the medical staff which fronted the asylum. Chronic patients were housed in the 'back wards', unless they laboured in the laundry, the kitchen, or one of the other workshops, in which case they slept close to their places of work to save time collecting them.[31] Selected wards equipped with sufficient padded rooms would be managed as 'refractory wards' which not only housed the disruptive and potentially violent, but were central to the privilege system as a constant reminder of the consequences of troublesome behaviour. To maximize efficiency in the distribution of supplies and circulation of inmates, the two-storey pavilions were arranged regularly around a huge, trapezoid corridor: a model seemingly originated at the Lancashire County Asylum, Whittingham.[32] The service departments, including the boiler house and the mortuary, were placed in the central area which divided the asylum into sides so that the distance between them and the wards was minimized.[33]

On the exterior, the palatial pretensions of earlier asylums had been superseded by drab functionality and grim solidity, not least because the Commissioners in Lunacy deprecated embellishment. Any architect tempted to soften the elevations with touches of decorative stonework was deterred by the likelihood of the Lunacy Commissioners referring back the design on grounds of extravagant inutility.[34] The prison and the poorhouse justified the cost of a forbidding, Gothic façade 'to symbolise on the outside, the terrors to be expected within, and thus to deter any potential evildoer from entering its portals'.[35] Such expense served no good purpose for institutions which, however punitive, repressive, and publicly loathed, were not supposed to deter or be seen for that matter. Even so, the total cost of Claybury, including the purchase of the generous, 270-acre site, was over £375,000.[36]

The path of least resistance

Hine's success in the Middlesex competition was to prove remunerative beyond the most optimistic expectations of subsequent business, as the LCC embarked upon a building programme which was almost desperate in its scale and momentum. Claybury opened in 1894 and once it had been filled, the LCC was managing five asylums providing 11,668 beds. By 1910 this had increased to over 19,000.

As soon as the LCC took office the Commissioners in Lunacy began pressing it for a sixth asylum,[37] to add to Banstead, Hanwell, Colney Hatch, Cane Hill, and the near completed Claybury, and to be of similar size. However, the new committee saw itself as progressive and was uninspired by the prospect of building yet another 2,000-bed institution. It therefore briefed a special Accommodation Subcommittee (1) to examine ways of providing for over 2,000 lunatics in several small asylums or in one or two of moderate sizes and (2) to consider various schemes 'showing the expenses and advantages of each plan'.[38] (Clearly rational planning models were not invented by postwar American political scientists, as we had all supposed.)

This evident shift in preference away from the 2,000-bed standard recurrently surfaced like an *idée fixe* whenever the main committee discussed asylum design. With equal regularity such discretion was overwhelmed by the pressure of numbers and subjugated to the imperatives of economy. Initially, hopeful that the demand would relent, the committee devised two short-term expedients. First it built temporary units in corrugated iron at Colney Hatch and Banstead augmenting the capacity of each by 300. These structures, which were lined with matchboard (ironically as it turned out), were approved by the Lunacy Commissioners on condition that they would be demolished after five years. Secondly, it contracted out nearly

3,000 of its charges to numerous public asylums as far afield as Exeter and Lancaster, and even in the private sector. The second was a costly measure given that other asylum authorities charged two or three shillings per inmate week above the economic cost, anxious to relieve a little pressure from their own local unions. For their part, the proprietary houses demanded up to nineteen shillings.[39]

Faced with mounting bills from other institutions and pressure from the commissioners, the committee commissioned Hine to design another 2,000-bed institution for a site at Bexley Heath in Kent.[40] Despite its striking similarity to the formula he had used at Claybury, Mr Hine negotiated a fee of £10,000 for his new scheme. The whole asylum faced south and the wards were stepped back 'to obtain the maximum amount of sunshine and prospect'. The inmate's view was enhanced by the trees with which the asylum was surrounded, and which also, in time, would serve to mask the place from the nearby public roads. Bexley provided ward accommodation on the basis of four clinical classifications: acute, infirm, epileptic, and chronic and working. There were three detached villas, one of which housed those inmates chosen to be farm labourers. Like all such institutions, it was designed to be self-sufficient and included a market garden, farm, water pumping-station and staff accommodation.[41] The total capital cost was £360,000. Notwithstanding its frustrations with the size of the institution, the Asylums Committee could at least console itself as Bexley realized a revenue cost of only eight shillings per in-patient week.[42]

With work on Bexley underway, the committee received another unwelcome communication from the commissioners, which pointed out that by the time Bexley opened in 1898, the requirement for places would have exceeded available capacity by over 1,000 and that a seventh asylum should be built.[43] Indeed with demand for places approaching eighty per week, the committee was alarmed and asked for a report. Its clerk obliged with arguments about demand having previously been depressed by shortage of accommodation and recent censuses showing a growth in the numbers of middle-aged people who furnished the majority of the registered insane.[44] Unfortunately these trends showed no sign of relenting so the Accommodation Subcommittee again advertised for sites, and were most encouraged to learn of a 1,050-acre estate, just outside Epsom, which was on the market for £35,000.[45] A site of this size could accommodate at least six asylums and therefore could potentially absorb the most pessimistic forecasts. It was also a bargain, given that the land at Bexley had cost £10,000 and that the subcommittee's brief had been amended in the light of the swelling budget, to emphasize the need for due regard to the burden on the ratepayers.

By the time it came to the attention of the Asylums Committee in 1896, the estate of Horton Manor had passed through a series of owners who had neglected both the estate and the manor house, which was by then rather dilapidated. The latest proprietor had deserted his draughty Epsom residence for the sunnier climes of southern Australia, and left instructions for his outstanding £36,000 mortgage on the estate to be redeemed. His agents gave good service and succeeded in bumping up his original asking price by obliging the LCC to gazump a second prospective buyer and pay £40,000.[46] The council had little to complain of, however, for it was subsequently advised to insure the existing buildings alone for £38,000.[47]

Attracted by the low revenue costs of Hine's Bexley design, the committee decided with increased reluctance to replicate it at Horton, earning the architect, who had now taken offices in Parliament Street, a further £6,000.[48] But before this work began, the committee resolved to place some of its contracted-out patients in a temporary asylum adjacent to the permanent site. The idea was to cluster iron units, of the type used at Colney Hatch and Banstead, around the old manor house. Perhaps in anticipation of opposition, the committee agreed the extra expense of lining these structures with plaster. By this time the Commissioners in Lunacy were promoting the kind of development which made architects such as Hine quite prosperous gentlemen. Such schemes were usually rubber-stamped. However, even this rather docile watchdog decided to bare its teeth at the proposal for the temporary asylum at Horton.

The plan was to house 700 female patients of all types and would be complete with all standard facilities. The manor house, suitably restored, would be converted into staff accommodation; all other buildings would be of the corrugated-iron type. The scheme was originally approved by the commissioners on the condition that it too would be demolished after five years. However, when the plan was costed, the committee was faced with a total capital outlay of at least £83,000, sufficiently close to the cost per bed of a large permanent structure to undermine the whole project on grounds of financial viability. The commissioners were therefore asked to extend the lifespan to between twenty-five and thirty years.

The effect of this rather ambitious request was to entrench the commissioners' position. They replied that they would only agree to a temporary scheme for 400 patients to be demolished after seven years, provided immediate work began on an eighth asylum. The committee appealed over the heads of the commissioners to the Home Secretary whose department proved more concerned with economy than standards of provision. The Manor Asylum was approved to house 700 for a fifteen-year period, provided that inmates were of the 'comparatively quiet and harmless class', and that conditions should maintain 'a high standard of suitability'.[49] Within two years of its 1899 opening, the Home Secretary also approved the addition of accommodation to The Manor for 110 male patients required for manual labour power.

Between 1893 (the year before Claybury opened) and 1900 the committee's revenue budget increased by 60 per cent.[50] As a consequence, it came under increased pressure from the council to restrict expenditure. Meanwhile there was no sign of the demand abating, implying the need for two more large units at Horton. So the committee embraced cost-cutting expedients wherever possible, including on-site brick manufacture and the use of glazed brick to line the corridors and staircases to save both on plaster and subsequent painting and cleaning bills.[51] It also resolved to maximize economies of scale by centralizing the supplies of water, gas and electricity for the entire estate, and sewage disposal.[52] On the same principle, a strip of land in the elevated and well-drained north-east corner of the estate was fenced off to serve as an unconsecrated burial ground for pauper patients. In drawing up their plans, the engineers were told to assume an eventual resident population of 12,000.[53] Subsequently, a rail link to nearby Ewell was built, to service the entire site.[54]

As building work on Horton and the central station progressed, the accommodation subcommittee had been examining the case for segregating male epileptics. Working colonies, on the 'cottage system', had been established on the continent of Europe for some time. They were purpose-built, self-contained asylums in which chronic lunatics, imbeciles, or epileptics were engaged in farm work and housed in free-standing villas, and thus differed from the Gheel Colony, which of course had its British admirers.[55] The Asylums Committee's chief engineer was dispatched to Europe to study these colonies and returned recommending the model of the Gaulkhausen Asylum near Cologne.[56] The LCC adopted this model for the housing of epileptics as its remit was of a scale which would make such a development viable.[57]

The thinking behind this scheme is illustrative both of the power that the less eligibility principle still wielded in late Victorian social policy, and of the fact that, whatever the official view, lunatics were not entirely protected from its rigours. As epileptic men provided much asylum labour power, they were firmly at the top of the social hierarchy of lunacy formulated by their keepers. As Dr Robert Jones, medical superintendent at Claybury and formerly of the great Earlswood asylum, contended:

> The insanity of the epileptic is different from that of the ordinary insane. The insane epileptics associate together and are sympathetic, the others solitary and egotistical. They are industrious and benefit to a marked degree by occupation and congenial industrial pursuits.[58]

The working epileptics were therefore to enjoy a higher standard of living than the common lunatic. They would live in autonomous single-storey villas scattered over a large open site. Indeed, one of the colony's three governing principles established by the committee dictated that any inmate failing to do his due share of work would be returned to the barrack asylum. The rest would enjoy 'as long as they worked, the ordinary freedom of a home, be spared the wearing of a very distinctive dress'[59] and earn further privileges if they worked exceptionally hard.[60]

Having considered erecting a metal-hut development on the site, the committee opted for brick-built villas to avoid further conflict with the Lunacy Commissioners. Each would house forty patients (about half the size of the standard asylum chronic ward) and would be staffed by a married couple, cast in the seemingly contradictory roles of houseparent and overseer of work. It was envisaged that the colony would sell a surplus of agricultural goods to generate an income to contribute to the upkeep of the place; although it proved in practice to be the most expensive asylum to maintain.[61] Women were precluded partly because the plan militated against the conventional division into 'sides' and partly because the work was considered unsuitable. At £70,000 for 325 beds, the cost of Ewell Colony, opened in June 1904, was relatively high.[62] It was probably the first villa-type institution built in England and would set the pattern for the mental defective colonies of the 1920s and 1930s.[63]

It will be gathered that the committee had used the Bexley design at Horton with some reluctance and so resolved to fend off pressure from the Lunacy Commissioners to replicate it again.[64] In 1897 a working party was briefed to study asylum design in Scotland, on the continent of Europe, and in the United States and Canada.[65] It finally reported in 1902, just as the committee began to plan its tenth asylum, again to be located at Horton.[66] The working party favoured the design of the Maryland State Asylum in the USA, where autonomous 200-bed ward blocks were positioned to look inwards on to large rectangular gardens. The units were connected by walkways, covered only overhead, which not only afforded pleasing views of the shrubs and herbaceous borders, but were also highly suited to the humid continental climate of the region. The committee greeted this recommendation with great enthusiasm and decided to erect a Maryland at Epsom. During the time necessary for commissioning the design, additional temporary accommodation would be provided at the manor.

Unfortunately the proposal never reached the drawing-board as the vehement opposition of the Lunacy Commissioners to yet more temporary units became insuperable due to a disastrous fire which destroyed the 320-bed temporary annexe at Colney Hatch in January 1903. Fifty-one patients lost their lives. The committee aborted a prepared appeal to the Home Secretary and was once again forced to accept a speedy expedient. Even so, some members held out for the Maryland proposal and the decision to use Hine's Bexley design was only carried on the chairman's casting vote.[67] To appease the dissenters, Mr Hine moved 500 beds from the main crescent into autonomous villas, each with its own unfenced garden, and planted a large garden on each side of the central service corridors separating the male and female sides. In addition, the corridors were left open at the sides, a feature which subsequent generations of patients and staff may have found somewhat less agreeable than their American counterparts, through the cold, wet, and windy Epsom winters. The new asylum was christened Long Grove after a strip of woodland on the site, and opened in June 1907. These adaptations naturally merited a review of the architect's fee, which was restored to £10,000.

Through the repeated engagement of the commissioners' consultant architect, the committee had at least avoided further disputes. As Sir John

Macdougall, a former chairman of the committee, later conceded, with a perceptible air of fatigue:

> We have always been pressed with much asylum work. I have never known the day when we were not building an asylum ... we have repeated and repeated, mainly from stress of time and going along the path of least resistance.[68]

The general rules

As noted earlier, each of the LCC's institutions was formally managed by its own subcommittee comprising members of the Asylums Committee. The degree of centralized management is striking. Apart from drawing up the General Rules and Regulations for Asylum Officers and Servants, maintaining accounts and keeping the statistical returns required by the Commissioners in Lunacy, the committee also administered a meticulous system of monitoring the supplies, the farm and workshop produce of each asylum, and the type of employment in which patients were engaged. Indeed it discharged its responsibility for the determination of patients' diet with such diligence that a standard weekly menu, including the size of portions, was fixed centrally, with each subcommittee having the discretion only to decide whether or not the bread was sliced prior to serving.

Within these tight parameters, the effective role of each subcommittee amounted to little more than to legitimize the decisions of the medical superintendent in whom 'paramount authority' was effectively vested.[69] The formal duties of the medical superintendent were legion. In addition to assuming full responsibility for the medical treatment of each patient and the determination of his or her recreation and employment, his administrative duties ranged from hiring and firing attendants and nurses, through to quite trivial matters such as the granting of permission for visitors to bring in babes in arms. Opinion varied as to whether or not these myriad responsibilities and the routine introverted lifestyle adversely affected the clinical work and morale of senior medical staff. Things had altered little by the 1920s, when the commission which answered Montagu Lomax's charges claimed that they did not and that, in any case, 'so many administrative questions are closely bound up with medical consideration'.[70] However, some years earlier, Dr Hawkes, assistant resident physician at Hanwell, presented a rather different picture. He argued that the mode of existence could not have been further than that pertaining in the outside world and encouraged 'the natural proneness of ordinary minds to work in a system of grooves'.

> A perpetual association with the most repulsive features of man's weakness, an atmosphere of moral miasma, an almost hopeless struggle, day by day, to retrieve or reset the broken fragments of reason, must more or less, one would think, in the course of time, affect even the brightest

> and strongest minds. The peculiar monotony of the life itself may also have an injurious effect on the mental characteristics of those who for a prolonged period are continuously exposed to the influence.[71]

But at least there was always the pension to look forward to.

Each large asylum employed around 270 nurses working twelve-hour shifts over a six-day working week. Like the medical officers they were required to be resident, and their movements were highly circumscribed, and sanctioned by the medical superintendent's office. Their responsibilities straddled those of the 'gaolers' who ran Hanwell when the *Lancet* Commission visited in the 1870s,[72] and those of modern nurses. The men wore the familiar blue military-style uniforms. At patients' mealtimes, they counted out cutlery and counted it back. The regulations literally obliged them to display huge bunches of keys, hanging by a chain from the waist.[73] At the same time, they were expected to maintain high standards of physical care, and to promote the moral welfare of their charges.[74] To teach these virtues, each medical superintendent ran training courses for the first professional qualification for mental nursing founded in 1891 by the Royal Medico-Psychological Association.[75]

Staff to patient ratios were good for the period, but very low by modern standards. For example, the total number of non-supervisory day staff on duty on any one day at Hanwell would have been about 200, or one attendant to every ten patients.[76] Given that the acute and refractory wards would have been relatively highly staffed, these figures clearly indicate that the great majority of patients must have been quiet and easily managed. Such low staffing establishments were viable only because they were supplemented by patient labour. The proportion of inmates employed in each asylum depended on the categories housed: Banstead and Colney Hatch, for instance, had high shares of chronic patients and therefore bigger pools of potential labour. In 1906 an average of 58 per cent of the LCC's asylum inmates were daily put to work, augmenting the workforce of the large asylums by 200 per cent. Of course employment was presented as 'one of the most beneficial agencies' in promoting the patient's recovery, or, in the case of incurables, for 'lending an interest in life'. The accounting made no attempt to measure the contribution of working patients to the running of each institution, although the Asylums Committee noted that 'considerable savings on the labour bill to the ratepayers'[77] were thereby generated. Work was routine manual labour, divided between the sexes as appropriate. Selected patients were taught trades partly because the asylum required a limited range of skills, but also, in the case of those who held out promise of recovery, to improve chances of successful adjustment upon discharge.

The heterogeneity of these institutions, alluded to earlier, was reflected in patient administration. With the exception of the Ewell Colony, the LCC asylums discharged a significant proportion of patients as 'recovered' or 'relieved', averaging around 35 per cent of the number of admissions over a year.[78] The 'revolving-door' was also well in evidence and readmissions were frequent. Standards of physical care were high, and throughout its first twenty years the LCC invested heavily in upgrading its older institutions. Conditions and diet were better than many patients could have been accustomed to in their outside existences, although the enforced temperance must have been a trial. Some asylums managed up to a fifth of their wards on the open door principle. Books, playing-cards, pianos, and billiard tables were provided in day rooms. In their annual reports, enthusiastic medical superintendents boasted of the elaborate programmes of entertainments they provided.

> The cricket team plays weekly matches throughout the summer, and a strong feature has been made of patients' matches. The football team has had a most successful season, only losing one game, viz. that played against the Fulham reserves, a fixture which it is hoped may be made an annual one, on account of the level of interest it arouses.... The fete given to celebrate the coronation was held on the 28th June, and was attended by 1,222 patients, who spent a most enjoyable day. In addition to ordinary amusements, steam roundabouts were provided, and, later on in the evening, a cinematographic exhibition was given to a large number of the female patients in one of the airing courts, this being repeated the following evening for the male patients. The annual sports were held on the 30th August, when an extensive programme of races etc. for both patients and staff was got through.... During the past winter, many efforts have been made to lessen the monotony of asylum life. Weekly dances have been held for the patients, in addition to the numerous dramatic entertainments which were provided.[79]

And so it went on, with lantern exhibitions, Gilbert and Sullivan, vaudeville shows, fancy-dress balls, supper parties, picnics, and organized walks. Of course the stark reality of incarceration overshadowed this image of social richness. The walking-parties were the privilege of the compliant, routed to avoid contact with the outside world and closely supervised by attendants ever wary of possible escape attempts.[80] The less trustworthy patients would be exercised, penned in by the latest escape-proof fencing, in airing courts adjacent to their wards. Inter-asylum staff sporting competitions flourished not least in order to keep participants fit, muscular, and well prepared for any emergencies on the wards. Each attendant carried a whistle with which to summon assistance for such incidents and only on these occasions were men allowed on to the female wards.

Chemical restraint was in regular, if infrequent use. The total amount dispensed suggests that drugs were employed to 'flatten' individual outbursts of disturbed behaviour, rather than to effect prolonged states of tranquillization. The more routine tranquillizers employed were the so-called strong dresses; garments in heavy canvas which restricted movement. Attendants also had resort to seclusion, subject to medical approval. Horton, for example, had twenty-six padded rooms. But again the returns suggest that they were not routinely used. The threat of it, whether expressed or covert, generally sufficed.

In his welcoming address to newly recruited attendants at Long Grove, Dr Charles Hubert Bond appealed to their sense of the romantic by invoking the spirit of Retreat as 'a beacon of enlightened reform which has never been extinguished'.[81] Raising his new subordinates' expectations by such talk was unfair, for in reality their careers were devoted to administering a custodial, insular, and rather tedious regime. Life on the wards was mostly quiet and uneventful. Attendants intermarried and bred the next generation, transmitting the asylum culture across time. The 60 per cent of new inmates who were never discharged resigned themselves to the routines of asylum life, and the downward spiral of crumbling personal identity, mental decrepitude, and the inevitability of burial as a forgotten pauper lunatic.

A mental hospital

In 1906, there had been general relief at the news that the increase in those the LCC had to accommodate was at its lowest for five years.[82] A decision on an eleventh asylum was therefore deferred until after Long Grove was commissioned. In the meantime the Asylums Committee embarked upon a long-cherished project which provided some temporary relief from its normal work.

In April 1889, the LCC established a working party to examine the case for a special acute hospital, which had been the focus of considerable debate during the 1880s and 1890s. It is clear from the working party's terms of reference that the intention was not to separate the treatment of acute insanity in general from the asylum network; far from it. The review took the narrow focus of the need for a hospital 'as a complement to the existing asylum system ... for the study and curative treatment of insanity'.[83] The working party was chaired by Brudenell Carter, an eye surgeon at St George's Hospital, who was vice-chairman of the council's Sanitary and General Purposes Committee, and included Carr-Gomm of the London Hospital, and the chairman of the Asylums Committee. It took evidence from sixteen senior national figures in medicine (Henry Maudsley was not among them) and examined the case with the firm conviction that the study and treatment of insanity was established as a field of enquiry for somatic medicine.[84]

This initiative was the logical progression from the profession's rationalization of the low cure rates in the asylum system as a whole. Since the theory of hereditary degeneracy had come to the rescue by proffering an explanation of the persistence of chronicity which was acceptable to ruling élites, alienists could argue that cure rates were bound to be depressed if measured against this 'great wet blanket which lies upon the whole thing'.[85] The other major plank in the platform was the need for scientific research and the associated critique of large asylums as stony ground for the seeds of enquiry. First, although there was no questioning the necessity for medical leadership, it had to be acknowledged that a good administrator was not necessarily a good scientist.[86] Secondly, medical superintendents of the large asylums were too preoccupied with all the endless administrative duties required by the job to pursue sustained enquiry.[87]

As there was certainly no question of doctors abandoning these administrative powers, what was required was a separate institution small enough to allow a substantial minority of selected, curable cases to be given the requisite individual attention in conditions which allowed research to flourish. A unique opportunity for the founding of a small, 100-bedded hospital and research centre for curable pauper lunatics existed in London where it could be associated with the great schools of medicine, and so the working party recommended.

Although sympathetic, the Asylums Committee soon became overwhelmed by the torrent of referrals from unions, and shelved the report. The advocates of research were consoled as the committee commissioned Hine to build a Central Pathology Laboratory at Claybury Asylum. Its first director, Dr (later Sir) Frederick Mott, built up an international reputation through his post mortem investigations, particularly into forms of insanity which originated in transmissible organic disease. Mott became a friend of the ageing Henry Maudsley[88] and at his behest succeeded in persuading the Asylum Committee to revive the mental hospital scheme in 1907 as the demand for asylum places abated and there was at last a degree of breathing space; Maudsley providing the incentive by offering £30,000 of his own money towards the cost of building.

Naturally, Maudsley supported the case for research. He was also convinced that the stigma with which certification and the asylum were associated in the public's mind was a major impediment to early treatment.[89] But beyond this, the project when complete would serve as a means for securing the initiation of alienists into the medical dynasty, which was otherwise proving difficult. Psychiatry's aspirations to the status of a recognized medical specialty necessitated daily intercourse and cross-fertilization with other branches of academic medicine. The greater the distance from what Scull identifies as the professionally contaminating effects of the pauper asylum, the more likely the success of the endeavour.[90] These ambitions are symbolized in the hospital's façade. 'Magnificence' may have been a 'fatal characteristic' in asylum design,[91] but it was wholly commensurate with the requirements of a prestigious London teaching hospital. In its final cost of £95,000, the 108-bed Maudsley Hospital at Denmark Hill represented a capital investment per bed nearly six times greater than at Horton and Long Grove.[92]

Normal service resumed

The building of the Maudsley has been presented as signifying the beginning of a new era of qualitatively different lunacy management 'in the community'.[93] This misconstrues the motives of its planners since the project was out of step with the contemporaneous, mainstream preoccupations of the Asylums Committee. For as work on the new hospital proceeded, the LCC had two other initiatives in progress which sustained sequestration as the overriding policy objective.

The first was the construction of the eleventh and the last great asylum built for London's insane. At first, the Asylums Committee decided that the residents of Epsom had suffered enough and began looking for a new site, only to be obliged by the Finance and General Purposes Committee of the main council to add a fifth asylum to the Horton Manor estate.[94] There had been time to commission a novel design on this occasion from the committee's own chief engineer.[95] Clifford Smith received only a fifth of Mr Hine's normal fee, for a design which was significantly more imaginative than the latter's LCC schemes. There was a central 'hospital' sector comprising the acute wards. Refractory cases were placed in wards 'much humbler in design and finish'. The quiet and harmless classes were housed in detached villas, geometrically dispersed across the forty-acre, fan-shaped ground plan. There were remnants of the design features of moral treatment institutes in the skeletal palladian façades and occasional grandly pillared portals of the villas. The administration block was fashioned as an early-nineteenth-century manor house. The asylum was left virtually complete when at the outbreak of the First World War the Treasury placed a moratorium on all public works not directly connected with the war effort. Further delayed by the need for repairs due to dilapidation caused by abandoning the scheme, and the postwar shortage of building materials, the asylum eventually opened in 1924 as West Park Hospital: the LCC having introduced the new designation in 1918, twelve years before the Mental Treatment Act made the change mandatory.[96]

The second major policy thrust arose from the implementation of the report of the 1908 Royal Commission on the Care and Control of the Feeble-Minded, to which the LCC's medical advisers and a former chairman gave the kind of evidence which inspired its recommendations. These were implemented in the 1913 Mental Deficiency Act which separately classified mental defectives for the purposes of confinement. The theory of congenital degeneracy was the medical interpretation of the ideology of social Darwinism which was finding increased favour amongst the English ruling élite:[97] in this sense British psychiatrists were evidently behind their European counterparts in adopting the theory.[98] However, by the early 1900s, it had become the foremost explanation of chronic lunacy, imbecility, and idiocy expounded by London's asylum doctors. The medical superintendent at Bexley was one of the most fervent proponents.

> There is a floating mass of degeneracy in the population which is constantly augmented by the victims of social vice and its satellites, syphilis and drink, and from this mass we derive the bulk of our asylum population.... Fortunately, the infant mortality among this class is

> very high. Marriage with members of insane stock is comparatively rare amongst the upper and middle classes, seldom amongst the intelligent working class, but with the degenerates, insanity does not appear to be considered a bar to matrimony.[99]

Britain escaped the worst consequences of the more frantic, maniacal manifestations of eugenics, unlike Europe and the United States where castrations were carried out. Instead, the sensible British approach adopted in the Act was to protect the national genetic stock by denying liberty to the congenitally degenerate through their social deportation to specially constructed working colonies. The continued expansion of the professional empire of the medical superintendent was thereby assured for another generation. In Hubert Bond's words, it was the 'most humane, economical and medically wise' solution.[100]

As soon as the Act took effect in 1914, the Home Secretary granted a further ten-year life span to the 'temporary' units at The Manor. After the First World War, and facing postwar economic stringency and shortage of building materials, the renamed LCC Mental Hospitals Committee added a few more brick buildings to the existing iron huts and created the Manor Certified Institution. The LCC was fortunate as an authority to share the responsibilities under the new Act with the Metropolitan Asylums Board, which was already well placed hygienically to put into store the bulk of the new legal classifications. Consequently, the Manor was the only mental deficiency institute opened by the LCC during this period. So all official reference to the place as the 'temporary asylum' disappeared, dispatched by the 1920 annual report's careful drafting:

> A large part of the fabric is of *semi-permanent structure*, a fact which has fitted the premises exceptionally well for use as an institution which must in the nature of things be experimental.[101] (emphasis added)

(The first 'temporary' units at the Manor were demolished in 1986 and the rest remain in use.)

The opening of West Park in 1924 marked the end of the metropolitan asylums building spree which had begun with Hanwell almost a century earlier[102]. In the two decades after the First World War, the corridors of the LCC mental hospitals (and occasionally of Westminster) were to resound with the claims of the therapeutic onslaught which, channelled and mediated through the Maudsley, were to precipitate the inexorable if lingering demise of the asylum. But that is another story.

Notes

I am grateful to Sheila Howells for her helpful comments on the text, and also to the staff of the Greater London Record Office and the Greater London History Library.

1 Care and maintenance of pauper lunatics was vested with county justices of the peace in quarter sessions by the 1853 Lunatic Asylums Act.
2 The Kent County Asylum at Barming Heath.
3 These institutions were legally designated as workhouses.
4 The Lunatic Asylum Act of 1853 was amended by the 1888 Local Government Act to enable a county council with several asylums to appoint one committee to manage and control them all.
5 For the full powers of a Committee of Visitors, and their accountability to the Commissioners in Lunacy, Lord Chancellor's Visitors and the Secretary of State, see the annual report of the London County Council for 1911, chapter xxviii, pp. 7–8. Or more generally see H.C. Burdett (1891) *Hospitals and Asylums of the World*, London: Churchill, vol. I, pp. 179–83.
6 G.M. Ayers (1971) *England's First State Hospitals 1867–1890*, London: Wellcome.
7 Gathorne Hardy, the president of the Poor Law Board, estimated that of the 25,000 to 30,000 inmates of the metropolitan parish workhouses, under 3,000 were able-bodied. Although Hardy sympathized with the lobby for a poor law hospital system (which included Florence Nightingale and Edwin Chadwick) he defended the Bill's implied added cost to the ratepayers by informing Parliament that the Bill's aim was to enforce the spirit of the 1834 Poor Law Amendment Act by ensuring the proper classification of paupers. This implied the separate accommodation of different classes so that the able-bodied could be 'subjected to such course of labour as will repel the indolent or vicious'. Hansard 3rd S., vol. 185, cols 157–61. See also S. Webb and B. Webb (1963 reprint) *English Poor Law History*, London: Frank Cass, Part II, vol. I, p. 319 and Ayers, *England's First State Hospitals*, pp. 17–18.
8 As the Lunacy Commission noted in 1859, 'stringent conditions (adopted to meet the able-bodied paupers of sound mind) are not only unnecessary for the insane, but are obviously very unjust and detrimental to them'. Supplement to (1859) Twelfth report of the Commissioners in Lunacy, HC 1859, p. 6.
9 In the five years up to 1867 there had been major outbreaks of diphtheria, typhus, cholera and yellow fever. Webb and Webb, *English Poor Law History*, p. 317.
10 The term was also applied to the isolation hospitals.
11 Initially at Hampstead, Stockwell and Homerton. See Ayers, *England's First State Hospitals*, p. 33.
12 'The cost of building need not, in general, much exceed one-half of that incurred in the erection of ordinary Asylums; and the establishment of Officers and Attendants would be upon a more economical scale than those required in the principal Asylums.' Supplement to (1859) twelfth report of the Commissioners in Lunacy, HC, p. 37.
13 A.T. Scull (1980) 'A convenient place to get rid of inconvenient people: the Victorian lunatic asylum', in A.D. King (ed.), *Buildings and Society*, London: Routledge & Kegan Paul, pp. 53–5.
14 (1909) Minutes of Evidence to the Royal Commission on the Poor Laws and the Relief of Distress, vol. IA, appendix V(17), Cmnd 4628, London: HMSO, p. 128.
15 Derived from figures for the population of England and Wales in the Minutes of Evidence . . . on the Poor Laws and the Relief of Distress, vol. IA, appendix V(19), p. 132, and for the County of London from G. Gibbon and R.W. Bell

(1939) *History of the London County Council 1899–1939*, London: Macmillan, p. 674.

16 By the end of the century a number of unions had grouped together to provide poor law infirmaries. The average cost per in-patient year in these institutions had reached £33 14*s* 8*d* by 1897 and rose further to over £41 by 1906. (1909) Minutes of Evidence ... on the Poor Laws and the Relief of Distress, vol. II, appendix XIII(B), Cmnd 4684, London: HMSO.

17 Evidence of J.S. Davy, assistant secretary to the Local Government Board, in (1908) Minutes of Evidence to the Royal Commission on the Care and Control of the Feeble-Minded, vol. II, HC, pp. 349–52.

18 Evidence of Sir John Macdougall, chairman of the LCC Asylums Committee 1902–3 and chairman of the LCC 1895–8, in Minutes of Evidence ... on the Care and Control of the Feeble-Minded, vol. II, p. 371.

19 A.T. Scull (1979) *Museums of Madness*, London: Allen Lane, p. 238.

20 Evidence of Sir John Macdougall, in Minutes of Evidence ... on the Care and Control of the Feeble-Minded, vol. II, p. 389. When pressed by the medical members of the commission to name names, on the grounds that otherwise, the statement was 'distinctly discreditable to the medical profession', Macdougall was forced to retreat and concede that he was expressing 'a pious opinion rather than fact'.

21 Not surprisingly, throughout the second half of the nineteenth century, the rate of pauperism fluctuated with the cycles of unemployment. However, the fluctuations in the former were by far the less dramatic partly due to the constantly accumulating morass of the non-ablebodied, but also to some extent because of the success of the workhouse in deterring the unemployed from seeking relief. See (1909) The Report of the Royal Commission on the Poor Laws and Relief of Distress, Cmnd 4499 London: HMSO, and the Minutes of Evidence, vol. 1A, appendix 5, p. 118.

22 See Lunacy Act 1890, section 24, subsection 6, in G.E. Mills and A.H. Poyser (1934) *Lunacy Practice*, London: Butterworth & Shaw, pp. 216–17.

23 The qualification was reduced to £5 in 1892, and abolished altogether two years later. George Lansbury himself began his political career on the Board of Guardians at Poplar, and subsequently became a member of the LCC. See Norman Longmate (1974) *The Workhouse*, London: Temple Smith, pp. 268–71 and Webb and Webb, *English Poor Law History*, part II, vol. I, pp. 232–3.

24 Annual report of H. Preston-Thomas, inspector for the union counties of Cornwall, Devon and part of Somerset. (1900–1) Thirtieth annual report of the Local Government Board, p. 123. His opposite number for the metropolis, H. Lockwood, held that workhouses were unsuitable even for the initial reception of lunatics; ibid., p. 349.

25 For a discussion of the principles of the Panopticon in relation to contemporary notions of humanism and philanthropy, as well as its impact upon asylum and prison architecture, see R. Evans (July 1971) 'Bentham's Panopticon: an incident in the social history of architecture', *Architectural Association Quarterly*, 3: 21–37.

26 The factory analogy was not lost on contemporary observers, of course, albeit to argue that the asylum had failed its primary purpose of reform. As Arlidge observed: 'In a colossal refuge for the insane, a machine so put together, as to move with precise regularity and invariable routine; a triumph of skill adapted to show how such unpromising materials as crazy men and women may be

drilled into order and guided by rule . . . a gigantic asylum is a gigantic evil, and figuratively speaking, a manufactory of chronic insanity.' Cited in Scull, *Museums of Madness*, p. 220.

27 See Scull, *Museums of Madness*, pp. 194–8.

28 Devon and Kent were two of a number of authorities which employed the same architect to build both the County Asylum and the County Gaol.

29 As well as the prestigious Middlesex commission, Hine won the competitions for his designs for the asylums at Dorset (1890), Ryhope, Sunderland (1891), the Isle of Wight (1893), Rauceby, Sleaford (1897). As his reputation developed, Hine was also invited by a number of counties to act as judge. See R. Harper (1981) *Victorian Architectural Competitions*, London: Mansell, p. 237. Following a spate of correspondence to its editor during 1893, *The Builder* implied that this success rate reflected more than George Hine's professional talents. It noted that in five competitions judged by one C.H. Powell, Hine had come either first or second, whereas in three other competitions that he had entered, where there had been three different assessors, he had not been placed. *The Builder* concluded from this that it seemed 'highly probable that if there had been distinct assessors in each of the first five competitions, the results would have varied to a corresponding degree'. (10 June 1893) *The Builder* 63: 441.

30 (1900) Fifty-fourth annual report of the Commissioners in Lunacy, HC, p. 10.

31 Separate accommodation for working patients was first officially recommended in 1856; (1856) Tenth annual report of the Commissioners in Lunacy, HC, p. 27.

32 Burdett, *Hospitals and Asylums of the World*, vol. II, p. 112.

33 Hine's ground plan for Claybury is reproduced in ibid., p. 158.

34 See (1856) Tenth annual report . . ., p. 26, and Suggestions and Instructions Issued by the Lunacy Commissioners, para. 36, in Minutes of Evidence . . . on the Care and Control of the Feeble-Minded, vol. IV, p. 415.

35 H. Tomlinson (1980) 'Design and reform: the "separate system" in the nineteenth-century English prison', in King (ed.), *Buildings and Society*, p. 112.

36 The site cost £37,895 and the building tender was £337,945 or just under £170 per bed. (1899) First annual report of the Asylums Committee, LCC, p. 91.

37 Greater London Record Office (hereafter GLRO) LCC Min 465, entry for 24 April 1890.

38 ibid., p. 437.

39 ibid., p. 205.

40 The site in Kent was convenient as, when built, Bexley could take the 500 residents of that county's Barming Heath Asylum for whom the LCC was paying inflated maintenance charges.

41 (1896) Seventeenth annual report of the Asylums Committee, LCC, p. 7. Bexley is also described (16 September 1898) in *The Builder*, vol. 75: 387, and full ground and site plans were reproduced and approved in the (1896) Supplement to the fiftieth report of the Commissioners in Lunacy, HC.

42 GLRO/LCC Min 566, p. 696.

43 GLRO/LCC Min 567, pp. 181–2.

44 (1897) Eighth annual report of the Asylums Committee, LCC, p. 11.

45 GLRO/LCC Min 564, p. 316.

46 GLRO/LCC Min 567, p. 397.

47 Sir John Macdougall's evidence, in Minutes of Evidence ... on the Care and Control of the Feeble-Minded, vol. II, p. 390.
48 Hine immediately hit a problem on the new site. Whereas the ground conditions at Bexley had been well drained and ideal for building, there was heavy clay under the Epsom Estate. Although this offered an opportunity to save money through on-site brick manufacture, extensive excavations were needed to sink the 20-acre foundations deep into the subsoil, to avoid the effects of contraction and expansion according to the wetness of the weather. It all added £20,000 to the cost. GLRO/LCC Min 567, p. 694.
49 ibid., p. 624.
50 From £362,450 to £579,500. Asylums Committee annual reports for 1893–4 and 1901–2.
51 GLRO/LCC Min 568, pp. 76–90.
52 A central station was erected which included a 400-foot well lined with iron tubing to prevent seepage of contaminated water, and an electricity switching station. Plans to build a gas works were abandoned once favourable terms had been agreed with a local company. Later, a central boiler house was added to heat all five institutions.
53 GLRO/LCC Minutes/Asylums Committee/Horton Subcommittee I, p. 58.
54 See A.A. Jackson (1981) 'The Horton light railway', *The Railway Magazine* 127 (966): 479.
55 Bucknill introduced a limited scheme for boarding out at Devon Asylum. See W.Ll. Parry-Jones (1981) 'The model of the Gheel Lunatic Colony and its influence on the nineteenth-century asylum system in Britain', in A.T. Scull (ed.), *Madhouses, Mad-Doctors and Madmen*, London: Athlone, p. 209.
56 W.G. Clifford-Smith (1901) *Notes of a Visit to Continental and British Asylums*, London: LCC.
57 Report on Housing of Epileptics, in (8 June 1898) GLRO/LCC Minutes/ Asylums Accommodation Subcommittee.
58 ibid.
59 (January 1896–February 1899) GLRO/LCC Minutes/General Purposes Committee, p. 61.
60 ibid., p. 387.
61 The separation of epileptics was later abandoned partly for this reason and the colony redesignated as an asylum for general, curable cases.
62 (January 1896–February 1899) GLRO / LCC Minutes / General Purposes Committee (meeting 8.12.1898).
63 Parry-Jones argues that the colony system never gained ground in Britain. See Parry-Jones in Scull (ed.), *Madhouses, Mad-Doctors and Madmen*, p. 212. Although this was true of the nineteenth century, it actually became the favoured model in Britain after the First World War.
64 The Commissioners in Lunacy wrote to the Committee in February 1903 pressing for a second replica of the Bexley design, to be sited at Horton; (1903) Fourteenth annual report of the Asylums Committee, LCC, p. 7.
65 GLRO/LCC Min 468, p. 74.
66 GLRO/LCC Min 571, p. 134.
67 ibid., meeting 17 February 1903.
68 Minutes of Evidence ... on the Care and Control of the Feeble-Minded, vol. II, p. 382.
69 (1906) Regulations setting forth the Duties of the Officers and Servants of the London County Lunatic Asylums, London: LCC, para. 32.

70 (1922) Ministry of Health, Report of the Committee on the Administration of Mental Hospitals, London: HMSO, pp. 32–3.
71 J. Hawkes (1871) *On the General Management of Public Lunatic Asylums in England and Wales*, London: Churchill, pp. 32–3.
72 J.M. Granville (1877) *The Care and Control of the Insane*, London: Hardwick & Bogue, vol. II, p. 26.
73 Regulations ... the Duties of the Officers and Servants of the London County Lunatic Asylums, paras 81–90.
74 'The attendants shall take pains to acquire a knowledge of the character of their patients, they shall pay constant attention to their food, dress, occupation, exercise, and amusement, and encourage them to good conduct, endeavouring to promote a return to the habits of neatness and order, and to obtain their confidence by friendly treatment and uniform attention to their comforts'; ibid., para. 137.
75 R.A. Hunter (1956) 'The rise and fall of mental nursing', *Lancet* 98–9.
76 For example, in 1906, Hanwell Asylum, with 2,151 inmates, employed 7 medical staff, 297 attendants (including night and supervisory staff), 149 general servants and 128 clerks, works and other staff; (1906) Seventeenth annual report of the Asylums Committee, LCC appendix G, pp. 202–12.
77 (1913) Twenty-fourth annual report of the Asylums Committee, LCC, p. 19.
78 The national average for 1909–13 was 33.5 per cent. Ministry of Health, Report of the Committee on the Administration of Mental Hospitals, pp. 66–7. Things had therefore barely improved since Granville found rates of 33.54 per cent at Colney Hatch and 30.31 per cent at Hanwell some four decades earlier. Granville, *The Care and Control of the Insane*, vol. II, pp. 128 and 194.
79 Annual report of G.J. Gilfillan, medical superintendent at Colney Hatch Asylum, in (1912) Twenty-third annual report of the Asylums Committee, LCC, p. 40.
80 'The routes taken by walking parties shall be those authorised by the Medical Superintendent, and it is desirable that as far as possible, quiet country roads should be chosen, towns and villages avoided. During the walk, the attendants shall be so stationed that the whole of the patients are under supervision, and no patient shall, under any circumstances be allowed out of sight.' Regulations ... the Duties of the Officers and Servants of the London County Lunatic Asylums (As to Patients' Walking Parties), facing p. 25.
81 Reproduced in (1957) *The Long Grove Sports and Social Club Magazine*, Long Grove Hospital Management Committee.
82 GLRO/LCC Min 571, p. 205.
83 (1890) Report of the Committee of the London County Council on a Hospital for the Insane, London: LCC, as reproduced in Burdett, *Hospitals and Asylums of the World*, vol. II, p. 159.
84 As it confidently asserted in the introductory remarks to its report, 'all the forms of insanity with which we are acquainted are the direct result of material changes affecting the instrument of thought, the brain, and ... in considering insanity with reference to preventive or curative treatment, these material changes are all that need to be taken into account.' ibid., vol. II, p. 164.
85 Evidence of Clifford Allbutt, Lunacy Commissioner, in ibid., vol. II, p. 195.
86 Evidence of Sir James Crichton-Browne, superintendent at Newcastle Asylum and one of the Lord Chancellor's Visitors, in ibid., vol. II, pp. 182–93.
87 Crichton-Browne provided an apt illustration by citing the case of one large

asylum where the patients were under the impression that the medical superintendent was actually the asylum architect simply because they never saw him unless there were problems with the ward chimney; ibid., vol. II, p. 195.

88 See A. Lewis (April 1951) 'Henry Maudsley: his work and influence', *Journal of Mental Science* 97: 259–77.

89 'Exaggerated apprehensions of danger and the common notion of insanity as a disgrace to be concealed or put out of sight, rather than a disease to be seen and wisely dealt with, are still responsible for much neglect of early attention.' H. Maudsley (1909) 'A mental hospital – its aims and uses', *Archives of Neurology* iv: 12. In order to allow the necessary voluntary admission to the Maudsley, which was legally a public asylum like any other, the council included provision in its General Powers Bill for the 1914–15 session of Parliament. (1915) First annual report of the Asylums and Mental Deficiency Committee, LCC, p. 13.

90 Scull, *Museums of Madness*, pp. 177–8.

91 Granville, *The Care and Control of the Insane*, vol. 11, p. 151.

92 This figure includes the costs of construction and site acquisition. Maudsley bequeathed a further £10,000 to add to his original donation. The LCC provided £55,000 of the total building cost of £95,000 and paid £10,000 for the site. These costs are somewhat at odds with the figure cited in K. Jones (1972) *A History of the Mental Health Services*, London: Routledge & Kegan Paul, p. 235.

93 Jones, *A History of the Mental Health Services*, pp. 226–35.

94 (1912) Twenty-third annual report of the Asylums Committee, LCC, p. 9.

95 Clifford Smith, *Notes of a Visit to Continental and British Asylums*.

96 Legally, it remained an asylum until the 1930 Act.

97 See P. Morris (1969) *Put Away*, London: Routledge & Kegan Paul, p. 18.

98 See I. Dowbiggin (1985) 'Degeneration and hereditarianism in French mental medicine 1840–1890', in W.F. Bynum, R. Porter, and M. Shepherd (eds), *The Anatomy of Madness*, London: Tavistock, vol. I, pp. 188–232.

99 (1906) Annual report of T.E.K. Stansfield in the Seventeenth annual report of the Asylums Committee, LCC, pp. 56–7.

100 Evidence of Dr (later Sir Charles) Hubert Bond, then medical superintendent of the Ewell Epileptic Colony (later of Long Grove and subsequently a Lunacy Commissioner) in the Minutes of Evidence ... on the Care and Control of the Feeble-Minded, vol. 1, p. 468.

101 (1920) Annual report of the LCC Mental Hospitals and Mental Deficiency Committee, p. 23.

102 A few villas were added here and there during the 1920s and 1930s.

CHAPTER TEN

Quarantining the weak-minded: psychiatric definitions of degeneracy and the late-Victorian asylum

Janet Saunders

From the middle of the nineteenth century the pauper lunatic asylum became the chief setting for the treatment of mental illness, part of a wider trend towards the adoption of institution-based responses to social deviancy and dependency, ranging from the penitentiary prison, workhouse, and juvenile reformatory to compulsory schooling.[1] Historians seeking to explain these changes have for almost two decades fallen into two camps: those espousing a broadly 'Whiggish' explanation in terms of progress and reform, and those offering various 'revisionist' interpretations emphasizing the functional role of the total institution to help maintain control in a society characterized by class conflict and the needs of the capitalist market economy.[2] Although the early excesses of this dialogue have now subsided in favour of less polemic approaches, the revisionist portrayal of the incarcerative asylum remains a powerful image.[3] The late nineteenth century has been tagged as the 'age of incarceration', in which the lunatic asylums, the 'museums of madness', had an important role to play. In the large public asylums built after mid-century the repression and custodial control inherent in the reformers' theory of 'moral treatment' soon gained dominance over therapeutic aims. Rehabilitation of deviants and treatment of the insane were superseded by a policy of 'quarantine', in which isolating problem people from society became a key role of the institution. Andrew Scull has suggested that the boundaries of insanity were stretched to encompass 'all manner of decrepit, socially inept and incompetent, and superfluous people', so that people living on the margins of acceptability became liable to incarceration in an asylum. Similarly, in penal policy, Michael Ignatieff points to changes from the 1860s, in which the prison came to be used not for reformation but for the penal 'quarantine' of an identifiable subpopulation of offenders.[4]

Yet this vision of the wholesale consignment of inconvenient people to institutions lacks clear evidence. More recently, it has been suggested that we do not know enough about who was admitted to asylums, and what precipitated their consignment there.[5] Who were these 'superfluous people' and how far did the asylum serve to quarantine them from society? With these questions in mind, we examine here the treatment of a group of inmates who were included by contemporaries in this 'marginal' population – the mentally retarded or subnormal. Social histories of the asylum have tended either to ignore the mentally retarded or to amalgamate them with the mentally ill, yet by implication the presence of the retarded, the 'socially incompetent', in asylum populations is an important part of the segregative analysis of the asylum's role.[6] Within the institutional setting of the 1860s and 1870s, psychiatric and penal professionals developed a notion of the 'weak-minded' as presenting a unique social problem and campaigned for their complete segregation from society in specialized instituitions. Yet their proposals for special segregation of the mentally handicapped were not implemented. We discuss the factors contributing to this rejection of a policy of segregation in the last quarter of the nineteenth century and the implications for our image of the incarcerative asylum and its inmates. A central question is whether the attitudes evident in the national debate about segregation and control of the retarded were reflected in local institutional practice. Much of the evidence used to illuminate this concern is drawn from my study of incarcerative institutions in Warwickshire, particularly of the records of the Warwick County Lunatic Asylum between the years 1851 and 1890. This evidence indicates that, at least with respect to the mentally subnormal, the asylums of the 1860s and 1870s were not serving to quarantine 'superfluous people' as successfully as Scull's interpretation would have us believe.[7]

Something should briefly be said about the terminology used to describe mental handicap in the late Victorian period. Three terms which need clarification are 'feeble-minded', 'weak-minded', and 'imbecile'. These were broadly used to refer to different gradations of 'imbecility of one or several of the faculties', as opposed to 'idiocy', which was reserved for severe conditions affecting all the faculties. During the second half of the nineteenth century the labels 'feeble-minded' and 'weak-minded' seem to have been interchangeable, the latter being more commonly used. Although they were occasionally used as descriptive terms for those who 'fell into a weak mind as a consequence of mania', their general usage was to describe congenital mental subnormality in reference to the less severely mentally handicapped.[8] In an early classification by Alexander Morison in 1824, imbecility was used to describe a condition of mental defect, both congenital and acquired. In the 1870s the term began to be restricted to congenital cases only, 'dementia' being substituted for mental weakness caused by disease. By this time, the medical profession was using a graduated classification of mental retardation, with 'idiots' at the lower range of ability, 'imbeciles' low to middle, and 'weak-minded' at the ability level closest to normality. Where the terms are used in this chapter, I have followed broadly these meanings.[9]

The perception of the 'weak-minded' as a problem population

The 1845 Lunacy Act provided for certification of idiots, lunatics, or persons of unsound mind. Thus in cases of mental subnormality it remained largely at the discretion of medical authorities as to who could be certified and who could not. Demands for the segregation and control of the mentally retarded as a specific group began to be heard from the late 1860s. Two groups of professionals saw the mentally handicapped as a problem: doctors in the prison medical service, and experts in psychiatry. Foremost in making these demands were prison surgeons. During the latter half of the century, changes in law and practice enabled offenders who were mentally ill or severely subnormal to be removed from prisons and sent to asylums, particularly in the case of serious offences brought to trial by jury.[10] However, these changes did not extend to the less severely retarded, most of whom remained imprisonable whenever they came into contact with the criminal law, outside the reaches of the Lunacy Commissioners. They became ultimately the responsibility of the prison surgeon who had to ensure that prisoners were fit to undergo prison discipline (in other words, solitary confinement) and who was able to order any necessary relaxation in discipline for particular prisoners. Two prison surgeons who were particularly influential in creating a stereotype of the weak-minded offender were James Bruce Thomson of Perth General Prison, and William Guy, medical superintendent of Millbank Prison in London from 1859 to 1866. Both were busy in the 1860s gathering data on mentally disordered prisoners. In a paper on the hereditary nature of crime, published in 1870, Thomson estimated that some 12 per cent of the inmates of Scottish prisons, exclusive of those sent to asylums as lunatics, were 'mentally weak in different degrees . . . apparently from congenital causes'. The figure was based on the number of cases placed on his registers for medical treatment on account of their mental condition.[11] Thomson's paper was widely read and of considerable influence.

More important, however, in the story of the weak-minded prisoner, was the work of William Guy, who from the 1860s mounted a personal crusade to confine the mentally retarded in separate institutions. When he became medical superintendent of Millbank Prison in 1859, Guy was already well known in the field of medical statistics, having given evidence before the Health of Towns Commission and written numerous papers on questions of sanitary reform, the health of bakers and soldiers and hospital mortality.[12] A leading light in the Statistical Society, Guy turned his attention to the health and mortality of convicts. In 1862 he published the results of a detailed census of the 7,170 inmates of the convict prisons, which included a cross-tabulation of the convicts' bodily and mental condition with their offences. He found that weak-minded, insane, and epileptic men and women were particularly disposed to crimes of arson and violence, and sexual offences. He also found that crimes of burglary and housebreaking were as common among the weak-minded convicts as among mentally 'normal' convicts. As he believed greater intellect was needed for these offences, Guy concluded that 'the able-bodied and intelligent housebreaker seeks the assistance of weak-minded men and women in his nefarious enterprises', and it was perhaps this which first impressed upon him 'danger of allowing persons of the imbecile class to remain at large'.[13] Millbank Prison was at that time the observation centre for all convicts suspected to be of 'weak or unsound mind' and Guy became absorbed in examining the incidence of insanity among criminals. In 1869 he carried out a statistical exercise to compare the degree of insanity among convicts with that among paupers in workhouses and with the population at large.[14]

Guy estimated insanity among the general population to occur in the ratio of about 1.67 per thousand, a very much lower figure than the 57 per thousand which he estimated to be the rate among convicts. He concluded that the convict population was much more liable to insanity than the general population. Yet his particular concern was the 'dark figure' of criminal weak-mindedness, which he reckoned to exist among the general population at about ten times the number of insane in prison. Guy's dark figure was made up particularly of the weak-minded and epileptic, who, he said, spent their lives roaming about the country, known as 'half-sharps' and 'dozeys', living by doles in the day time, sleeping in the casual wards of workhouses and taking part in criminal activity. Guy's solution to the problem of these roaming criminal imbeciles was to round them up and certify them as insane, increasing the number and size of lunatic asylums to cope with all these extra cases. Thus, Guy suggested, the lunatic asylum would become the substitute for the workhouse, the hospital, and the prison.[15] In much the same way, Dr Thomson in the following year suggested that transportation and long sentences might lessen the numbers of hereditary offenders.[16]

These prison surgeons' concern with weak-mindedness might have passed unnoticed among the plethora of Victorian statistical investigations had it not been for the dilemma of penal theory in the 1860s. The optimism that had accompanied the adoption of the separate system in the 1840s barely survived beyond the 1850s. Within a decade of the adoption of the new system it became clear that the model prisons were not reforming criminals.[17] The demise of transportation meant that some new policy was needed. In 1863 a Royal Commission investigated the operation of the penal servitude and transportation acts and a Select Committee reported on the state of discipline in the local gaols. Both recommended stronger measures. With the added incentive of the garotting panic of 1862, imprisonment was given an explicitly deterrent slant by the 1862 Prison Act.[18]

Yet even deterrence seemed to lack the power to curb crime. Penal writers and the annual reports of the police and prison departments persistently confirmed that offenders were returning to prison again and again. Incorrigible offenders were legion, particularly in the case of petty offences, where sentences were short enough to allow criminals to accumulate a string of committals. In this atmosphere of defeat the suggestion that such offenders were by their very nature irreclaimable must have seemed an attractive proposition for despairing penologists.

Both Thomson and Guy were adamant that the weak-minded were recidivists and vice versa. Thomson singled out as of low mental ability the 'habitués who go out and into prison now and then, who live by crime and have been born in crime'.[19] Part of the link between the weak-minded and recidivism was a real one. Some of the most frequently convicted local prison inmates were the alcoholics, often diagnosed by prison doctors as of weak mental capacity. Similarly itinerants, another frequently reconvicted group, were sometimes mentally retarded people without family support, who found it impossible to get work or housing.[20] By the late 1860s habitual offenders were beginning to be described in medical and biological terms. At the Exeter meeting of the British Association in 1869 Dr Wilson read a paper entitled 'The moral imbecility of habitual criminals as exemplified by cranial measurements'. Wilson had examined and measured the heads of around 460 prisoners and concluded that habitual criminals were cranially deficient.[21] Such investigations formed part of the growing scientific debate on the question of progressive degeneration, which was carried on with vigour in the general mood of psychiatric pessimism that was pervasive throughout Europe by the 1870s.[22]

The theory of progressive degeneration had first been elaborated in 1857, when the Frenchman Morel outlined a four-stage transmission of inherited defects leading eventually to idiocy and insanity.[23] However, in the 1870s the psychiatric writer most responsible for introducing degeneracy theory into the debate about habitual criminals in Britain was Henry Maudsley. Maudsley used the findings of the prison doctors to support the theory that mental illness was largely inherited and that a tendency to insanity could not be controlled by the will of the individual. Implicit in Maudsley's theory was the idea of progessive degeneration through inherited defects of constitution:

> When the insane temperament has been developed in its most marked form, we must acknowledge that the hereditary predisposition has assumed the character of deterioration of race, and that the individual represents the beginning of a degeneracy, which, if not checked by favourable circumstances, will go on increasing from generation to generation and end finally in the extreme degeneracy of idiocy.[24]

Thus the mentally deficient and the criminal were linked in that they represented merely different points along the slippery slope towards idiocy. For Maudsley the existence of habitual criminals was proof of this 'tyranny of organisation'; 'they go criminal as the insane go mad, because they cannot help it'.[25] Maudsley's theory seemed all the more plausible in that it offered evolutionary explanations of moral and mental deficiency.

Darwin's *Origin of Species* was published in 1859 and although comments on human evolution were limited in this work, the following years saw a growing acceptance of evolutionary theory and debate about its implications for human character and society. Thus social Darwinism was well under way by the time Darwin published his own thoughts on human evolution in *The Descent of Man* in 1871.[26] By then it was generally believed that human nationalities could be graded on a developmental scale.[27] Criminals, the weak-minded, and paupers were seen as atavistic throwbacks or cases of arrested development typifying lower stages of human evolution.[28] Studies of the family histories of persistent offenders were widely used to substantiate the theory. Thomson recounted stories of criminal families to show how 'the lower forms of mental disease such as silliness and imbecility' alternated in 'degenerate' families with idiocy, epilepsy, eccentricity, and crime.[29] Even without the more well-known American studies such as that of the Juke family, published in the mid-1870s, English theorists already had a long-established body of information to support their ideas.[30]

That biology might explain habitual crime was appealing to prison administrators and criminologists perplexed at the failure of deterrent imprisonment. An important convert to this biologism was Sir Edmund DuCane, chairman of the directors of convict prisons and head of the Prison Commission. By 1875 DuCane was convinced that crime was to a great extent 'connected with mental inferiority of some kind, whether as cause and effect or as accompanying one another'.[31] From his own experience, DuCane claimed that physical stigmata denoted both habitual criminals and habitual vagrants and that aspects of the 'criminal character' resembled more closely the behaviour of primitives than that of civilized races. Such characteristics were 'wandering habits, utter laziness, absence of forethought or provision, want of moral sense', and what he described merely as 'dirt'. Deterrence could not reform the members of this 'separate caste' and DuCane supported Dr Guy's opinion that the best solution was to remove such persons to custodial institutions. There they would be contained and prevented from leading their depredatory lives at large and also from 'propagating their kind'.[32]

The new pessimism was evident in the proceedings of the commission which investigated the workings of the Penal Servitude Acts in 1878, of which William Guy was a member. The most fruitful evidence from Guy's point of view was that given by William Hardman, chairman of the Surrey Quarter Sessions, who commented on the 'low physical and moral type' of offender regularly appearing before him. He agreed that a new type of institution, 'something between a workhouse and an asylum', was needed to confine these 'imbeciles'. The committee discussed the possibility of allowing two doctors to certify imbecility, as ground for detaining an offender in one of the proposed asylums beyond the term of a prison sentence. Hardman pointed out, however, that there would be public opposition to such extension of medical discretion. 'There is a great deal of nonsense talked about the liberty of the subject in this country', he declared.[33] In their report, the commissioners concluded that weak-minded criminals formed a large proportion of the habitual criminal class, thus providing official endorsement of Dr Guy's image of the habitually criminal imbecile.

Weak-minded inmates in prison, county asylum, and workhouse

As the local prisons were brought under the control of the Prison Commission in 1877, opinions about weak-minded convicts were naturally extended to the inmates of the county and borough prisons. How does the tenor of the national debate compare with treatment of weak-minded prisoners at the local level? The 1865 Prison Act laid down that each prison was to have its own doctor, who was to inspect all prisoners on entry to prison. Particular attention was to be given to the prisoner's mental health, partly because it might break down under the solitude, but also to enable the prison authorities to defend themselves against accusations that weak-minded inmates had been made so by prison discipline.[34] Comments on weak-minded inmates are scanty in prison records before 1865. Before regular inspection was introduced the prison chaplain was probably the official best placed to recognize mental disability. At the local prison in Shrewsbury the chaplain kept a journal from 1856 to 1861 in which he noted particulars of 191 prisoners received into the prison. Seven of these were described by him as being of 'weak intellect', 'dull', or 'half-witted' but none was subsequently removed to the local county asylum.[35] Such a piece of evidence is rare. In Warwickshire, prison records were limited to the chaplain's and surgeon's reports to the quarter sessions, and these yield no mention of weak-minded prisoners.

However, the records of the Warwick County Asylum contain those of criminal cases admitted from the prison and help to illuminate practices there. Altogether thirty-four out of 146 'criminal lunatics' admitted to the asylum between 1852 and 1890 were described as weak-minded or imbecile by the asylum staff. Several of them had been managed within the prison as weak-minded prisoners before insanity was certified. In these cases there is no evidence that discipline had been relaxed. A young woman said to be weak-minded on admission to prison was set to work in the washhouse, until she became noisy and troublesome, running screaming around the laundry yard. Another girl described by the asylum doctors as of 'deficient cranial development' and 'imbecile expression' was punished in prison for a similar outbreak, insanity only being suspected when the punishment failed to produce any effect.[36] The picture which emerges is one in which feeble-minded prisoners were subjected to normal prison discipline. Sometimes their inability to conform to that discipline was sufficient to allow a certificate of insanity and transfer to an asylum. One of the few circumstances which warranted a relaxation of the separate system was when prisoners became suicidal. A young woman committed for assault who developed a 'peculiar reserved manner' in gaol and talked of destroying herself, was never allowed to be alone in her cell. Placing suicidal weak-minded prisoners in association with other prisoners was recognized practice, and became so common at Millbank Prison that the authorities suspected most convicts who attempted suicide to be attempting to get out of separate confinement.[37]

The effect of imprisonment on offenders' mental health should not be discounted, and it was one of the topics examined by the 1878 Commission on the Penal Servitude Acts. Dr Campbell of Woking Prison admitted that when the separate system had first been introduced and rigidly enforced it had a deleterious effect on the minds of the prisoners. It is likely that some of the so-called feeble-minded convicts were in fact old offenders who had served repeated sentences under solitary or separate confinement, and who had been mentally damaged by it. The governor of Maidstone Gaol believed that separate confinement could cause insanity even when no tendency had existed before imprisonment, but other governors were less enlightened. The governor of Portland Prison attributed all the insanity which occurred in the convict prisons to 'the habit of perpetual never-ending self-abuse' among the convicts.[38] In its conclusion the commission found that the weak-minded created special disciplinary problems; they were subject to sudden outbursts of temper and strange and eccentric acts of violence; they were a source of irritation to the ordinary prisoners and were often encouraged by them to be insubordinate and violent to the wardens. The prison authorities felt that often, for the sake of prison discipline, they had to punish weak-minded prisoners for offences which were not the full responsibility of the weak-minded themselves. Part of the problem was that the weak-minded could not be relied upon to respond rationally to the penal regime with merely grudging acquiescence and suppressed protest.[39] They were more likely to express their feelings openly, as the chaplain of Parkhurst Prison explained:

> You never know what they will do or say to you. I am very careful in my public ministrations to say nothing which will give them any cause of excitement. A man will get up and say 'That is me, Sir.' When I have been using our church prayer, the collect for unity, peace and concord, I have heard a man say 'There is no peace here; look how I have been punished', and that man has to be removed quietly.[40]

Clearly such outbursts as these threatened to upset the balance of discipline within the prison at any time and could easily spark off more serious actions by other prisoners. It is tempting to speculate whether the label of weak-minded was not in some cases merely a label for individuals who doggedly refused to give in and accept their role as repentant sinners quietly working out their punishment. The sources, however, allow only the conclusion that people labelled as weak-minded represented a perpetual problem for the prison authorities, and were viewed as a distinct category of deviant, requiring new institutional provisions.

How were mentally handicapped people viewed and treated in other institutions? The casebooks and admission forms of the Warwick County Asylum suggest that it was chiefly the most severely mentally handicapped adults who were certified and sent to the asylum, and even then only those who became violent or exhibited delusions. In 1861 when five 'idiots' were admitted to the county asylum, Dr Parsey, the superintendent, commented that 'only such idiots as are found to be unmanageable in their own homes, or union houses, are sent here'.[41]

Nevertheless by the late 1860s the number of severely mentally handicapped patients at the Warwick County Asylum was interfering with the treatment of the other inmates and creating problems of classification and organization. In 1867 it was decided that all the harmless cases should be removed to a new building, where the cost of their care would be cheaper, at the same time creating space in the main asylum for private patients. The new 'Idiot Asylum' which opened in 1871 was to provide accommodation for the 'idiots and imbeciles from the unions and workhouses', presumably to extend to those on outdoor relief as well as indoor relief.[42] This could, in theory, have taken in many of the weak-minded as well as the more seriously handicapped, but only the worst cases from the workhouses were sent in. A separate case note volume for the Idiot Asylum was kept between 1871 and 1884, in which the case histories of patients transferred there from the main asylum were copied up from earlier case books and new admissions entered. The staff assessed the 'improvability' of each patient on entry to the idiot asylum, and the case notes show that many of the adult inmates were given some training in the school, despite pessimism about how much they might benefit from it. Notes concerning the capabilities of patients transferred from the main asylum indicate that prior to 1871 little attempt had been made to discover what they could do, or to increase their abilities. In the new asylum these abilities were utilized in the service of the institution. In 1873 less than half of the ninety-one inmates of the idiot asylum received school instruction, but nearly three-quarters of them were capable of some sort of employment: on the farm, in the laundry, knitting and sewing and at simple trades, or fetching and carrying about the asylum. It was estimated that the work of at least half of them was of real value to the institution, but no comment was made of its value to the idiots themselves.[43] Apart from the work done by the inmates at Warwick's idiot asylum, the superintendent's annual reports contain very little comment on treatment there. In the 1870s and 1880s asylum superintendents still saw insanity as their chief concern. Many of them, like Parsey of the Warwick Asylum, had trained in the era of optimism; inmates for whom they could only offer custodial care were an unfortunate necessity, but not the main business of a county asylum.

Despite Parsey's insistence on the low ability of idiots admitted to the Warwick Asylum, definitions of idiocy were somewhat elastic. A young woman admitted in 1872 was described as dumb, but she understood perfectly when spoken to; another who was deaf and dumb could answer questions when written on a slate. In 1876 twenty-two of the idiot asylum's inmates were described as dumb.[44] Despite this clear stretching of the boundaries of insanity, it is also evident that mere weak-mindedness did not justify long-term detention. Two weak-minded women, 'criminal lunatics' who had come to the asylum from the local prison, were discharged within six months as recovered, although one was described as 'still very simple' and the other as exhibiting no mental peculiarities apart from 'a certain amount of probably natural weakness'. Their committal to prison and transferral to the asylum took place in the 1870s when concern over the fertility of weak-minded women and the inheritance of mental defect was growing. Their discharge, however, indicates that incarcerating weak-minded people was not a major function of county asylums. There are numerous instances of other inmates who fell neatly into Dr Guy's stereotype of the criminally inclined weak-minded, but who were discharged as not insane. In 1877, for example, a Prussian baker was admitted from the prison who told the superintendent that he had not followed his calling lately but had gone about the country playing a concertina and often got drunk. He had been in asylums before and in gaol many times, and had apparently spent the past fourteen years wandering about the country. He was nevertheless discharged recovered in 1878. It is difficult to put inmates into categories from case note descriptions such as 'simple-minded', 'drunkard', 'irregular character' and the like, but it is clear that inmates described in these ways were likely to be discharged if there was some improvement in their behaviour or if no evidence of delusions or of severe handicap could be found.[45]

The workhouse was the more likely home of mentally retarded people who could not subsist or be supported outside an institution. Many were numbered among the harmless and chronic lunatic cases who were retained in workhouses long after the establishment of the county asylums, kept there primarily because it was cheaper to provide workhouse insane wards than to pay for expensive asylum care.[46] Attempts to induce guardians to send lunatics to asylums, such as a subsidy introduced in 1874, merely resulted in an influx into the asylums of all the chronic cases, whose difficult nursing care could be offloaded on to the asylum staff.[47]

In the workhouse as in the asylum, the variability of classification makes it difficult to discover how many inmates were insane, idiot, or weak-minded at any one time. In Warwickshire, the Coventry workhouse was the only one to contain a separate ward for the insane, but all the county unions retained some cases in the workhouse. The Lunacy Commissioners' report for 1851, for example, stated that there were sixteen insane inmates at Coventry. The 1851 census enumerators' books for the workhouse reveal a finer classification of four lunatics, two idiots, one imbecile, five 'weak-minded' and two inmates with fits. On the other hand, Warwick Union Workhouse relief lists of the 1860s and 1870s used only the word 'insane' to denote mental defect, and the 1871 census of the workhouse allows the identification of 'imbeciles' only. Without the kind of detailed descriptions given in the Coventry case it is not possible to ascertain whether these figures included the 'weak-minded' at all. Only one of the imbecile cases listed for Warwick workhouse could be later located in the register of the County Idiot Asylum. Four cases were retained in the workhouse into the 1890s, although one of them was only twenty years old in 1871 and might have benefited from the 'training' available at the asylum.[48]

Most of the mentally retarded in workhouses were probably not classified separately from the other occupants. In 1849 the Poor Law Board had expressly stated that a weak-minded pauper must either be classed as a lunatic and treated as such, or not a lunatic and therefore requiring no special treatment in the general workhouse.[49] It seems the Lunacy Commissioners approved of this policy. Reporting in 1859, they commented that a number of the pauper lunatics in workhouses were weak-minded rather than insane and were thus properly kept in the house, rather than an asylum. By way of example they cited the case of a woman, the sole 'lunatic' inmate of Aberayron workhouse in Wales:

> She is reported to be weakminded, and if so is properly kept in the workhouse, more especially as she has three illegitimate children. She has three times returned in a state of pregnancy, after having been discharged, or rather, I believe, insisted on her discharge.[50]

By the early 1870s, however, ideas were beginning to change in favour of asylum detention. A medical handbook advised doctors that weak-minded persons with 'strong sexual propensities' should not be allowed to remain in the workhouse, but should be certified and removed to an asylum.[51] Such advice was probably of little effect in the face of the guardians' preference for workhouse over asylum provision, and the fact that many of the retarded were not certifiable as insane. In London the Metropolitan Poor Act of 1867 provided for the establishment of two asylums at Leavesden and Caterham for over 1,000 inmates each, which were to take idiots and imbeciles from the metropolitan workhouses. Only certifiable lunatics could be transferred there, however, and it was not until 1903 that it was felt necessary to issue a special order for the transfer of children who were mentally defective, but not certifiable, to the two asylums. Outside London no similar alternative to the workhouse or lunatic asylum existed. Most of the retarded remained in workhouses as ordinary inmates. Towards the end of the century, when Poor Law officials began to protest about the lunatic presence in the workhouse, they could still refer to 'gibbering idiots' and imbeciles who were said to cause great distress to the other inmates.[52]

It was acknowledged by contemporaries that weak-minded persons were useful in the workhouse. Those not severely handicapped proved valuable able-bodied workers as the house became less and less like the institution envisaged in 1834 and more akin to an infirmary.[53] The weak-minded were employed in laundry and domestic work, even as helpers in the care of lunatics and young children, until this latter duty was ended by a directive in 1868.[54] The Lunacy Commissioners gave their approval to this exploitation of the weak-minded in their report for 1867, commenting on their suitability for this sort of work.

> For the most part they are harmless, tractable and readily disposed to work; and with a little encouragement and superintendence often become extremely industrious and useful. In some of the smaller workhouses where there are few or no other able-bodied inmates, most of the garden and outdoor labour is performed by males of this description; and the females are very frequently employed in household work, in the kitchen and scullery and in the washhouse, where being under the eye of the matron, they are active and obedient servants.[55]

Certainly the guardians would have been reluctant to lose such willing and inexpensive workers to the county asylums.

Evidence from Warwickshire showed another side to this docile image of weak-minded paupers in the workhouse. The mentally retarded and other handicapped people, such as the deaf, who were often mistaken for mentally deficient, did not always accept their position unquestioningly, and as permanent inmates could be a source of trouble for the authorities. The insane paupers were liable to the same rules of discipline as the able-bodied inmates, and were frequently punished or brought before magistrates for violent or disruptive behaviour.[56] Paupers were often sent to prison for breaches of workhouse discipline, and nine of the Warwickshire criminal lunatics had been initially imprisoned in this way. Some of these people were mentally retarded, several others were epileptics or alcoholics who had damaged workhouse property during a fit, and one was an old man suffering from general paralysis. One middle-aged man was described as a congenital imbecile, although he could read and write. Following the death of his parents he had managed to support himself by doing odd jobs. Occasionally he had to fall back on the workhouse and on one such occasion he absconded without leave and stole something from a boat on the way. He was sent to prison for two and a half months, where, according to the surgeon, the solitude led to delusions and insanity. All of these were part of the amorphous group of the marginally insane who were forced into the workhouse through lack of work, food, or friends to care for them.[57]

The weak-minded and segregative control

The toleration of weak-minded inmates in asylums and workhouses as useful, if occasionally troublesome, workers, contrasts sharply with the organizational and disciplinary problems they were seen to present in local prisons. Within the convict system, a degree of segregation was implemented by concentrating feeble-minded prisoners at Woking Prison, although even there they were mixed with other prisoners.[58] When the Prison Commission took over the local prisons in 1877, it could not cope with all the extra weak-minded inmates in this way, and it is from this time that the problem of how to deal with them, and the question of whether they should be in prison at all, assumed new proportions and urgency.

By the end of the 1870s this campaign was reaching its climax. In 1879 Dr R.M. Gover, Guy's successor at Millbank Prison, became Medical Inspector of Government Prisons and began to collect data concerning the number of weak-minded offenders received into the local prisons each year. His report for 1879–80 contained a return of 541 cases of weak-minded and imbecile prisoners convicted during 1879. Governors had been asked to give their opinion as to whether such offenders were frequently reconvicted. Although the return provided inconclusive evidence that the weak-minded were habitual criminals, the commissioners ignored this in their report. They suggested that means should be devised to ensure that proper care be taken of persons whose 'imbecility or low mental power has conduced to their becoming criminals and who for the same reason cannot be deterred by remembrance of past punishment from repeating their crimes and suffering the penalties'. Again the claim was made that the weak-minded were used by other criminals to help them commit crimes and thus avoid detection themselves, to emphasize the danger of neglecting the issue.[59]

An opportunity to investigate the matter more fully came when the Commissioners in Lunacy and asylum superintendents renewed their campaign to remove criminal lunatics from county asylums. The psychiatric lobby wanted separate institutions to be provided for offenders certified insane while serving sentences, claiming they were difficult patients to control and contain in county asylums.[60] DuCane recommended that in order to do the question justice, a full inquiry was necessary, particularly since it presented an opportunity to examine the whole question of disordered offenders who were habitually criminal. In a letter to the Home Secretary, DuCane made it clear that his solution to this problem was long-term detention of such people.

> A very considerable proportion of our criminal population consists of people mentally affected or deficient in some way or another, and many of them are criminal because they are lunatic or imbecile. These persons commit crimes, sometimes grave, sometimes paltry, get sentenced to short or long periods, discharged and then begin again as a matter of course, and perhaps breed others like themselves to supply criminals for the next generation. Either they have no friends or their friends will not or cannot look after them. It would be to the interests of society if these people were confined and taken care of and it would not fail to be a benefit to them to be removed from a life passed either committing crime or suffering from having done so.[61]

The scene was set for an extension of institutional control to the mentally handicapped. The Departmental Committee which was established in 1881 to enquire into the subject of criminal lunacy included among its considerations whether 'special provisions should be made for the care and custody of imbeciles who are habitually criminal?'[62] The committee members included Edmund DuCane and William Guy, and also Dr Arthur Mitchell, one of the inspectors of the Scottish Board of Lunacy, who proved to be an important contributor to the outcome.[63]

Much of the questioning of Guy and DuCane was aimed at collecting evidence to support the segregation of feeble-minded habitual criminals, but from the outset it became clear that the subject was a difficult one. How exactly to define this group was the first major obstacle. There was disagreement among the witnesses as to a precise definition of the terms 'weak-minded', 'imbecile', and 'idiot', although most agreed that these conditions were recognizable to medical men or those with experience of the weak-minded and insane.[64] It was clear that any identification and segregation of the weak-minded would rely heavily on the discretion of doctors, who were already under public criticism for their subjective and sometimes even ridiculous criteria for the diagnosis of lunacy.[65] This also meant that it was difficult to estimate the number of cases that might have to be dealt with. The witnesses simply agreed that there were 'many' cases in the prisons, workhouses, and asylums.[66]

Guy and DuCane were joined in their concern to segregate criminal imbeciles by W.G. Campbell, one of the Commissioners in Lunacy. They argued, first, that the weak-minded were hard to manage in existing institutions because they were treacherous, unpredictable, and dangerous; secondly, that because of their recidivism they needed a greater degree of control than other offenders; and thirdly, that special imbecile asylums should be established so that criminal imbeciles would be segregated 'in some safe place where they could work for their living', and where they would be prevented from 'propagating their kind'.[67] William Guy pointed out that some precedent for the detention of imbeciles already existed under the 1853 Lunacy Act's provision for lunatics found 'wandering at large', as it was chiefly imbeciles who fell into this category.[68] Guy was less clear about the numbers of imbeciles to be dealt with. He advocated that immediate provision should be made for the 231 imbeciles already undergoing imprisonment as convicts. This, however, was only the first step in the ultimate incarceration and control of all the mentally deficient who were likely to commit crimes, and Guy's estimate of their numbers ran into many thousands. He implied that they made up a large proportion of the 108,000 persons known to the police as thieves, vagrants, habitual drunkards, and prostitutes, and also that the majority of the 23,000 persons prosecuted for wilful damages each year, were imbeciles. Ultimately it was for these numbers of people that his scheme was intended.

The members of the committee, however, were not drawn solely from the prison service. Opposition to Guy's scheme came particularly from Dr

Mitchell, who, from the 1860s, had been advocating care of the insane within the community as an alternative to the asylum system.[69] As Deputy Commissioner in Lunacy for Scotland, his ideas were largely based on the system applied by the Scottish Lunacy Commission by which mentally deficient and other harmless lunatics were either subsidized to remain with their families or were boarded out to 'kindly guardians', who were paid to provide the imbecile with a home, food, care, and clothing.[70] Mitchell explained that under this treatment they became more good-natured, less irritable and mischievous, and 'being dressed like ordinary people of the working class, the old village fools seemed at once to disappear from the villages without having really left them'.[71] This practice had become an established part of Scottish care of the insane and a return of 1867 showed that over a quarter of Scotland's lunatic poor were cared for in this way.[72]

Mitchell's ideas were set out in a lengthy memorandum to the commission. Essentially he was opposed to the detention of mentally disordered people by the prison department outside the control of the Lunacy Laws, and rejected broadening the category of lunacy. What he found most disturbing was Guy's insistence that such sequestration of weak-minded offenders should be for life. Not even under the Lunacy Laws were people banished to an institution for life, at least in principle, and Mitchell was disturbed that only the opinion of two prison medical officers would be justification for permanent detention. Mitchell realized that the full unfolding of Guy's scheme would involve the segregation of far greater numbers of weak-minded offenders than those already in prison, and he pointed out how expensive this would be.

Perhaps Arthur Mitchell's most important criticism, however, was his challenge of Dr Guy's characterization of the imbecile. The stereotype of the criminal imbecile was based largely on the prison doctor's experiences of imbeciles in prison, who, Mitchell insisted, represented only a handful of the weak-minded as a whole and were quite different from those met with in other institutions and at large. Such people were all too often neglected and led hard and miserable lives. Unable to earn a living they frequently had little choice but to wander, beg, and steal. Such habits did not indicate any instinctive desire to do so; 'they are not naturally restless thieving vagabonds'. Against the experience of the prison doctors Mitchell substituted his own. He asserted that many of the cases he had witnessed in asylums, prisons, boarded-out and at large, were as likely to commit crimes or become dangerous as he was himself.[73] Mitchell cast doubt on the criminality of the weak-minded, the accuracy of the prison medical officers' diagnoses of imbecility, and the claim that they were difficult and dangerous prisoners. Even the recidivism of the weak-minded was disputed. Mitchell re-examined the return of weak-minded prisoners in the local prisons for 1879, and discovered what the Prison Commission had chosen to ignore: that fewer than half of the governors reported that weak-minded offenders were frequently reconvicted.[74]

Mitchell's case was strengthened by the evidence of his witness, Dr John

Sibbald, who, as Commissioner in Lunacy for Scotland, also had a long connection with the Scottish system of care.[75] Between them Sibbald and Mitchell succeeded in casting enough doubt on the criminal imbecile question to make it impossible for the commission to come to a firm conclusion. 'It was not foreseen', the final report stated 'that the question would present itself under so many aspects and assume such a breadth and importance.' A particular problem was the possible cost of institutionalizing the weak-minded. The commissioners accepted Guy's argument that the cost would be offset by increased public protection and a reduced burden on the Poor Law, but they hesitated to make recommendations which would increase taxes. A positive result from the prison lobby's point of view was the commission's agreement that a serious problem existed, a conclusion which Dr Mitchell had tried to dismiss. However, the report stated that there was no existing legislation which could be applied to this 'new class of persons' and that the question of special provision should be reserved for fuller investigation by a separate commission.[76] The rest of the report was devoted to the difficulties of providing for 'criminal lunatics' proper.

The prison doctors' narrow characterization of the mentally deficient as habitually criminal was a crucial factor in the failure of their proposal for greater control, because it proved to be a stereotype that was easily demolished by experts with other experience. Writers like Guy and Maudsley had created between them the phantom of the 'habitual criminal imbecile' who haunted the prisons, asylums, and vagrant wards, threatening the whole of civilized society with criminality and degeneracy. Yet when it came down to it, the habitual criminal could not be adequately identified as weak-minded; neither could criminality be proved to be the natural instinct of the imbecile. When the Scottish advocates of community care of the weak-minded presented their alternative experience of mental handicap, the prison lobby's call for greater incarceration was shelved indefinitely.

The question did not resurface for consideration for another twenty years. In the years following the 1881 report, the Prison Commissioners continued to complain of their burden, but were obliged to make the best of it. Provisions were made to concentrate weak-minded, epileptic, and suicidal prisoners, whose sentences were longer than two months, in selected prisons. All that could be done with other weak-minded offenders was to keep them in special association cells, away from the rest of the prisoners, but still within the prison.[77] In other institutions the detention of the weak-minded continued unchanged.

In the workhouses and asylums, weak-minded inmates presented less of a special problem than in the prisons. In many ways their presence was of benefit to these institutions. In the asylums, mentally retarded inmates who could not be discharged fell into the category of long-term inmates, a group which posed problems for the asylum's image as a curative institution.[78] This image, however, was more seriously damaged by the chronically mentally ill. The retarded could at least be presented as receiving 'training' and education in the asylum, which they could not receive in any other available institution. Idiot departments and idiot wards, with their emphasis on improvement of the seriously retarded and utilization of the working capacity of the less retarded, should be seen as an attempt by the asylum doctors to salvage some of their curative expertise and image from the advance of the custodial asylum filled with chronic cases. In the workhouses, too, the weak-minded seem to have fulfilled a need: supplying the institution with able if not always willing workers, to offset growing numbers of elderly and non-ablebodied inmates.

This may well explain why the national debate seems to have had no noticeable effects on the attitudes of local asylum authorities in Warwickshire. Dr Parsey, superintendent of the county asylum, had his mind already made up in 1867 when he seconded a motion to establish a private idiot asylum in the county.[79] When idiots were let loose, he stated, they were a source of much crime, degradation, and mischief. In an asylum they could become useful workers but whenever he had made an attempt to send any of them back to society they had deteriorated and had to be readmitted.[80] Yet such opinions were not reiterated in Parsey's annual reports, and in practice he continued to discharge such patients throughout the later decades of the century. His successors, Dr Sankey and Dr Miller, were similarly silent and no change of policy seems to have occurred. From the 1880s the term 'congenital mental deficiency' appeared in the annual tabulations of types of mental disorder in admissions to the institution, but the only distinction made within the category was between patients with epilepsy and those without. In 1899 three cases who would have fitted into William Guy's characterization of criminal imbeciles were discharged as not insane enough to warrant detention. Dr Miller commented that one of these, 'a girl who might be considered by some to belong to the type of moral insanity', was observed for several weeks but 'her actions and conduct seemed to be simply that of a cunning and crafty criminal'.[81]

Conclusions

Increased segregation and specialized control of the mentally handicapped were far from inevitable in the latter half of the nineteenth century. An important implication of the campaign to quarantine the weak-minded must be that the lunatic asylums of the 1860s and 1870s were not performing the function of isolating 'superfluous people' and 'marginal elements' as well as historians of the asylum have assumed. To some extent the prison lobby's campaign itself was in keeping with a trend towards a policy of quarantine. One of DuCane's explicit concerns was to keep habitual criminals out of circulation as a preventive measure in the repression of crime.[82] Yet this trend was not paralleled across the institutional spectrum. Examination of the treatment of the weak-minded at the level of the local institutions shows that one reason for the prison lobby's failure to get its view accepted was that weak-minded inmates simply did not present a major problem for other institutions. Concern with the control of the mentally handicapped was confined in this period to a small group of scientific 'experts' and social investigators, especially those connected with the institutions where 'deviance' could be studied. 'Scientific entrepreneurs' like Guy and Maudsley found converts among the prison controllers and high-level asylum administrators but the appeal of their concrete proposals for more confinement remained fixed within that small circle of professionals.

As a stereotype the image of the criminal imbecile did not entirely fade away after 1881. The debate had drawn sufficient attention to the 'criminal imbecile' to secure for him a place in late Victorian perceptions of the 'criminal class'. Stedman Jones has described the development of middle-class anxieties about the existence of a 'residuum' of all types of socially inadequate people subsisting from crime, indiscriminate charity, and casual labour, and forming an especially large group in the metropolis.[83] This image, fuelled by social Darwinist ideas about the degeneration of the urban poor, had by the 1880s almost replaced older theories about a more specifically 'criminal' class. Beside the threat of racial degeneration and the existence of a potential 'mob', the criminality of the degenerate, which Guy and DuCane had tried hard to make into a major issue, seemed less important. After 1881, the question of the weak-minded criminal and the mentally deficient generally became subsumed in the broader debate concerning the degenerate poor of the residuum. The language of psychiatric Darwinism had become part of the jargon of social investigators and reformers, but the debate had gone beyond merely psychiatric concerns and the frustrations of institution administrators. The tenor of Booth's *Darkest England and the Way Out*, which was published in 1890, demonstrates this change:

> there will still remain a residuum of men and women who have, whether from heredity or custom, or hopeless demoralisation become reprobates. . . . There are men so incorrigibly lazy that no inducement you can offer will tempt them to work; so eaten up by vice that virtue is abhorrent to them, and so inveterately dishonest that theft is to them a master passion . . . it must be recognised that he has become lunatic, morally demented, incapable of self-government, and that upon him therefore must be passed the sentence of permanent seclusion from a world in which he is not fit to be at large. . . . It is a crime against the race to allow those who are so inveterately depraved the freedom to wander abroad, infect their fellows, prey upon Society and to multiply their kind.[84]

During the years between the 1880 commission on criminal lunacy and the Mental Deficiency Act of 1913, the eugenic arguments hinted at in the earlier debate were increasingly brought to bear on the question of the mentally deficient. In the new discourse, however, the locus of concern was shifted from the prisons and the habitually criminal imbecile to the workhouses and their transient weak-minded inmates, feeble-minded women in particular. Here was a clear contrast with the arguments before the 1890s, which planned incarceration for chiefly male mental defectives, identified by their propensity for crime and vagrancy. It has been convincingly argued by Simmons that it was the identification of feeble-minded women as the chief culprits in the spread of mental deficiency which above all secured the passage of segregative legislation for the weak-minded in 1913.[85] This later image of mental deficiency, of feeble-minded women who passed in and out of the workhouses, leaving their illegitimate and assumedly defective children in the care of the Poor Law authorities, proved to be a far more compelling one than that of depredatory male offenders, habitual inmates of prisons.

The failure of the campaign to confine the mentally handicapped which occurred in the last quarter of the nineteenth century suggests that we must be wary of overstating a policy of quarantine in this period. It is clear that although the boundaries of insanity were potentially wide, asylum superintendents were not keen to detain people who were merely weak-minded, and continued to discharge them throughout a period of increasing fears about social degeneracy. It is important to note too that at the local level philanthropy was still important in the provision of care facilities, that families of all classes still preferred to look after their own wherever possible, and that general apathy was more characteristic of broader public opinion.[86] The wrongful confinement of the sane commanded more interest in that respect than did the plans of scientific entrepreneurs to make confinement more effective and wide-ranging.[87] Only to those administrators whose job it was to confine the insane and offenders was it of importance that their task was difficult or their role paradoxical. In the latter part of the nineteenth century, too much division existed among these 'experts' to allow any one group to dictate changes in the use of incarceration. Only the broadening of the debate about feeble-mindedness and the causes of social deviancy outside its institutional setting, which took place as the eugenics movement gathered steam at the end of the 1890s would bring about deliberate extensions of the custodial system and a more conscious discussion of the ideology of segregation.[88]

Notes

1 A valuable collection of discussions concerning these developments can be found in M.J. Wiener (ed.) (Winter 1981) 'Humanitarianism or control: a symposium on aspects of nineteenth-century social reform in Britain and America', *Rice University Studies* 67, 1.

2 The lines of this debate are carefully assessed in Wiener, 'Humanitarianism or control'; and also in A. Scull (1983) 'The historiography of Anglo-American psychiatry', and M. Ignatieff (1983) 'State, civil society and total institutions: the critique of recent social histories of punishment', both essays collected in S.

Cohen and A. Scull (eds), *Social Control and the State*, Oxford: Martin Robertson. In these essays both Scull and Ignatieff have sought to modify an emphasis on the custodial nature of the asylum and penitentiary systems. However, the 'social control' perspective which informed their earlier standpoints still very much sets the questions for current investigation. See, for example, J. Walton (1985) 'Casting out and bringing back in Victorian England: pauper lunatics, 1840–70', in W.F. Bynum, R. Porter and M. Shepherd (eds), *The Anatomy of Madness*, London: Tavistock, vol. II.

3 A starting-point for sociological study of the nature of the total institution was provided by E. Goffman (1968) *Asylums: essays on the social situation of mental patients and other inmates*, London: Pelican; enduring images of the Victorian prison and asylum are evoked in M. Ignatieff (1978) *A Just Measure of Pain*, London: Macmillan, and A. Scull (1979) *Museums of Madness*, London: Allen Lane.

4 Scull, *Museums of Madness*, p. 256; A. Scull (1977) 'Madness and segregative control: the rise of the insane asylum', *Social Problems* 24: 347; Ignatieff, *A Just Measure of Pain*, p. 204.

5 J. Walton (1986) 'Poverty and lunacy: some thoughts on directions for future research', *Society for the Social History of Medicine, Bulletin* 38: 64–7.

6 Where care of the mentally handicapped has been studied separately from that of the mentally ill, segregation is seen as only one aspect of treatment, alongside, for example, special education: J. Ryan and F. Thomas (1980) *The Politics of Mental Handicap*, London: Pelican; P. Potts (1983) 'Medicine, morals and mental deficiency: the contribution of doctors to the development of special education in England', *Oxford Review of Education* 9, 3. More recently, social historians have begun to deal with mental retardation in its own right, informed by the debates which have taken place about the asylum and mental illness: P.L. Tylor and L.V. Bell (1984) *Caring for the Retarded in America: a History*, Westport: Greenwood.

7 For fuller details of this work and the use of case histories see my thesis: J. Saunders (1983) 'Institutionalised offenders: a study of the Victorian institution and its inmates, with special reference to late-nineteenth-century Warwickshire', University of Warwick PhD thesis.

8 A. Morison (1824) *Outlines of Mental Diseases*, Edinburgh: McLachlan & Stewart pp. 102–9: D.H. Tuke (1882) *Chapters in the History of the Insane*, London: Kegan Paul & Co. p. 300; W. Norwood-East (1936) *Medical Aspects of Crime*, London: J & A Churchill p. 133.

9 H.G. Simmons (1978) 'Explaining social policy: the English Mental Deficiency Act of 1913', *Journal of Social History* 11: 393–5; usage of these terms is exemplified in the Report of the Commission on Criminal Lunacy, Parliamentary Papers (PP) 1882 XXXII (841), Evidence of Dr Sibbald, q.1759, and Dr Orange, q.454–517.

10 For the fullest administrative history of crime and mental disorder, see N. Walker (1968) *Crime and Insanity in England*, Edinburgh: Edinburgh University Press, vol. 1; N. Walker and S. McCabe (1973) *Crime and Insanity in England*, Edinburgh: Edinburgh University Press, vol. 2.

11 J.B. Thomson (1870) 'The hereditary nature of crime', *Journal of Mental Science* XV: 487–98.

12 *Dictionary of National Biography*: 'William Augustus Guy 1810–1885', statistician, editor of Jnl Statistical Society 1852–6 and president 1873–5.

13 W. Guy (1875) *Results of Censuses of Population of Convict Prisons in England Taken in 1862 and 1873*, London, pp. 14, 29; W. Guy (1869) 'On insanity and crime', *Journal of the Statistical Society* XXXII: 172, in which he refers to cases of his own observation of the corruption of the weak-minded by criminals.

14 His description of the 'pauper community' provides some insight into his bias in regard to social disadvantage. The 'class of paupers' Guy believed to be 'a morass which holds the stagnant waters from running streams, made up of the children of vice or misfortune; of the able-bodied adults who cannot find work or will not exert themselves to obtain it; of all the sick from all classes of society who have failed, or refused to make any provision for the future; and of aged persons, the worn-out culprits of society mixed with a few victims of misfortune. This strange community naturally attracts to itself the idiot, the imbecile and the lunatic ... among the class of paupers then we may expect to find insanity in all its forms at a maximum; and it cannot but prove instructive to compare this exceptional class with the convict population.' Guy, 'On insanity and crime', 168.

15 ibid., 167, 187. Guy estimated that around 160 per 1,000 of paupers aged between 20 and 45 were insane, around three times the proportion among convicts.

16 Thomson, 'Hereditary nature of crime', 9, 14.

17 The chaplain of Warwick New Prison, for example, commented sadly at the end of 1861 when the one-year-old prison had failed to diminish the number of prisoners. 'Instances have already occurred where parties have returned two or three times.' Warwick County Record Office (hereafter WCRO), Chaplain's Report to Quarter Sessions, Michaelmas 1861.

18 For further discussion of this decline in optimism and the onset of deterrence see Ignatieff, *A Just Measure of Pain*, pp. 200–4; J. Davis (1980) 'The London garotting panic of 1862', in V.A.C. Gattrell, B. Lenman, and G. Parker, *Crime and the Law: a social history of crime in Western Europe since 1500*, London: Europa, pp. 193–7, 209.

19 Thomson, 'Hereditary nature of crime', 3; Guy, 'On insanity and crime', 167.

20 For a contemporary view of the connection between mental handicap and the vagrant life see J.H. Brenten (1861) *The Tragedy of Life*, London: Smith Elder & Co., in which stories of 'Waffling Will' and 'Wandering Geordie' stress the dangers of allowing such 'poor imbeciles' to remain at large.

21 Referred to in W. Tallack (1871) *Humanity and Humanitarianism*, London: F.B. Kitto p. 18; Dr Campbell, medical officer of Broadmoor Special Hospital in the 1870s, made further observations of the brain size of criminals and concluded that the brains of criminals were smaller than those of ordinary adults: E. DuCane (1875) 'Address on the repression of crime', *Trans. Nat. Assoc. Prom. Soc. Sci.*: 305.

22 For studies of the idea of progressive degeneracy in the national contexts of France and Italy, see I. Dowbiggin (1985) 'Degeneration and hereditarianism in French mental medicine 1840–90: psychiatric theory as ideological adaptation', in Bynum, Porter and Shepherd (eds), *The Anatomy of Madness*, London, vol. I; D. Pick (Spring 1986) 'The faces of anarchy: Lombroso and the politics of criminal science in post-unification Italy', *History Workshop* 21.

23 B.A. Morel (1857) *Traité des dégénérescences physiques, intellectuelles et morales de l'espèce humaine, et des causes qui produisent ces variétés maladies*, Paris.

24 H. Maudsley (1874) *Responsibility in Mental Disease*, London, pp. 46–8.

25 For a fuller discussion of Maudsley's ideas see V. Skultans (1979) *English Madness*, London: Routledge & Kegan Paul, pp. 131–4. The phrases quoted here are from extracts from Maudsley's writings quoted in V. Skultans (1975) *Madness and Morals*, London: Routledge & Kegan Paul, pp. 189, 192.

26 G. Jones (1980) *Social Darwinism in English Thought. The Interaction between Biological and Social Theory*, London: Harvester.

27 Jones, *Social Darwinism in English Thought*, p. 147.

28 Thus Maudsley pointed to the appearance of 'remarkable animal traits and instincts' in the insane and mentally deficient and made comparisons of the brains of idiots with those of apes and chimpanzees: H. Maudsley (1870) *Body and Mind*, (1873) Gulstonian Lectures for 1870, London: Macmillan, pp. 43–7; DuCane, 'Repression of crime', 302.

29 Thomson, 'Hereditary nature of crime', 9–12.

30 For example, the Rev. J. Clay, 'The criminal statistics of Preston Gaol', cited in L.O. Pike (1876) *A History of Crime in England*, London: Smith, Elder & Co. p. 668; R.L. Dugdale ([1877] 1975) *The Jukes* (first published as part of the 30th annual report of the Prison Association of New York; reprinted New York: AMS Press, Inc).

31 DuCane, 'Repression of crime', 302–3.

32 Public Record Office (PRO): HO45/71439.

33 Report of the Penal Servitude Acts Commission: PP 1878–9 XXXVII, q.5078, q.8000, q.12626–32, q.12663–74.

34 U. Henriques (1972) 'The rise and decline of the separate system of prison discipline', *Past and Present* 54: 86.

35 Shropshire County Record Office, Shrewsbury Prison Chaplain's Journal, QS/ Box 53.

36 WCRO, Warwick County Lunatic Asylum (hereafter WCLA) Criminal Lunatics, my case numbers 068 and 056. (For reasons of confidentiality specific case numbers cannot be quoted.)

37 WCLA Criminal Lunatics, my case number 034; Report of the Directors of Convict Prisons for 1859, PP 1860 35 (2713) p. 471; F.W. Robinson (1864) *Female Life in Prison*, London: S. Low p. 239.

38 Report of the Penal Servitude Acts Commission, PP 1878–9 XXXVII, evidence of Dr Campbell, q.7020; Maidstone Prison Governor, q.4814; Portland Prison Governor, q.2326.

39 For a discussion of overt and suppressed protest carried on by Victorian prison inmates see Ignatieff, *A Just Measure of Pain*, pp. 10, 178.

40 Penal Servitude Acts Commission, PP 1878–9 XXXVII, q.8745.

41 WCLA report for 1861, p. 7.

42 WCRO (December 1867) report of Committee on the Establishment of an Asylum for Idiots, QS 43/2.

43 ibid., and WCLA reports for 1873 and 1875.

44 WCLA, Idiot Asylum Casebook, case no. 87; WCLA report for 1876; WCLA Criminal Lunatics, my case number 027.

45 WCLA Criminal Lunatics, my case numbers 094, 101 and 106; also WCLA report for 1865.

46 According to R. Hodgkinson's study of the workhouse insane, in 1869 when there were over 25,000 lunatics in county asylums, there were still some 11,000 cases in the workhouses: R. Hodgkinson (1966) 'Provision for pauper lunatics, 1834–71', *Medical History* 10: 146–53.

47 WCLA, superintendent's reports 1878 and 1882.
48 WCRO, Warwick Union Indoor Relief Lists (CR51); PP, Lunacy Commissioners 6th annual report (1851), appendix A, p. 46; WCLA, casebook (CR1664/618).
49 S. Webb and B. Webb ([1910]1963) *English Poor Law Policy*, London: Longman; reprinted 1963, London: Cass, p. 123.
50 PP, Lunacy Commissioners, supplement to 12th report (April 1859), Appendix p. 39.
51 J.T. Sabben and J.H.B. Browne (1872) *Handbook of Law and Lunacy*, London: J & A Churchill, p. 96.
52 Webb and Webb, *English Poor Law Policy* (1963 edn), pp. 225–7.
53 In 1867, Edward Smith, the medical officer of the Poor Law Board, observed that able-bodied people were seldom found in workhouses during the greater part of the year and that the inmates were almost solely the aged and infirm, the destitute, sick and children. Poor Law Board, 20th annual report, 1867–8, quoted in Webb and Webb, *English Poor Law Policy* (1963 edn), p. 134.
54 E. Smith, Dietaries for the Inmates of Workhouses, Report to the Poor Law Board, PP sess 1866 35, p. 24; Webb and Webb, *English Poor Law Policy*, (1963 edn), p. 125, draws attention to this 1868 directive.
55 Further Report of the Commissioners in Lunacy 1847, PRO/PR104, p. 258.
56 Hodgkinson, 'Provision for pauper lunatics', 148; PP, Lunacy Commissioners Report for 1858, p. 29.
57 WCLA Criminal Lunatics, my case numbers 112 and 145; WCRO Warwick Board of Guardians Minutes, October 1871. See also Saunders, 'Institutionalised offenders', chapter 6, which examines the social profiles of the inmate population of the prison, asylum, and workhouse in Warwickshire.
58 Walker and McCabe, *Crime and Insanity*, vol. 2, p. 41.
59 PP, Prison Commission, 3rd report, 1879–80, p. 7, and appendix no. 10, pp. 28–30.
60 As note 10. See also J. Saunders (1981) 'Magistrates and madmen: segregating the criminally insane in late-nineteenth-century Warwickshire', in V. Bailey (ed.), *Policing and Punishment in Nineteenth-Century Britain*, London: Croom Helm.
61 PRO HO45/71439 August 1879.
62 Criminal Lunacy Commission, Report, p. 19.
63 The chairman was Leonard H. Courtney (1832–1918), Professor of Political Economy at University College, London 1875–6, said to be 'among the ablest and most advanced doctrinaire Liberals' (*Dict. Nat. Biography*).
64 Criminal Lunacy Commission, q.1757–9, q.453–4, q.567, q.679–96.
65 P. McCandless (1974) 'Insanity and society: a study of the English lunacy reform movement 1815–70' University of Wisconsin PhD thesis, pp. 188–202.
66 Criminal Lunacy Commission, q.553, q.1226, q.1824.
67 Criminal Lunacy Commission, e.g. Guy's questioning of witnesses 1763–6, 820, 535; Campbell's question 1768 and DuCane's questions 679–96, 837–53, 1900–29, and q.1032.
68 Criminal Lunacy Commission, appendix B, memorandum 1, 'The "insane" and the "imbecile"', p. 162.
69 A. Mitchell (1864) *The Insane in Private Dwellings*, Edinburgh; A. Mitchell (1868) 'The care and treatment of the insane poor', *Journal of Mental Science* 13: 472–97.

70 See McCandless, 'Insanity and society', 558–9.
71 Criminal Lunacy Commission, A. Mitchell, 'Notes on the return of lunatic, imbecile or weakminded prisoners in convict prisons', appendix A 10, p. 147.
72 McCandless, 'Insanity and society', 558–9.
73 Criminal Lunacy Commission, appendix B, memo 2, pp. 164–7.
74 Criminal Lunacy Commission, appendix A, return no. 13, p. 150.
75 Criminal Lunacy Commission, q.1768.
76 Criminal Lunacy Commission, Report, p. 19.
77 Prison Commission, 8th report, pp. 13–14; the Departmental Committee on Prisons 1895, PP 1895 LVI, reiterated in its report the connection between crime and degeneracy; p. 48.
78 P. McCandless (1979) 'Build! Build!: The controversy over the care of the chronically insane in England 1850–70', *Bull. Hist. Med.* 53: 553–74.
79 It was not felt appropriate within the confines of this chapter to examine the provision of a public subscription asylum for 'idiots above the pauper class' in Warwickshire. See my thesis, 'Institutionalised offenders', where the issue of private asylum care is examined alongside the public institution.
80 Midland Counties Idiot Asylum, report of a meeting, 5 January 1869.
81 WCLA Report 1899–1900, p. 16.
82 PRO HO45/71439.
83 G. Stedman Jones (1971) *Outcast London*, Oxford: Oxford University Press, pp. 281–336.
84 General W. Booth (1890) *In Darkest England and the Way Out*, London: Salvation Army pp. 204–5.
85 Simmons, 'Explaining social policy', 393–5.
86 In Warwickshire, the establishment and support of the public subscription 'Middle Class Idiot Asylum', was characterized by statements as to the mercy of placing idiots in an institution, not a need by society for their confinement. It was persistently difficult to raise subscriptions from a generally disinterested public, to the extent that the building was always underfilled because funds were lacking. Saunders, 'Institutionalised offenders', 299; Walton's work on the Lancaster Asylum has emphasized that families used the asylum as a last resort only: Walton, 'Casting out and bringing back'.
87 P. McCandless (1978) 'Liberty and lunacy: the Victorians and wrongful confinement', *Jour. Social History* 11: 369.
88 See the collection of papers in (1983) *Oxford Review of Education* 9, 3; particularly D. Barker, 'How to curb the fertility of the unfit: the feebleminded in Edwardian Britain', pp. 197–211.

CHAPTER ELEVEN

The lunacy profession and its staff in the second half of the nineteenth century, with special reference to the West Riding Lunatic Asylum

Richard Russell

The therapeutic failure of the Victorian lunatic asylum is now a recognized fact. Death-rates ran at around 40 per cent on admissions and the other 60 per cent were by no means all permanently recovered. Indeed, around a quarter of these were not actually discharged at all but simply moved on to other institutions, in many cases to another lunatic asylum. Each new admission could look forward to a mean average stay of about three years with only a fifty-fifty chance of getting out (dead or alive) in less than one.[1]

This picture did not improve as the century wore on. The only change was that the size of the overall asylum population steadily grew, much to the concern of the rate-paying public and the dismay of the Commissioners in Lunacy, who concluded in their thirty-first report, 1876, that only 7.22 per cent of insanity was actually curable. The popular magazines such as *Cornhill, Contemporary Review* and *The Nineteenth Century* were filled with articles that spoke of a rising tide of insanity sweeping the country, which the lunatic asylums were entirely powerless to stop.

In the face of this it needs to be asked how the medical profession operating in this area was able to survive. Certainly it could not be said to have flourished in the latter part of the century, but it did undergo developments which set a pattern for the future.

Perhaps the best starting-place is to realize that the provision of cures was not the only element in mental physicians' discourse. There were other activities, other *raisons d'être*, through which they justified their existence and built the groundwork of their profession. In pursuing these activities the upper strata of the lunacy profession grew more remote from the practicalities of everyday asylum life, causing a shift in the effective obligations of the lower ranks, whose job it was to attempt to restore some sort of normality to the patients in their care. This in turn had consequences for the whole of psychiatric development.

The development of asylum doctors and superintendents into a profession took place in two main areas: in the pages of the professional journal and through the profession's own organization, with its attempts at educational standards and entry-control. Underpinning both was the asylum itself, which was the linchpin of the whole enterprise. In these two areas individual doctors made their bids for advancement, trying to make their personal best out of less than promising circumstances.

At first sight nowhere seems less promising than the asylum, with all its negative achievements at the therapeutic level. However, these huge and bleak institutions afforded more rewarding activities than simply the attempt to treat insanity directly. Within their walls lived, or existed, many hundreds of inmates who could be counted, tabulated, and subdivided in many interesting ways, in accordance with the fashionable practice of statistics. Figures on admissions, discharges, and deaths were, of course, already regularly kept. But other information about the patients could also be treated in this way. Tables were drawn up on the marital status, age, religious persuasion, and occupation of inmates. More pertinently perhaps, 'type of insanity' and 'probable cause of insanity' were carefully quantified.[2]

No conclusions seem to have been drawn from all this statistical activity, yet it was clear that the upper echelons of the profession believed the activity to be valuable. In 1869 a special committee was appointed to look at such matters and recommended a standardized procedure of book-keeping, regularized classification of cases, a standard form of case book and a plan of treatment under the separate heads of 'nourishment', 'bodily disorder', and 'brain function'.[3] Four years later J.A. Campbell wrote:

> There can be no reasonable doubt that if these tables are accurately kept in the different asylums, they must, from their exactitude and uniformity, become the material from which the history of insanity in this country will be drawn.[4]

This was a truism, of course, since mental physicians had cornered the field of relevant information, but subsequent history testifies to its unproductiveness either for our understanding of insanity or for the well-being of the patients. The reams of statistical tables continued to appear as if this were a ritual process that would one day mysteriously lay bare the facts of insanity. As D.J. Mellett recently remarked:

> Assembling of information was dangerously near to becoming an end in itself.[5]

If tables of statistics marked the limit of doctors' researches amongst the living, they found themselves more in their element with the dead. With a mortality rate of 40 per cent the asylum could provide easy meat for the dissector's scalpel. There was no legal objection to such examination without a coroner's order[6] provided no relative objected so not surprisingly post-mortems became a regular feature of the asylum's medical activity.

Here in the mortuary mental physicians attempted to find evidence for their long-held assertion that insanity was indeed a disease of the brain. The results of massive programmes of brain-dissection were often published. In 1876, W.G. Balfour at the Hampstead Asylum revealed the results of over 700 post-mortems and concluded that 640 of these showed signs of brain-lesion. The remaining 60, he presumed, had similar lesions which current techniques were unable to detect.[7] However, in attempting to relate these findings to actual behaviour in the living he was reduced to crude surmises in which his anatomical knowledge was of no assistance:

> An unhealthy idea, *however generated* [emphasis added], will surely produce in the nerve cells through which it passes, an unhealthy condition, which, if not remedied, will sooner or later lead to a permanent change in these cells, and they in turn will corrupt others.[8]

Thus Balfour produced, through asylum post-mortem activity, a justification of medical intervention which entirely avoided the question of insanity's actual generation, or original cause. It also avoided the question of its treatment in the living. An ex-patient, citing a text book by Voisin, commented,

> [The book] states that in simple insanity he finds certain alterations in the grey matter of the cerebellum, consisting of minute apoplexies, effusions of haematin and haematosin into the lymphatic sheaths, infarctions, atheroma, capillary dilations, and necrosis of vessels, and certain changes of cerebral cells. Quite so. It may all be very true, but I can offer no suggestions as to medical treatment based on these remarkable assumptions.[9]

The Journal of Mental Science

The lunatic asylum, as well as being a necessary research base, was also the launching-pad of the mental physicians' own journal, which began life simply as *The Asylum Journal* in 1853. From the beginning it was rooted in the new county asylums built under the 1845 Lunacy Act and, despite a change of name to the *Journal of Mental Science*, was able to provide the aspiring asylum doctor with an arena in which he could float ideas, publish letters and research papers, and generally attempt to build up his career. In the process the *Journal* helped to establish the profession as a credible branch of medical science.

In its earlier years it also provided a route into the profession at all levels – from superintendent to cook – and was a forum for the development of all facets of asylum life. However, during the first ten years of its publication it fell into the exclusive hands of the profession's upper echelons and no longer served an all-round purpose. A split was growing between the higher and lower sections of the lunacy 'business'.

This capture of control by the top end of the profession can be seen in the *Journal's* early history. It was started not by the Association of Medical Officers of Hospitals for the Insane (AMOHI) (which had been in existence since 1841) but as a private initiative by J.C. Bucknill, the AMOHI being a small affair with only a handful of members able to attend meetings.[10]

The new journal was at first a modest publication. It consisted of sixteen royal octavo pages and cost sixpence. For the first fourteen issues it was biquarterly; then in 1855 it grew to 128 pages, became a quarterly and changed its name to the *Asylum Journal of Mental Science*. This growth presumably reflected the great interest (and financial support) shown by mental physicians. Two years later the *Journal* grew again to 156 pages and in 1858 dropped the word 'Asylum' from its title along with the parochial connotations that went with the word, and became simply the *Journal of Mental Science*. In 1861, with funds increasing, the printing was transferred from a provincial printer to a superior firm in London.

The earlier issues had a down-to-earth, almost homely feel. The editorship seems close to the readership. On the back page there were job advertisements: an 'experienced cook' was wanted in Devon for £20 per annum;[11] a 'clinical assistant' was needed in Oxfordshire,[12] at a salary of £70 per annum plus board. Even the top jobs were advertised on the back page. After the suicide of Dr Grahamsley at Worcester, a new medical superintendent was sought, with an advertisement offering £350 per annum, furnished lodgings, coals, candles, washing, and vegetables from the garden.[13] There were letters from doctors offering practical tips on managing the routine work of the asylum. One from James E. Huxley at Maidstone, for example, advised the use of dilute sulphuric acid to clean the urine from the floors of 'wet and dirty wards'.[14]

However, these homely items soon disappeared as the *Journal* grew to become a weighty and (hopefully) influential quarterly. Quite rapidly it divorced itself from direct asylum involvement, not just by dropping the reference to it in the title but also by its selection of contents. The first issue of the newly named *Journal of Mental Science* opened with a leading article entitled, 'Hamlet: a psychological study'. There followed a discussion of Tuke's paper on the diagnosis of general paralysis of the insane, a paper by Dr Davey on the relationship between insanity and crime, and another by Dr Huxley on relations between the Lunacy Commission and the superintendents of various asylums. There was the second part of a study of warm and cold baths in the treatment of insanity (a somewhat academic work) and a report of the AMOHI annual meeting. The final section contained accounts of two inquisitions of lunacy (a rare procedure involving those who were both insane and very wealthy), a reply to a newspaper attack on privately owned asylums, reviews – 'The ganglionic nervous system' by James George Davey among them – and a letter from a doctor regretting that local residents at seaside resorts objected to the presence of asylum inmates, since it lowered the rateable value of the properties. Lastly there were notices of appointments (obviously the applications had gone on elsewhere) including, interestingly, a notice that a 'Dr H. Maudsley [has been appointed] Assistant Medical Officer at the Essex County Lunatic Asylum, Brentwood'.[15]

The career of Henry Maudsley was not unconnected with the development of the *Journal of Mental Science* and its increasing remoteness from those nearer the bottom end of the profession. From his new, if modest, position he was able to interest the editor, J.C. Bucknill, in his ideas on matters physical and mental. His first paper was published one year later, by which time Maudsley was already medical superintendant at the Manchester Royal Lunatic Hospital. It was 'The correlation of mental and physical force; or man a part of nature',[16] which revealed his philosophical inclination and evolutionary views on the human mind that were to be so characteristic of his subsequent writing.

This great concern with the theoretical was much in keeping with the editor's own approach. Gone were the handy hints on washing floors. Issue 32 carried 'Consciousness as a truth-organ considered', by the Rev. W.G. Davies, chaplain of Abergavenny Asylum, speculations on the 'Causes of mental disease' by American doctors, a report on the new Jamaican asylum and an account of the religious revival in Belfast.[17] Number 33 carried a lengthy article by Maudsley on the psychology of Edgar Allan Poe.[18]

The editorship of the *Journal* was transferred in 1863 to C. Lockhart Robertson, a frequent past contributor.[19] This same issue carried a third article by Maudsley, 'Considerations with regard to hereditary influence', which spells out his strongly pessimistic view of the curability of insanity.[20] Although none of his writing concerned the treatment of patients or the organization of asylums, these articles of Maudsley's were not without their significance both to him and to the profession. With the following issue, number 45, he became joint editor, along with Robertson. [21] Henceforth the *Journal* was to become truly the home of medical theory and speculation, whilst practical and administrative matters to do with the asylum itself, the cutting-edge of the profession's dealings with insanity, were dropped altogether.

The struggle for careers

As the *Journal* passed into the hands of the profession's élite, who were themselves already opting out of asylum involvement (Maudsley, for example, left asylum work at this time to become a physician at the West London Hospital),[22] it ceased to be a significant arena in which the bulk of asylum doctors could contest for advancement. Instead, it was the asylums which remained the base for the making of ordinary careers. Most of the appointments recorded in the asylum reports show movement within the asylum framework rather than into or out of it, though there were new arrivals and a few departures from asylum work, especially at the lower levels.[23] Thus when Dr Ernest Bevan, second assistant, Male Department, at the West Riding Lunatic Asylum was promoted to senior assistant medical officer, Female Department, his place was filled by Dr Arthur Ronnie, the asylum pathologist and assistant medical officer.[24] New appointments were commonly made from staff in other asylums, as was Dr Richard Millar, West Riding's senior clinical assistant, who left to take up a better position at the Sussex asylum.[25]

This order of things remained true of medical education in lunacy. There had been courses of lectures instituted over the years by individuals, such as Alexander Morison (1823), John Conolly (1842) and Thomas Laycock (1860s), but these were all extremely few and far between. Asylum experience and 'in-house' lectures were practically the only sources of specialist knowledge. Not until 1885 did the mental physicians' own organization, the Medico-Psychological Association,[26] persuade the General Medical Council to introduce a Certificate in Psychological Medicine. This required three months' residence and a course of lectures. However, nobody applied for the first examination.[27]

Nevertheless, asylum education was beginning to influence the wider medical world by the 1880s and 1890s, though only to a small degree. Dr Bevan Lewis, superintendent at the West Riding Asylum, was appointed lecturer on mental diseases to the Leeds School of Medicine in 1885, following his own successful lectures within his own institution. He reported that

> the experience of this Summer's Session has impressed me with the fact that the teaching capabilities at the Asylum might be widely extended. At present the Asylum Museum [still going strong] shows numerous desiderata in the way of models, diagrams, anatomical and microscopic preparations and these we shall be able in time to supply at a trifling outlay and by our own individual resources.[28]

The asylum was also able to supply the resources of its own pathology laboratory where not only anatomy but also vivisection was available as a teaching aid.[29] Bevan Lewis felt confident enough in 1890 to offer a postgraduate course of lectures to medical practitioners throughout the West Riding, which was well attended,[30] and before long he found that the courses he was giving at Leeds attracted a growing interest, with 'an exceptionally large class of 40 students' in 1894.[31] It was during these years of growing interest that the British Medical Association itself adopted 'Mental Disease' as a separate section in its annual meeting for the first time. Dr Hack Tuke gave the very first address to this new Psychological Section in 1888.[32]

The overall inadequacy of specific educational qualifications was a major reason for the profession's inability to regulate the entry of newcomers. There was some control at the top end, through the devices of the MPA, but the operations of the upper reaches were already somewhat remote from the asylum floor. Down in the hectic day rooms and corridors, where patients outnumbered medical staff by hundreds to one, new men were working the wards, over whom the more exalted levels of the profession held only partial sway.

There was some regulation, of course. Gone were the days when asylums were open to men of great character and influence – men such as Ellis, Conolly, and even Maudsley in his way.[33] The new generation of asylum doctors followed a more prosaic route, usually via a university degree from either Edinburgh or London. The new clinical assistant at the West Riding Asylum in 1882 was an Edinburgh graduate.[34] So was Dr Paterson, who left his post of clinical assistant to become assistant to the State Criminal Lunatic Asylum at Broadmoor.[35] The West Riding's new clinical assistant in the Male Department in 1886 was a Bachelor of Medicine and a Master of Chemistry at Edinburgh,[36] while the man who replaced Dr Paterson was a graduate from London.[37]

At first sight this new blood does not seem to have brought a great deal of challenge to the system in the nineteenth century. On the surface all seems calm. Possibly this reflects the tight grip held by the few at the top. Maudsley and Lockhart Robertson controlled the *Journal* very effectively and only significant contribution to research rather than to asylum practice would have made much impact there. Prominence in those fields was more likely to come from those working in neurology, or clinical psychology, than from people doing day-to-day medical work in the asylum. At least, the profession's own records, and particularly the *Journal*, show no great sign of impending change.

However, this does not necessarily mean that there was no change, only that such change as there was went largely unrecorded. This would not be surprising since now that the *Journal* had grown remote from everyday practice and the top men in the field were all busy with academic and clinical work there must have developed a sizeable body of day-to-day routine which informed the lower levels of asylum work. Whatever was established from previous practice would have been passed down by existing staff to new recruits – either explicitly or by example in the wards – without the aid of official published sources. This body of orally transmitted 'know-how' would not have made much impression on the sources which a historian is bound to examine, yet it would have been subject to all the influences of the approaches and attitudes brought to the job by successive new members of staff. We should be aware therefore that under the appearance of calm there may have been changes which only became apparent much later.

This possibility suggests that we should look more closely at the employment structure among the lunatic profession and at the tensions which normal asylum functioning created. For it was here that, lacking any clear professional guidelines on ethical conduct or expectations, the second generation of medical men may have been quietly altering the nature of the business.

The superintendent

Without doubt the system reserved its greatest benefits for the medical superintendent, particularly if he was a man with a taste for the exercise of personal authority. This was the legacy of earlier reforms, and especially of the notion of 'moral treatment' in the sense of using the influence of the sane mind upon the insane as a way of affecting recovery. From this, it was argued,

> it follows . . . that one man must be placed at the head of the establishments . . . and that his mind must pervade the whole establishment.[38]

Despite the decay of moral treatment into virtually anything that was not an administration of some obviously physical remedy, such as drugs or (rarely) electrolysis, this particular tenet of the 'moral' approach remained strong. Personal authority, vested in the superintendent, was the arbiter of a rigid social system that embraced every aspect of asylum life. There could be 'only one captain of a ship', said Charles Mercier, reworking a familiar metaphor. He

> must be before all things a man of strong character, a man of dominist will, who can impose his will on others and compel obedience by the sheer force of his own strong nature.[39]

With the asylum under such a regime the inmates could not subvert its routines with their madness.

But the 'dominist will' affected more than just the behaviour of the inmates. The superintendent's power to choose a medical officer was his alone (though officially the appointment was made by the local Committee of Visitors). It was not unknown for personal considerations to enter in, with the superintendent avoiding any undue challenge to his authority by selecting

> a companionable chap . . . a good-humoured, pleasant, patient gentlemanly fellow, with no conspicuous ability, and no very firm strength of character[40]

much to the irritation of ambitious young doctors, who felt themselves discriminated against for their more recent and superior knowledge, which might show the older superintendent in a poor light.[41]

Such was their hold on the profession, however, that such criticisms were very rarely made public. In print, such drawbacks as the young doctors referred to were put down to the unfortunate habits of individuals and the system of personal authority was upheld. Indeed, not surprisingly perhaps the superintendent was regarded as personally responsible for all the work of recovery that went on in the asylum, if not as the single-handed champion of all that lunacy reform stood for. 'It is one of the happy circumstances', wrote Daniel Hack Tuke, the flat-footed visionary and apologist of the asylum system, connected with the great movement which has taken place in this and other countries, that men have arisen in large numbers who have proved themselves equal to the task. We witness the creation of an almost new character – the asylum superintendent.[42]

Superintendents needed all the build-up they could get. The money was not all it might be for someone in a position of such authority. Bevan Lewis, on his appointment in 1884 to 'medical director' of the West Riding Asylum, could draw a salary of just £600 p.a. This was increased to £800 in 1892 and to £1,200 in 1910. His successor, Shaw Bolton, was appointed at an annual salary of £1,050.[43] Along with the post went a large house, full board, and the pick of the stores for the superintendent's table. All this compared favourably with the income of the average general practitioner, who in 1910 could gross £832 in provincial work,[44] and was some four to five times the sum which lesser ranks in the asylum could command.[45]

In return for this the superintendent was bound to a remarkably imprecise set of services. His *medical* duties were left undefined by any clause in the Lunacy Acts or by any official guideline. Some writers did go so far as to recommend a timetable, but this was only very general. Charles Mercier proposed that the superintendent should be in his office not later than nine o'clock:

9.00 – 10.30	Signing reports and notices. Correspondence.
10.30 – 1.00	Tour of the wards, accompanied by the medical officer.
1.00 – 2.00	Inspection of inmates' lunch, then takes his own.
2.00 – 5.00	Interviews with patients brought to him by the head attendant. Tour of any remaining wards. Inspection of staff.
After dinner	Social functions. Surprise visit to the wards.[46]

Such a timetable would, of course, still allow the superintendent to maintain his contacts with the rest of his profession. This would involve visits to local (and not so local) medical men, a scrutiny of the literature and perhaps a paper of his own for the *Journal of Mental Science*. Also, there were meetings of the MPA and other such professional associations to be maintained. In such a manner he no doubt hoped to find employment in private medicine as a visiting physician or perhaps as a consultant for the Commissioners in Lunacy. This would help to offset the modest advantages of a professional situation that did not offer great opportunities for further advancement.

The medical officers

The subordinate officers felt the difficulties of further advancement keenly. They were a growing breed. From the original practice of employing only one assistant per asylum, the appointment of several men in different positions had become so commonplace by 1888 that the MPA set up a four-man committee to represent this 'large and growing body'.[47]

The committee promptly sent a questionnaire to all asylums asking for numbers, terms of service, and salary-levels. It was not pleased with the results. At the quarterly meeting in November 1889 Drs Dodds, Strahan and Greenlees (the fourth man, Dr Wiglesworth, having died just previously) presented their case.

There were, they said, essentially two levels of subordinate medical staff: the senior officers who were of long standing and experienced in their speciality having spent on average six years in it, and the junior officers, less dedicated and less experienced. These junior men, they argued,

> are in great part birds of passage, who take an asylum appointment merely to gain very useful experience, or in order to spend the time necessary to acquire that grave and senior look deemed essential to the private practitioner. They use their asylum appointment as others do resident hospital and infirmary appointments. They have from the first no intention of remaining within the speciality, and after a brief experience betake themselves to other and more attractive fields. These juniors receive from £80 to £120 or more per annum. So far as we have heard, there is neither complaint nor ground for complaint here.[48]

For the junior staff there is no voice raised, either at the MPA or in the *Journal*. Yet whatever the validity of the criticisms they made against these 'birds of passage' the senior staff did have a valid grievance. They wanted parity with officers of similar standing in other public medical services. Army and navy surgeons, they pointed out, could get £280 a year and a gratuity of £1,000 after ten years' service, yet the average salary for asylum officers was only £161.[49]

They had other complaints too. The increasing workload in the already bulging asylums meant that medical officers were sometimes doubling for the superintendent while being expected also to cope with extra clerical duties. They felt their skills were undervalued, and they resented the high esteem in which the superintendent was held while their own efforts went unappreciated.

> The recognition of such seniors as responsible physicians would undoubtedly do away with the pious fraud at present perpetuated on the public, viz. that the Superintendent is in all cases the physician who marks the symptoms in the sick in body and mind and treats those symptoms as they appear.[50]

But the senior officers were skating on thin ice.

> This is delicate ground, on which we will not venture further.

Such was the power of the superintendent's authority within the MPA that the committee preferred to proceed on a more tactful note. 'Our position,' they said,

> is not that our superior officers [i.e. the superintendents] are too highly paid – the reverse is often the case – but that assistants as a class are underpaid.[51]

As for the burden of clerical work, there should be a class of junior clerks to remove the 'millstone of clerical work' from their necks. Asylums should be smaller, they concluded, with assistant staff more highly regarded, and lastly, yet perhaps not insignificantly, the committee asked that medical officers be allowed to marry.[52]

In truth, the life of a senior medical man was not enviable. Normally he would live in the asylum, in a room provided with the usual board and washing facilities.[53] His income was modest. Ernest Birt, the house surgeon at West Riding in 1880, received £130 p.a. This increased to £180 in 1884, £210 in 1890, £260 in 1901 and £300 in 1905. The deputy chief assistant was appointed in 1885 on a salary of only £64, which increased to £100 in 1890.[54]

There was slender hope of advancement from positions such as these. Charles Mercier commented that he

> sees the best years of his life slipping away from him without any advancement of his interests or improvement in his prospects.[55]

The usual escape route was to drop asylum work altogether and go into private medicine.[56] Hardly surprising, then, that so many young men were 'birds of passage' under these conditions, and one can understand the hostility shown towards them by those with dedication, or without alternative means, who remained for years the widowers of lunacy.

Nurses and attendants

Below the level of the junior officers, far beneath the consideration of any professional committee, lay the substantial body of men and women who actually held the asylum system together. If medical officers felt themselves poorly paid at £161 per year, the asylum nurses and attendants had a far worse time of it. In 1890 a nurse was appointed to the West Riding Asylum at £17 per year, with board and lodging.[57] The rate had risen from £15 in the 1870s and from a meagre £12 or £13 in the early 1860s. Male attendants could get double that figure, even though they were not allowed to marry and so were not supporting a family.[58] The terms included also a clothing allowance and laundry facilities. On top of this it was possible to obtain an allowance of ten shillings a year for good conduct and extra money after long service, but few stayed long enough to benefit from this.

The turnover of staff among nurses and attendants was rapid, particularly for the men. Most male attendants worked in the asylum for around two to three months, though in Wakefield this short time-scale may have been partly the result of the mining boom in the 1870s. Even so, most women spent similar periods in work, though several did remain for one or two years.[59]

The work itself was arduous. Much of it resembled that of a domestic servant. There was a great deal of cleaning and polishing to be done, as well as fetching, carrying, dressing, bed-making, and serving meals.[60] But also they were expected to bear the brunt of attending to patients' welfare by providing exercise, amusement, employment, supervision, and a general state of cleanliness.[61] Such 'medical' duties included keeping the air fresh and warm, maintaining records of the patients' progress, and taking body temperatures.[62] Nurses and attendants were also expected to know how to apply cold dressings and poultices, fomentations, enemas, and suppositories, and to give baths of various kinds, as well as the technique of packing a patient in a wet sheet to control manic excitement.[63]

The working conditions were exhausting. Maintaining cleanliness among a great many incontinent, or 'wet and dirty', patients was as unwholesome a task as can be imagined, while the general disposition of many of the others left much to be recommended. Nurses and attendants could expect to work for most of the day and sometimes at night, although night nurses were becoming more common during the century.[64] Even so, the average number of hours per week was still around seventy in 1912.[65] Sometimes coverage at night would be achieved by changing the shift patterns; day shifts starting at midday after night duty, or finishing at 3 p.m. before night duty, as at Colney Hatch.[66] Shifts might even be run together with only four hours' rest after a twenty-hour stretch, as occurred at Lancaster in 1896.[67] More often, 'night' shifts would include 'light work' during the day with staff working from 10 a.m. until 2 a.m. the next morning, with only four hours' break in the afternoon.[68]

Even when asleep the nurses could not always escape duty since they were commonly expected to use a room adjoining a ward[69] and were frequently kept awake by the noise made by disturbed patients.[70] Staff could normally look forward to one afternoon off each week, one or two Sundays in the month and seven days during the year,[71] although at some asylums a little more time off seemed to be allowed.[72] The rest of the time they lived, of course, within the walls of the institution.

There was some improvement in conditions over the years, though this was only slight. Provision for a private mess-room was growing in the 1880s, suggesting that staff were getting a little more spare time. In 1887, Bevan Lewis, the superintendent of the West Riding Asylum, ordered a reading and recreation room to be built.

> At present, after duty hours, if the weather be increment [*sic.*] or if the nurses do not desire to leave the building, she has no resource other than returning to her bedroom, which in all cases is too small and confined even as a sleeping-room.[73]

Further evidence of increasing spare time is the spread of games and music lessons and brass band competitions between 'rival' asylums, usually a mixture of staff and patients meeting at a local pub.[74] Such developments were only in keeping with universal trends, however, and did not disguise the fundamental hardships of the job.

In immediate charge of attendants and nurses was the head attendant, who acted as the link between the ordinary staff and the medical officers. His job was largely to oversee the general administration and to supervise up to 300 or more patients. It was he who first inspected new inmates and presented a medical report to the doctor in charge. It was the head attendant, too, who acted as go-between for patients who wanted to speak to the medical superintendent.[75] At the West Riding Asylum he was a man of 63 and received an income significantly higher than his subordinates.[76] Charles Mercier outlined his duties thus:

7.30	Breakfast.
8.00	Back on the wards.
10.30	Tour of inspection.
1.30	Dinner. Supervision of wards and airing courts.
5.00	Patients' tea.
10.00	Masterlock all communication doors.[77]

There is no mention of his role in staff management and little, if any, work exists which examines the head attendant in relation to medical development or the life of asylum inmates.

Profession and staff

Relations between the attendants as a whole and the medical staff, particularly the medical superintendent in view of his immense authority in the asylum, showed some curious mixture of expectations. Superintendents ran their asylums with a firm measure of control. This is perhaps to be expected in such a paternalist regime in which many of the male attendants were drawn from the army or from agricultural labour and the nurses largely from domestic service.[78] It is further suggested by the fact that 91 out of the 567 male attendants employed at the West Riding Lunatic Asylum between 1860 and 1880 were sacked by the superintendent for reasons varying from 'dishonesty' to being found 'drunk',[79] though this may simply reflect the poor calibre of the staff they were employing.

The work itself, however, brought its own insecurities and consequent need for vigilance. Of the male attendants working at the asylum between the above years nearly 4 per cent (21 in all) were dismissed for 'cruelty' to patients, though among the females the figure was around 1.4 per cent (a total of 8). This accounted for about one-third of all dismissals.[80]

The magnitude of such acts of cruelty and their origins are not easy to ascertain but the strictures against any kind of physical abuse of a patient were particularly strong. The Commissioners in Lunacy in particular vigorously condemned any such thing, since the abandonment of 'mechanical restraint' and the barbarities that had resulted from the practice was the cornerstone of the public asylum's new 'humanitarian' regime which it was their duty to uphold. Thus in 1891 one attendant found himself instantly dismissed for 'forcibly pushing' a patient,[81] while a certain John Owen was not only sacked but prosecuted and fined for 'striking a patient'.[82]

The consequences of such criminal conviction were often extreme. An attendant in the Northwood asylum was fined £15 for assault, but because he had no money he was sent to prison for two months instead.[83] Another attendant found guilty of taking a patient into a bathroom and striking him was fined £5. He also could not pay and so was sentenced to one month with hard labour.[84]

Acts of cruelty such as these were no doubt inexcusable, but to be fair to the attendants, who were ill-trained and uneducated, the awkwardness of some inmates conspired with the strictness of asylum regulations to produce some very difficult conditions that had unfortunate results. In 1880, for example, a jury heard how a 31-year-old crippled man, 'noisy, restless, incoherent and of faulty habits' was put in a bath with the taps running and the plug left out, as a means of cleaning his soiled body. The patient cried out and was removed back to bed and medical assistance summoned. The medical officer found signs of scalding which were 'not severe' around the legs and buttocks. Nevertheless the patient, 'being feeble', died ten hours later apparently from shock. 'It was calculated that the heat of the water was about 120°F.' The commissioners felt it was their duty to commit one of the two nurses involved for manslaughter. The assize jury rejected the charge.[85]

Yet alongside such fierce regulation the medical superintendents as professional men regularly extolled the virtues of the 'good' attendant and ascribed to him a high place in the pantheon of medical remedies for insanity. Nursing was seen as a vital part of treatment.

> The nurse who can enter most closely into the mind of her patient, who can probe her feelings with instinctive readiness, and adapt her circumstances to the varying moods presented, is, indeed, a valuable auxiliary to the medical [officer].[86]

> The condition of a patient is materially promoted or retarded by the activity or supineness of the Attendant.[97]

What medical men seemed to be looking for was nursing staff who possessed

> a quiet, calm, gentle demeanour, free from the least flurry, a constant cheerfulness and brightness unruffled by any of the patients' vagaries, an absolutely even temper, great patience and forbearance.[88]

What they got instead of such paragons of humanistic virtue were staff who were

> coarse, harsh, passionate, indifferent, untrustworthy, intemperate; having no higher conception of their office than that of gaoler.

They were 'lazibodies' and the 'outcasts of other trades'.[89]

Why was such a discrepancy perpetuated? Significantly, while the medical superintendents railed against the mass of attendants who fell short of their high ideals, they did very little to correct the situation. The Commissioners in Lunacy had called for higher wages to attract 'persons of quality',[90] yet rates of pay set at £16 p.a. for women and £30 for men were described by superintendents as 'liberal' in 1881,[91] and no one was anxious to raise them.

Neither was much effort made to improve the level of training among attendants. One or two superintendents had set up special courses in the early days of public asylums[92] but nothing of a general character was mooted until a letter in the *Journal of Mental Science* in 1870, to which there was no immediate response. Then in 1876 T.S. Clouston began a series of lectures to the Medico-Psychological Association on the importance of training good attendants, to which there was equally no great response. Not until the enterprise of Campbell Clark in 1883, proposing competitions and prizes for essays written by attendants on matters of insanity, was any enthusiasm shown. It then consisted in the compiling of *A Handbook for the Instruction of Attendants on the Insane*, published by the association in 1885. Finally, systematic training and examination for attendants began in 1890, under pressure from similar schemes in the large teaching hospitals.[93]

It seems probable that the regular attacks upon the quality of asylum attendants was masking a deeper failure, that of the asylum system itself. The more 'moral treatment' developed into a round of exercise, useful employment, diverting entertainment, and general institutional routine, the more the nursing staff were regarded as central to the therapeutic process.

> The attendants are the backbone of a lunatic asylum. The happiness and welfare of the patients while they are in the asylum depend far more on the character and conduct of the attendants than on those of all the rest of the asylum staff put together.[94]

Yet the medical profession could not allow its own expertise to be eclipsed and would only accept the value of their own 'ideal' attendant as useful in the medical process. In effect they elevated the 'good attendant' to the level of a myth that represented, yet now ironically came to stand in place of, the powers of asylum-based medicine itself. When the reality of the asylum's failure became obvious it was easy to point the finger at the shortcomings of the very human and ordinary nursing staff, and so avoid facing up to the greater ineffectiveness that existed at the higher reaches of the lunacy profession. Similarly, when the medical men found that the asylum system, with its institutional pressure and its authoritarian structure, could not be run without violent mishap it was the nurses and attendants who carried the can.

Yet the nursing staff were indeed the backbone of the asylum. At all the upper levels of the profession medical men had reached an impasse. At the very top the big names in lunacy had removed themselves altogether from asylum work, while medical superintendents angled for publication in the *Journal* and an outlet into research work or more lucrative private practice. Lower down the profession the medical officers were stuck in their asylum laboratories, dissecting brains and administering a daily routine of medication to the inmates. Aspiring young men looking for a respectable income in medicine passed in and out, making scarcely any impact on the institutional routine. Only the nursing staff handled the inmates at any properly human level, coping with them day-to-day and carrying the main burden of the process of reformation which was supposed to bring about their recovery.

For a brief time during the later part of the nineteenth century it seems reasonable to suppose that the nursing staff were the most vital part of the whole asylum business. As yet not brought under closer professional control by the collusion of senior mental physicians with the feminist-inspired British Nursing Association in 1897,[95] or by the educational initiatives from above aimed at re-vamping their image – and personal status – from 'attendant' to 'mental nurse',[96] their attitude and changing social perspectives could have had significant consequences for treatment and professional relations.

This is an area which clearly needs more research. Yet it may be that the asylum system upon which the whole lunacy profession rested, which preserved the superintendents and senior medical officers in a species of medical redundancy, was being slowly transformed by new ideas brought from below, by the nursing staff, whose origins and attitudes the men at the top were not fully able to control.

Notes

1 (1872–90) Admissions Registers, Wadsley Asylum, Middlewood Hospital, Sheffield. (1860–90) Admission Registers, West Riding Lunatic Asylum, Wakefield PRO, C85. (1890) Annual Report of the West Riding Asylum Committee, Wakefield PRO. These figures can be found in greater detail in my PhD thesis (1983) 'Mental physicians and their patients', Sheffield University.

2 As they were, for example, in the annual reports of the Mapperley Asylum, Nottingham, for 1891, which includes all the tabulated material referred to here.

3 Report of the Committee appointed at a meeting of the Medico-Psychological Association, held at the Royal College of Physicians, Edinburgh, 1869. See (July 1870) *Journal of Mental Science* 74: 223–32.

4 J.A. Campbell (April 1873) 'Unity in public reports', *Journal of Mental Science* (hereafter *JMS*) 85, XIX: 67–8.

5 D.J. Mellett (July 1981) 'Bureaucracy and mental illness', *Medical Histroy* XXV, 3: 235.

6 See 6th and 7th, William IV, C89.

7 W.G. Balfour (April 1874) 'Pathological appearances observed in the brains of the insane', *JMS* 89, XX: 49–60.
8 ibid., 59–60.
9 'Sane Patient' (1879) *My Experience in a Lunatic Asylum*, London: Chatto pp. 96–7.
10 A. Walk (1953) 'The centenary of the Journal of Mental Science', *JMS* 99: 633. There was at the time of its launch another journal supplying the same market, Forbes Winslow's *Journal of Psychological Medicine*, and many AMOHI members subscribed to this journal. Bucknill was able to draw on the interest in lunacy created by the 1845 Lunacy Act to gain the willing consent of AMOHI members for his own venture. After placating Forbes Winslow in 1857 by electing him president of the AMOHI, the association won his support for the new journal and the *Journal of Psychological Medicine* was closed down.
11 (1854) *Asylum Journal* 6: 96.
12 ibid., 4: 64.
13 ibid., 7: 112.
14 ibid., 9: 143.
15 (October 1858) *JMS* 27, V.
16 (1859) *JMS* 31, VI; and chapter 6, by Trevor Turner, in this volume.
17 (1860) *JMS* 32, VI.
18 (1860) *JMS* 33, VI: 328–69.
19 (1863) *JMS* 44, VIII: title-page.
20 ibid., 482–513.
21 ibid., (1863) *JMS* 45, IX: title-page.
22 A. Walk, (1976) 'Medico-psychologists, Maudsley and the Maudsley', *British Journal of Psychiatry* 128: 22.
23 Quarterly reports of the West Riding Lunatic Asylum (hereafter QRWRLA), Wakefield PRO, C85.
24 ibid., 20 January 1885.
25 ibid., 30 July 1885.
26 Originally an initiative by the energetic Samuel Hitch in 1841, who created the Association of Medical Officers of Hospitals for the Insane as part of his asserted campaign against the use of physical restraint in the treatment of the insane. The AMOHI changed its name in 1865. See A. Walk and D. Lindsay Walker (1961) 'Gloucester and the beginnings of the R.M.P.A.', *Journal of Mental Science* 107: 603–32.
27 Aubrey Lewis (1967) *The State of Psychiatry; essays and addresses*, London: Routledge & Kegan Paul.
28 QRWRLA (30 July 1885), Wakefield PRO, C85.
29 QRWRLA (19 March 1891), Wakefield PRO, C85.
30 QRWRLA (23 June 1892), Wakefield PRO, C85.
31 QRWRLA (21 June 1894), Wakefield PRO, C85.
32 QRWRLA (26 September 1889), Wakefield PRO, C85.
33 Aubrey Lewis (in *The State of Psychiatry*) has some interesting things to say about Maudsley's almost total lack of qualifications and his unpremeditated arrival into the world of lunacy following his rejection from the East India Company.
34 QRWRLA (26 January 1882), Wakefield PRO, C85.
35 QRWRLA (20 January 1885), Wakefield PRO, C85.
36 QRWRLA (29 October 1885), Wakefield PRO, C85.

37 QRWRLA (29 January 1885), Wakefield PRO, C85.
38 J.T. Arlidge (1859) *On the State of Lunacy and the Legal Provision for the Insane, with observations on the construction and organisation of asylums*, London: Churchill, p. 122.
39 Charles Mercier (1894) *Lunatic Asylums, their Organisation and Management*, London: C. Griggin & Co., pp. 196–8.
40 ibid., p. 245.
41 Dr Dodds, Dr Strahan and Dr Greenlees (1890) 'Assistant medical officers in asylums: their status in the speciality', *Journal of Mental Science* 52, XXXVII: 48–9.
42 D.H. Tuke (1882) *Chapters in the History of the Insane in the British Isles*, London: Kegan Paul & Trench, p. 462.
43 Staff Wages Book, Stanley Royd Hospital Museum, Wakefield (hereafter SRHM).
44 M.J. Peterson (1978) *The Medical Profession in Mid-Victorian London*, Berkeley: University of California Press, p. 217.
45 Staff Wages Book, SRHM.
46 Mercier, *Lunatic Asylums*, pp. 243–4.
47 Dodds, Strahan and Greenlees, 'Assistant medical officers in asylums', 43.
48 ibid., 44.
49 ibid., 46–7.
50 ibid., 48.
51 ibid., 50.
52 ibid., 52.
53 Staff Wages Book, SRHM.
54 ibid.
55 Mercier, *Lunatic Asylums*, p. 246.
56 ibid., p. 246.
57 Staff Wages Book, SRHM.
58 Register of Attendants, SRHM.
59 ibid.
60 Arlidge, *On the State of Lunacy*, p. 105.
61 In many ways this provision was all that remained of the once noble concept of 'moral treatment' (see Russell, 'Mental physicians and their patients'). It is notable that all such work fell to the nursing staff to perform.
62 (1886) *Handbook for the Instruction of Attendants on the Insane*, American edn, Boston, Mass.: Medico-Psychological Association, pp. 61–73.
63 ibid., pp. 101–2.
64 (1857) Eleventh report of the Commissioners in Lunacy, p. 46; (1859) Thirteenth report of the Commissioners in Lunacy, pp. 64–5; QRWRLA (29 January 1885).
65 Mick Carpenter, (1980) 'Asylum nursing before 1914: a chapter in the history of labour', in C. Davies (ed.), *Rewriting Nursing History*, London: Croom Helm.
66 (1859) Thirteenth report of the Commissioners in Lunacy, pp. 65–7.
67 (1896) Fiftieth report of the Commissioners in Lunacy, pp. 27–8.
68 (1859) Thirteenth report of the Commissioners in Lunacy, p. 68.
69 ibid., p. 64.
70 Mercier, *Lunatic Asylums*, p. 286.
71 ibid.
72 QRWRLA (20 June 1888).

73 ibid. (27 October 1887).
74 Mercier, *Lunatic Asylums*, p. 287.
75 (1860) 'A descriptive notice of the Sussex Lunatic Asylum, Haywards Heath', *Journal of Mental Science* VI, 33: 255.
76 Staff Wages Book, SRHM.
77 Mercier, *Lunatic Asylums*, pp. 280–3.
78 'A descriptive notice', 257.
79 Register of Attendants, SRHM.
80 ibid.
81 Minutes of the meeting of the Commissioners in Lunacy (11 September 1891), PRO MHSO.
82 ibid. (6 March 1876).
83 ibid.
84 ibid.
85 (1880–1) Forty-fifth report of the Commissioners in Lunacy, p. 62.
86 W. Bevan Lewis (1899) *A Text-Book of Mental Diseases: with special reference to the Pathological Aspects of Insanity*, 2nd edn, London: C. Griggin & Co., p. 462.
87 (1859) Thirteenth report of the Commissioners in Lunacy, pp. 61–2.
88 Lewis, *Text-Book of Mental Diseases*, p. 462.
89 (April 1866) *Journal of Mental Science* XII: 44–5.
90 (1859) Thirteenth report of the Commissioners in Lunacy, pp. 62–3.
91 (1881) Annual report of the Nottingham Borough Asylum, Mapperley Hospital Library.
92 Most notably Alexander Morison at Surrey in 1843, and W.A.F. Browne at Crichton Royal in 1854.
93 See A. Walk (1961) 'The history of mental nursing', *Journal of Mental Science* 107: 1–17.
94 Mercier, *Lunatic Asylums*, p. 284.
95 F.R. Adams (1969) 'From association to union – professional organisation of asylum attendants, 1869–1919', *Brit. Journal of Psychiatry* 20: 11–26.
96 Mark Finnance (1981) *Insanity and the Insane in Post-Famine Ireland*, London: Croom Helm, pp. 181–2.

CHAPTER TWELVE

The wages of sin: the problem of alcoholism and general paralysis in nineteenth-century Edinburgh

Margaret S. Thompson

Late-nineteenth-century psychiatrists tried to disentangle the threads that caused mental illness – heredity, life's passages, social factors, dissipation. This chapter examines the 'wages of sin' and the threats posed by dissipated behaviour to mental and physical health. The correlation between alcoholism and promiscuous sexuality intrigued Scottish doctors and social reformers – yet they failed to recognize the causal link between syphilis and general paralysis of the insane, or to connect the medical, epidemiological, historical, and cultural clues that suggested the relationship. It points out how shocking the discovery of the spirochete for syphilis was to Victorian Scots, many of whom regarded venereal disease as a just punishment for sexual promiscuity and an indicator of social decay. Finally, it relates the dilemma of the psychiatrist, Dr Thomas Smith Clouston, who remained a prisoner of his assumptions, culture, and environment – very much a figure of his time.

One of the many questions that is beginning to be addressed in the history of psychiatry is why the optimism about cure at the beginning of the nineteenth century gave way to pessimism at the century's end.[1] Scots perceived madness to be increasing during the transition from agrarian to industrial society – one complex social and medical dilemma that prompted social reformers and doctors to probe correlations between public and mental health, behaviour, and environment. Dr Thomas Smith Clouston (1840–1915), physician-superintendent of Morningside and first official Clinical Lecturer in Mental Disease at Edinburgh University (1879), was the acknowledged doyen of Scottish psychiatry. The teaching appointment linking academic and clinical psychiatry gave him an unrivalled professional reputation. His *Clinical Lectures On Mental Diseases* went through six editions between 1884 and 1906 and was the recognized textbook on psychiatry for medical students. In addition, his numerous scholarly articles and books on the 'new' subject of 'mental hygiene' amplified his views and aimed to educate the public on prudent and prophylactic lifestyles.[2] Towards the end of the century Clouston was forced to confront contemporaneous concerns about increased numbers of pauper insane, heredity, syphilis, drug and alcohol abuse.

People who indulged in 'dissipated behaviour' were responsible for their mental state. Sin and sexuality were inextricably linked in the Scottish consciousness. The following chapter discusses Morningside's inmates who were labelled as 'sinners' in a statistical analysis between 1874 and 1894. It analyses the diverse diagnoses, prognoses, and outcome as psychiatrists pondered the effects of alcoholism and promiscuous sexuality and the complex interrelationships among psychiatrists, asylums, inmates, and local cultural milieux.

By 1894 the Royal Edinburgh Asylum (Morningside) had grown in numbers from six inmates when it opened in 1813 to an impressive institution which housed 800 inmates from all social classes. Under the Lunacy (Scotland) Act of 1857 Morningside was given authority to admit patients from all classes of the city's diverse population.[3] The Act mandated that Clouston treated patients from paupers to the very rich. The asylum's extensive Gheel model, which emulated the best features of the famous and controversial Belgian village where the insane were cared for in a home-like atmosphere, comprised elegant homes and villas exclusively for the wealthy (East House).[4] West House treated middle-class and pauper inmates. Private patients (9 per cent) paid on a sliding scale according to income. Charity cases (11 per cent) were given financial assistance from a special charity fund started in the 1850s to help impoverished middle-class, genteel individuals avoid the stigma of pauperism and segregate them from 'vulgar, unrefined paupers'. Paupers comprised the majority of inmates (80 per cent), the fees of the latter paid for by the parish of birth. Each addition had been designed by Clouston to reflect the appropriate social class of its inmates with great care and attention to environmental detail.[5]

Clouston was a somaticist in theory, but his varied interests included blood lines, class lines, sexual differences, and social totems and taboos. From the beginning of his tenure in 1873 he sought to distinguish between harmful or self-destructive behaviour and that which was prudent and prophylactic. He was never the reductionist who believed only in heredity. In fact, he believed strongly that predisposition to madness could be 'counteracted by suitable environments' and praised environmental theories as the most sophisticated in contemporary thought;[6] he was, therefore, a behaviourist and an environmentalist. His treatment, apparently at variance with his somaticism, makes his Scottish behavioural programme interesting Clouston's updated interpretation of 'moral therapy' eschewed education and religion. Rather he stressed cultivation of self-discipline, self-sufficiency, and independence.

Clouston stressed the relationship between a healthy mind and a healthy body. 'Mental hygiene' required moderation, a judicious balance of work and play. In addition to recommending prudent personal behaviour,

Clouston advised against excessive study in the young, and deviance from the straight and narrow – dissipation, sexual excess, or 'self-abuse'. Good mental health demanded adherence to Victorian moral values, duty, continence, and self-control.[7]

Clouston thought that it was pointless to blame inmates whose insanity was 'caused' by various somatic diseases, epilepsy, senile dementia, 'idiocy', 'hereditary propensity', or a vast array of complex economic or social factors. These inmates would fall under the heading of the 'deserving poor' mandated for care under the 1857 Lunacy Act. Moreover, he was well aware of the dislocating effects of industrialization, malnutrition and poverty on the lives of working-class patients, particularly poor married women. 'Virtuous' West House women (82 per cent paupers) indicated that physical disease, social and economic dependency, inability to cope, and lack of support systems necessitated their care.[8] The collective picture of 60 per cent of non-dissipated West House males (80 per cent paupers) shows that they were physically sick, old, 'suicidal', 'dangerous', 'maniacal', severely depressed, senile or brain damaged, helpless and dependent. For Clouston, who dealt primarily with a deprived urban population, 'incurability' was a given fact. His gospels of work, play and fitness – regimes of rest and nurture – were germane for Edinburgh's impoverished paupers.

On the other hand, inmates who indulged in 'dissipated behaviour' were responsible for their condition. The question of moral judgement becomes crucial. Alcoholism remained a chronic problem. 'Debauchery' and 'licentiousness' often led to syphilis or general paralysis. Sexual activity and a chance encounter with the wrong person could precipitate dire consequences – the ultimate determinant of disease.

Since dissipation precipitated many mental problems inmates labelled 'sinners' form the most complicated group in the asylum to analyse. Who among Morningside's inmates suffered from alcoholism, syphilis, and general paralysis? Class and gender show significant differences. Forty per cent of West House men were alcoholic, syphilitic, or both. By contrast only 17 per cent of their female counterparts suffered from these same diseases.

The 'wages of sin' took their toll on rich inmates too. In East House 20 per cent were alcoholics (27 per cent of the men and 12 per cent of the women); 22 per cent of men had syphilis. Combined syphilis and alcoholism made life miserable for another 7 per cent of men and their families. Significantly, syphilis was not diagnosed in wealthy East House women.

Contemporary social ideas on sex, marriage, and the family warned doctors that dissipation threatened the sacred institution of marriage. Temptations available in society included drunkenness and sexual licence provided by the pub and the prostitute. This kirk and doctrinaire Presbyterianism were the traditional agents of social control of sexual behaviour. Since the sixteenth century church leaders had preached against 'whoremasters and harlots' and recognized the connection between drink

Figure 12:1 Alcohol and syphilis in West House inmates

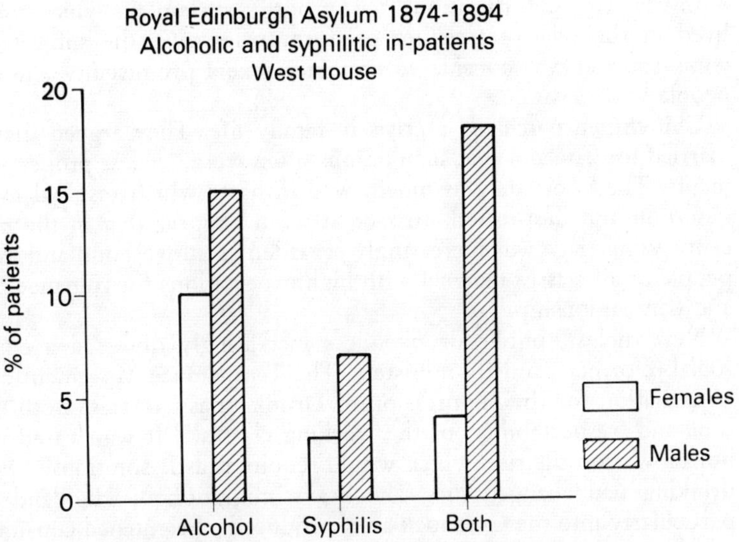

Figure 12:2 Alcoholic and syphilitic East House inmates

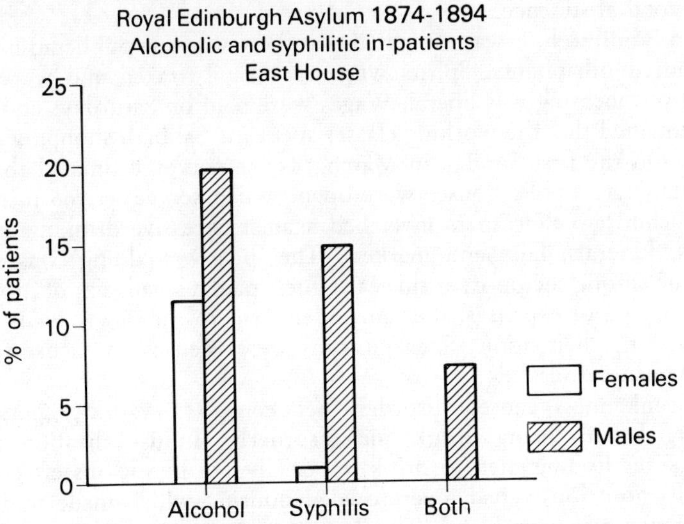

and sexuality.[9] In the nineteenth century kirk sessions remained obsessed with the 'sin of fornication'.[10] The bothy system, in which young men lived in the relative freedom of dormitories, was the subject of frosty comment and was considered to foster sexual promiscuity among young people.[11]

Churchmen perceived a crisis in family life. They argued that the rich married too late and that such unions often were loveless property arrangements. The poor, they assumed, wed in haste which resulted in frequent desertion and destitution. In fact, it would appear that in the nineteenth century marriage was increasingly regarded as a love-bond and that young people of all classes married with high expectations for romance, intimacy, and companionship.[12]

Nevertheless, public drunkenness increasingly obsessed a coalition of social reformers, mostly ministers. The Temperance Movement created an 'Association for the Suppression of Drunkenness' to raise both the moral tone and 'respectability' of the working classes.[13] It was feared that alcoholism was on the rise, which would require drastic solutions.[14] Fashion in drinking had changed too. The heavy migration of Highland workers, particularly into the Greenock area, produced a heightened consumption of whisky as distinct from beer, which had been the eighteenth-century poor man's tipple. The rich had in the past drunk claret. Now whisky became popular. Determined to suppress vice, some reformers increasingly pushed for total abstinence.

In Edinburgh, it was estimated that there was one public house for every hundred inhabitants. Spirits were not heavily taxed and were relatively cheap. Licensing was liberal. Wages were paid on Saturdays and reformers maintained that the working classes spent the Sabbath shopping and drinking. On the first Sunday in March 1853, a survey estimated that approximately 312 public houses were open, which served 41,796 men, women, and children. Reformers inveighed against excessive drinking at christenings, funerals, fairs and markets. The 'penny wedding' was in current vogue among the poor; at this each guest paid a small sum of money. After the paying of expenses, the remainder went to the newly weds to help in furnishing their home. Such customs were used as an excuse for a 'Bacchanalian carousal'.[15]

Drunkenness caused disorder. Between 1852–3, 6,047 persons were charged with being drunk and disorderly. Industrialization intensified pressures leading men to drink, especially the pernicious effects of Scotland's notoriously bad, overcrowded housing which made public houses attractive gathering places. The 'howff' or local pub had been a traditional social centre in Scottish culture, the consulting-room of doctors, the haunt of lawyers and poets in the capital. It was the hub for gossip and cheer in the country. Moreover, drinking patterns and habits were changing, reflecting higher class barriers. The poor increasingly drank in public houses; the rich in the privacy of home.[16]

The Forbes-Mackenzie Act of 1853 legislated the closing of pubs on

Sundays and limited drinking hours during the week. Other temperance strategies included limiting the number of licences and attempts to educate the young. Such measures aimed to help protect dependent women and children to cope with alcoholism's attendant miseries – domestic violence, child abuse, neglect, and economic destitution.[17]

The social, moral and medical effects of excessive drinking perplexed nineteenth-century Scottish psychiatrists. Contemporary medical opinion was divided as to whether alcoholism was a disease, in which case the victim needed sympathetic attention, care and treatment, or a sign of depravity. In the latter case moral opprobrium was justified. Whether drunkenness 'caused' poverty, or destitution resulted from drinking, was another debated question. Clouston claimed that alcoholism was a factor in 15 to 20 per cent of all cases of insanity nation-wide.[18] He argued that in some cases the alcoholic was insane but that in others alcoholism was 'a bad habit, or even a vice'.[19] Moreover, he believed that children of alcoholics risked potential 'degeneracy', sometimes as 'predisposition', sometimes in 'definite forms'. They could inherit 'idiocy, stuntedness, ugliness, deformity, deaf-mutism, sterility, incapacity for high education and immorality'.[20] The social consequences of alcoholism would in an ideal future become 'practical wisdom' for doctors and alcoholism would be an important part of medical study. The psychiatrist would become a powerful 'prophylactic guardian' of the 'physical and mental well-being of the people, and the high priest of authority for the regulation of the conditions of life'.[21]

Prevention was vital for youngsters at risk to head off potential weakness, imbecility, neurotic tendencies, and proneness to 'nervous affections'. Otherwise, they would become addicted to drink at an early age and the process would be irreversible. Whisky would 'fly to the brain' and they might develop delusional insanity or sink into dementia. Clouston prescribed fresh air, minimal study, and total abstention. 'Teetotalism in his case', Clouston averred of the youngster, 'should be a law of being' to offer him a fair chance in life. But if the 'original constitutional powers' were not too far weakened, 'Nature's law of striving to attain her average' could intervene and preserve mental health and bodily soundness. Nevertheless, periods of development and 'decadence' (old age) required solicitous attention. Clouston defined five forms of alcoholic insanity.

delirium tremens
chronic alcoholism
mania a potu
alcoholic degeneration
dipsomania.[22]

Yet Clouston devoted only seven pages of his *Clinical Lectures* (1884) to alcoholism, which suggests personal distaste for the subject.

Clouston disliked treating alcoholics in Morningside since after their initial desperately ill stage, they rapidly became ambivalent to treatment and 'resisted cure'. Moreover, they upset other inmates who felt degraded by associating with drunkards. He argued that alcoholics should be treated in separate institutions exclusively for inebriates. He supported the 'Habitual Drunkard's Act' of 1879 and the Inebriates Act of 1888 – legislation that was never successfully implemented.[23]

Yet, some doctors and bureaucrats treated alcoholics with barely concealed contempt and despised the cunning, duplicitous inebriates who coaxed or bribed workmen to smuggle whisky into institutions. One poorhouse overseer claimed that

> Every inmate, male and female, and suspicious visitor are searched on entrance, but for all that it [whisky] commonly finds its way in. Sometimes a bottle of whisky by pre-arrangement is found in the boundary wall in an old boot or shoe. Sometimes it has been brought in, in the inside of a fish, a loaf of bread, or in the hollow of a turnip.[24]

He maintained that they were the 'worst description of lunatics to grapple with'.[25]

In spite of ambivalence and frustration, Clouston had no option; he was legally obliged to admit and treat alcoholics. Ideally, alcoholics should be treated on an island where 'whisky is unknown'. Then work, supervision and strategies to 're-develop the conscience' would be attempted.[26] Within Morningside inebriates were dosed with stimulants such as strychnine and the 'continued current' if 'brain stimulation' did not preclude such treatment. Rigid abstinence and a regular, controlled 'physiological' life in the open air, preferably employed in garden work, were prescribed. Such a regime could cure a first attack but after two or three bouts alcoholism was considered to be chronic and incurable.

Statistical analysis of West House inebriates shows that sex and class revealed significant differences. Among paupers the figures were similar (11 per cent males and 10 per cent females). Among charity and private patients, numbers were negligible. The explanation for the absence of middle-class inmates may be that their families chose uninspected 'retreats' for alcoholic relatives – a point to which we will return later.[27] In East House 27 per cent of males were alcoholics, as were 12 per cent of the women.

Paradoxically, in spite of Clouston's contention that chronic alcoholism was 'incurable', 66 per cent of alcoholic men were discharged as 'cured' and had the highest probability of 'cure' among any group of West House inmates. Clearly, subjective clinical criteria, obvious only to the attending physician, were used to determine who, among alcoholics, was 'cured'.

In fact, however, after alcoholics had 'dried out' they were the only group among Morningside's inmates that could realistically be returned to a society which, Clouston admitted, tolerated them. Most alcoholic men discharged as 'cured' were married and could be cared for by their wives.

A typical case was that of a 41-year-old innkeeper who had been a hard drinker for years. He was sleepless, restless, and had paranoid delusions

Figure 12:3 Alcoholic Inmates by Sex and Class

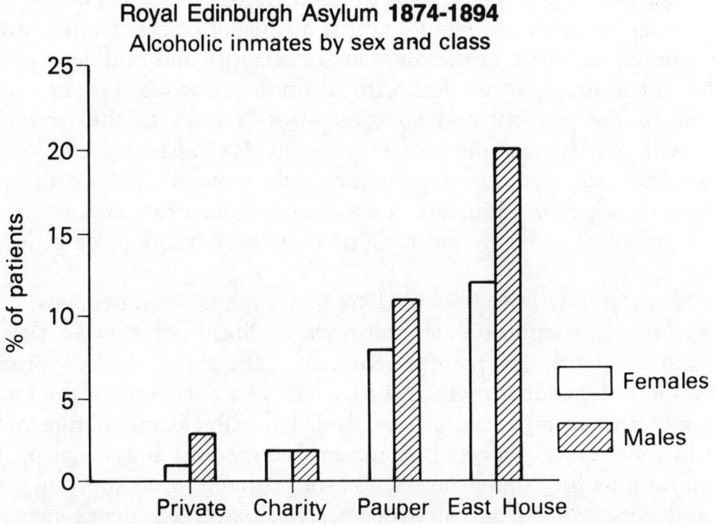

that his wife poisoned his food and kept men in cupboards in the house. He made an unsuccessful suicide attempt, and on admission was 'insanely suspicious, hallucinating', tremulous, unable to write or talk.[28]

He was treated with bromide of potassium and steel, and a diet of liquid custards made with six pints of milk and ten eggs a day, in addition to solid food, plus long walks in the open air three times a day. Since he attacked others and tried to throw himself out of windows, a constant attendant was assigned. Three months later he was unimproved, refused to read, play games, interest himself in anything or anyone or speak unless spoken to. After six months he slowly began to recover. But his prognosis was poor. Clouston maintained:

> A chronic degeneration of the whole brain plasma has begun. The intellectual power, the power of application, origination and independent energising are weakened, the delusions of suspicion are apt to persist, the morals and self-respect are apt not to be regained, lying, stealing and cowardice are indulged in. The affection for wife and children is impaired. Those symptoms run on for a year or two, and then we have dementia supervening.[29]

Clouston testified as an expert witness on 21 November 1894 to the Departmental Committee on Habitual Offenders, Vagrants, Beggars, Inebriates and Juvenile Delinquents. His position on alcoholism shows Clouston's strong and common-sense views. He claimed that there were no accurate statistics on dipsomania and alcoholism and refused to acknowledge alarmist reports of increased alcoholism among wealthy women. Moreover, he argued that families of dipsomaniacs could choose to have them institutionalized in uninspected 'retreats', some of which were managed by 'quacks'. They would thus avoid the stigma of certification (being labelled insane) and would retain control of their finances.[30] His testimony underscores the increase in the numbers of wealthy and middle-class families who chose this way to deal with alcoholic relatives. He was equally conscious of the poverty and constant stress factors in the lives of the 39 per cent married pauper women within Morningside. Unlike other psychiatrists who stigmatized poor alcoholic women as more disgusting than male drunkards, Clouston, with compassion, excused these women who sought solace in drink and claimed they were 'more to be pitied than condemned'.[31]

The 1895 commission concluded that in spite of repeated government investigations, legislation on alcoholism was a 'dead letter' in Scotland and underlined the depth of a painful problem.[32] The sheer numbers of inebriate or alcohol-dependent men, and to a lesser extent women, the fact that the disease affected all social classes, added to the chronic nature of alcoholism in most cases, reflected an intractable medical and social problem. The implications for family misery, loss of production, waste of money on drink and personal self-destructiveness, even perceived 'degeneracy' were all issues of concern. Clouston remained ambivalent towards inebriates.

Yet, while alcoholism inspired a public campaign and widespread discussion, venereal disease, another source of untold human misery, was hidden in silent shame. Nevertheless, the link between drunkenness and venereal disease posed further problems for all medical men.[33] All of these complex issues were to become more perplexing, involved, and difficult before the medical enigma that surrounded venereal disease was resolved.

Psychiatrists did not understand the specific causal link between syphilis and general paralysis in the 1880s. Nor did they realize that general paralysis was the tertiary phase of syphilis. They did recognize that syphilitics showed certain behaviours, including 'loose ways, immoral habits', and were often drunkards as well. Syphilis was increasingly cloaked in a conspiracy of silence for the general public – as opposed to social reformers – because of the constraints of Victorian prudery and the stigma attached to venereal disease. Nevertheless, the subject intrigued Scottish doctors and clergy.[34]

Since prostitutes were considered to be the principal locus of venereal infection 'the fallen woman' became the object of study. In 1841 William Tait, an evangelical doctor, estimated that there were approximately 800 prostitutes in Edinburgh. While deploring the morals of 'fallen women', Tait argued that the basic cause of prostitution was economic.[35] His study *Magdalenism: An Inquiry into the Extent, Causes and Consequences of Prostitution* (Edinburgh: 1841), admitted that many additional 'part-timers' and 'sly' prostitutes augmented their meagre wages during university term-time by drifting in and out of prostitution.[36] Edinburgh housed approximately 200 brothels, the average number of women in each was three. In a population of 137,899, therefore, there was one full-time prostitute for every eighty men.[37] Tait was adamant about the horrendous effects of syphilis and described the gruesome consequences of 'licentiousness' and sexual indulgence, particularly if men associated with prostitutes.[38]

By the 1850s William Acton, a London venerologist-surgeon, argued in his book *Prostitution Considered in Its Moral, Social and Sanitary Aspects in London and Other Large Cities with Proposals for the Mitigation and Prevention of Its Attendant Evil* (1857, revised in 1870) that such pessimistic views were outmoded. The drunken slut had been replaced by fashionable, 'pretty, elegant' young women, with more self-respect. Some were eminently respectable, and after a brief career in prostitution returned to a 'regular mode of life'. The turn-around in the prostitute's fortunes, he argued, was due to the fact that syphilis when 'properly treated' was now rarely fatal.[39]

Nevertheless, Acton supported the Contagious Diseases Acts passed in the 1860s to protect Britain's soldiers from diseased prostitutes in English garrison towns.[40] The Acts codified the sexual double standard. While prostitutes were medically inspected and incarcerated if found to be infected, clients – with the exception of soldiers and sailors – went uninspected, uncensured, and untreated.

The Acts never applied in Scotland but the issues that inflamed the debate were central to nineteenth-century Victorian consciousness – the protection and stability of the family unit, retaining the ideal of 'pure womanhood', versus civil liberty, social control, regulation of vice, and state regulation of prostitution.

Clouston the psychiatrist saw syphilis and general paralysis as two distinct diseases, which he described in two separate chapters of his *Clinical Lectures On Mental Diseases* (1884). He wrote of syphilis as a distinct somatic disease.[41] He claimed to be at a disadvantage in describing the precise natural history of syphilis because he dealt only 'with the brain symptoms', an omission that suggests little communication between psychiatrists and other doctors. Nevertheless, Clouston recognized four forms of syphilitic insanity:

1) secondary syphilitic insanity
2) delusional syphilitic insanity
3) vascular syphilitic insanity
4) syphilomatous insanity.

'Secondary syphilitic insanity', occurring during the second stage of the disease, coincident with the eruption, was curable and rare.[42] In these cases, after the disappearance of syphilis, patients recovered mental health. 'Delusional syphilitic insanity', Clouston averred, stemmed from 'slight brain starvation from an obscure syphilitic irritation that has become arrested'.[43]

'Vascular syphilitic insanity' and 'syphilomatous insanity' had clear definite pathology.[44] The former depended on the 'poison to affect the blood-vessels of the brain and cause slow arteritis, with diminished blood-carrying capacity and consequent slow starvation of the cerebral tissue. By contrast, syphilomatous insanity depended on the tendency of the poison to affect the connective tissue, neuroglia, membranes and bones and to cause pressure, irritation direct and reflex, and inflammation in the convolutions.'[45]

General paralysis was described as a somatic disease with distinct physiological, pathological, and psychological characteristics which could be triggered by a diverse list of causes such as 'brain exhaustion, irritation, excesses in drinking, sexual excess, over-work, over-worry, syphilis or injuries'.[46]

Clouston defined general paralysis of the insane as

> A disease of the cortical part of the brain, characterized by progression, by the combined presence of mental and motor symptoms, the former always including mental enfeeblement and mental facility, and often delusions of grandeur and ideas of morbid expansion or self-satisfaction; the motor deficiencies always including a peculiar, defective articulation of words, and always passing through the stages of fibrillar convulsion, incoordination, paresis and paralysis; the disease process spreading to the whole of the nerve tissues in the body; being as yet incurable, and fatal in a few years.[47]

General paralysis was tragic since it attacked individuals in their prime (mostly men aged 25 to 50), had no apparent correlation with 'hereditary propensity' to madness, and was fatal. The puzzling killer was 'the most terrible of all the modern diseases of modern life',[48] which had no respect for class distinctions, although it ravaged more men than women.

Clouston divided the natural history of general paralysis into three stages. First patients showed fibrillar tremblings, slight incoordination of facial and speech muscles, together with mental exaltation and excitement. The second stage was characterized by increased muscular incoordination and paresis with mental enfeeblement. By the tertiary phase patients had almost inarticulate speech, and finally 'paralysis with mental extinction'.[49]

General paralytics were difficult patients. By the second stage they were incontinent, and had delusions of grandeur and staggering gait (locomotor ataxia). In the tertiary stage speech was impaired or totally absent and they required water-beds and careful nursing to prevent leaking urine from creating bed-sores. Clearly, as the dreary picture indicates, it was impossible to nurse these individuals in poor homes. Yet, Morningside's nurses showed little overt repugnance to these inmates. General paralysis was treated as an irrevocable consequence of 'dissipated habits' – unpleasant, but necessary to be dealt with for the family's sake. Significantly, in his *Clinical Lectures* (1884 edition) Clouston maintained, 'I do not think there is any proof that it [general paralysis] is syphilitic in origin.'[50]

In his 1887 *Physician's Annual Report*, Clouston noted that the incidence of general paralysis was decreasing, due to the current economic depression.[51] In hard times he believed that men spent less money on drink and prostitutes. Shortly after Clouston's 1887 guess, however, the disease was documented to be on the rise.[52] Numbers of cases grew consistently every year. We cannot be sure if the increase was due to better diagnosis, more honest reportage by doctors, or greater willingness of families to institutionalize victims.

Doctors were placed in the difficult, anomalous social role of curing the patient ostensibly without passing moral judgement on his behaviour or sexual conduct. Distinctions between 'responsibility for risk', determinism and destiny, heredity and free will, became subjects of discourse. Henrik Ibsen (1828–1906), the Norwegian playwright, confronted the issue in his play *Ghosts* (1881), and captured how the complexities, ambiguities, and problems of venereal infection impinged on family life.[53] His heroine Mrs Alving's choice not to leave her debauched, venereally diseased husband early in her marriage led to the 'innocent infection' of Oswald, their only son. In the wrenching final scene Oswald, rapidly succumbing to blindness, insanity, or both, begged his mother to help him commit suicide.

The asylum was the final resting place for some victims afflicted with venereal disease, either caused by their own 'dissipated habits' or, as in *Ghosts*, by what was called at the time 'hereditary taint'. Yet venereal disease was still tricky to diagnose with precision because of the long periods of remission. Since there was no medical consensus as to aetiology in either syphilis or general paralysis, it was statistically difficult to discover or prove and impossible to treat effectively.

Given the pressures to adhere to Victorian respectability it is obvious that the confused, complex issues of venereal disease posed difficult ethical issues for medical men. There was no reliable cure and the confusion between the two diseases compounded the problem. Moreover, sin and sex were inextricably linked in the minds of many contemporary Scots, particularly the censorious Free Church clergy.[54] Asylum inmates who were victims of general paralysis of the insane would inevitably be labelled with the double stigma of being both mad and bad. The debate on sexuality and prostitution was a moral issue that doctors could not avoid. How did physicians deal with these diseases, and the ominous increase in the numbers of victims?

Recent historians claim that some American doctors did not tell patients that they suffered from venereal disease to protect them from social stigma.[55] Nor did they inform the wife of the husband's venereal infection, under the aegis of doctor-patient confidentiality.[56] An infected wife could become sterile or the foetus could be infected with syphilis. As early as 1837 the French virologist Philippe Ricord had discovered specific differences between syphilis and gonorrhoea through a series of experimental inoculations from syphilitic chancres, and was the first to explicate primary, secondary, and tertiary syphilis.[57] Alfred Fournier in France was the first to describe how these infants were predisposed to newborn blindness. In addition they could develop meningitis, mental retardation or hydrocephalus among other constitutional defects.[58] The tragic social consequ-

Figure 12:4 Syphilitic Men and Alcoholic and Syphilitic Men

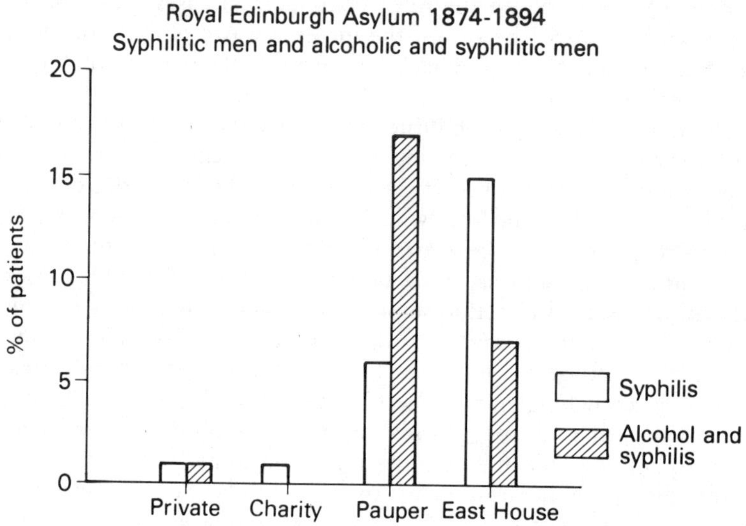

ences of venereal disease increasingly became the doctor's moral, ethical, and medical dilemma late in the nineteenth century.[59]

Since the 'wages of sin' were associated with such ominous but diverse prognoses, Morningside's inmates with a history of syphilis or combined alcoholism and syphilis form a complicated picture. Who were the patients affected by these diseases? Again, class and gender show significant differences.

Only 3 per cent of West House women (9 cases) had syphilis, and 4 per cent had combined syphilis and alcoholism (12 cases), a very small proportion of women. In East House there was one case of tertiary syphilis – a 29-year-old London governess from an ultra-respectable family who had a reputation for impeccable personal behaviour. Admitted for 'softening of the brain', within twelve months she was dead. Most likely she was a case of congenital syphilis or had a 'hereditary taint'.

Since venereal disease was much more prevalent among men I analysed all men, including East House men who suffered from syphilis, or combined alcohol and syphilis.

Out of the total male population sample, 17 per cent of paupers were both alcoholic and syphilitic, as were 7 per cent of East House men. Among East House men 15 per cent had a history of syphilis, compared with 6 per cent of West House paupers. Again, numbers and proportion of West House private and charity male cases were negligible. West House private males tended to be middle-class professionals, doctors, lawyers, businessmen, and farmers. Charity cases were impoverished and genteel, frequently teachers, students, or tradespeople fallen on hard times because of the financial drain of long-term mental illness.

It is clear that among Morningside inmates rich men and male paupers show more evidence of the effects of sexual dissipation than charity or private male cases. Like alcoholic inmates, it may be that middle- or upper-class families chose to nurse victims of general paralysis of the insane at home.

Nevertheless, these findings based on class and sex corroborate other historical evidence that lower- and upper-class men were more sexually promiscuous, while middle-class men tended to be more continent.[60] They affirm the double standard of sexual morality. Moreover, they point out the social necessity of the prostitute and commercial sex as an 'outlet' for male sexual frustration and underscore her role as scapegoat. The final irony was that venereally diseased men did sometimes infect their 'pure' wives and 'taint' their children.

Nevertheless, among West House men who suffered from syphilis, alcoholism, or both, 47 per cent were discharged as 'cured' while 27 per cent died (7 per cent with syphilis, 20 per cent alcoholic, and 7 per cent with both). Equally, among West House women diagnosed as having syphilis or alcoholism or both, 49 per cent were discharged as 'cured', while 31 per cent died (12 per cent with syphilis, 14 per cent with alcoholism, 6 per cent with both).

It is clear that inmates with alcoholism or 'social diseases', as venereal infections were euphemistically called, were a source of frustration and exasperation to psychiatrists. Doubtless these cases were discharged as rapidly as possible, as soon as either spontaneous improvement or remission occurred.

It was not clear why so many alcoholic and syphilitic inmates were being discharged as 'cured'. Clouston apparently chose not to believe – in face of mounting evidence – that syphilis was the necessary precursor of general paralysis. That reality put him in an embarrassing position in Presbyterian Scotland of being in charge of an inmate population, a large proportion of whom incurred the double stigma of being mad in addition to being 'promiscuous', or dissipated.

The epidemiology of general paralysis was revealing. It was a city disease, seldom found in the Highlands, and rarely discovered in Ireland, which perhaps indicates that the Catholic Church was capable, through sexual repression, of saving its flock from its ravages.[61] By contrast, a Dr Thomas Dowse claimed that out of 10,000 inmates in the Central London Sick Asylum three-fourths were victims of 'acquired or hereditary (congenital) syphilis',[62] numbers which made Clouston 'shudder' as the significance became obvious.

Early in the 1890s in the new Central Pathological Laboratory of the Scottish Asylums, housed in Morningside's grounds, Dr Ford Robertson sought to solve the enigma of general paralysis of the insane.[63] In 1902 Robertson requested additional funds to support more comprehensive research in physiology, pathology, and bacteriology, hoping to discover the aetiology and find treatment for general paralysis, which he believed was caused by an organism which he called *Bacillus paralyticans*.[64]

Table 12:3 *Deaths from General Paralysis in Scottish Asylums, 1865–1911 Asylyms*

	Average of Five Years								
	Average Number of Pauper Patients Resident			*Average Yearly Number of Deaths of Pauper Patients from General Paralysis*			*Proportion of Deaths of Pauper Patients from General Paralysis per 1,000 of Average Number Resident*		
	M	F	Both Sexes	M	F	Both Sexes	M	F	Both Sexes
Group 1 – Asylums serving large towns: Aberdeen District, Dundee District, Edinburgh (Royal and District), Woodilee, Gartloch, Hawkhead, Kirklands, and Paisley. Years 1907–11.	2,426	2,305	4,731	89	23	112	36.8	10.1	23.8
Similar group for 1900–4.	2,214	2,279	4,493	74	21	95	33.4	9.2	21.1
Group 2 – Asylums serving districts having populations largely urban and industrial: Ayr, Fife, Lanark, Midlothian, and Stirling. Years 1907–11.	1,606	1,495	3,101	38	8	46	23.8	5.3	14.9
Similar group for 1900–4.	1,710	1,768	3,478	36	8	44	21.1	4.5	12.7
Group 3 – Asylums serving districts chiefly agricultural and pastoral: Aberdeen Royal, Argyll, Banff, Dumfries, Elgin, Haddington, Inverness, Montrose, Perth, and Roxburgh. Years 1907–11.	1,771	1,881	3,652	17	4	21	9.4	2.3	5.7
Similar group for 1900–4.	1,442	1,542	2,984	11	2	13	7.6	1.3	4.4

Source: *Fifty-fifth Report of Lunacy Commissioners in Scotland* (1912), p. lxxiii.

The numerical increase in general paralytics was analysed by Scotland's Lunacy Commissioners in 1875, 1895, 1901, 1906, and 1912. In their fifty-fifth report (1912) scientific investigation corroborated what had long been conjecture and growing conviction.[65] It was now accepted scientific fact that prior syphilitic infection was the necessary precursor and determinant of general paralysis. Still, there remained unanswered questions. Among syphilitics only a small proportion developed general paralysis. There could be a latency period of ten or even twenty years between initial infection and the terminal phase. Moreover, ordinary anti-syphilitic treatment apparently had no beneficial effect in these cases. Finally, the disease affected four times more men than women.[66]

Lunacy Commissioners reported some good news. The Registrar General's Report of 1910 claimed that general paralysis caused a mere 0.3 per cent of all reported deaths. The number may be artificially low if medical complicity in hiding true diagnoses was commonplace in Scotland.[67] In asylums, however, general paralysis was responsible for about 14 per cent of inmate deaths. Moreover, both the numbers and the proportion of general paralytics had increased consistently since statistics had been recorded.

Ironically, Morningside itself had the dubious distinction of being the Scottish asylum that showed the greatest proportion of inmates in whom general paralysis was a principal or contributing 'cause' of insanity. The point is not that Edinburgh citizens were more promiscuous, for only 26 per cent of East House inmates were Edinburgh-born. The significance lies in the fact that Morningside accepted syphilitic inmates and victims of general paralysis. It underscores the importance of understanding policy-making decisions in given institutions and acquiring a knowledge of admissions policy.[68]

The discourse on syphilis and the discovery of the spirochete fed into debates on moral and sexual conduct. The truth about the aetiology of general paralysis produced an irrevocable change in attitude to victims of venereal disease, and to prostitutes. Doctors increasingly debated their ethical responsibility to society and to virtuous members of the 'weaker sex' who were still generally perceived to be passive, asexual victims of male lust. Some doctors now believed it was their moral obligation to provide sex education for young people as a prophylactic measure.[69] Hysteria against the 'social evil', male promiscuity, the double standard, the 'white slave trade' and the potentially dire effects of venereal disease on racial 'degeneration' fed into the nascent eugenics movement.[70]

Since prostitutes were increasingly seen as diseased troublemakers, mentally unstable 'unnatural women', their deviant social role became even more controversial.[71]

Over the period of analysis 3 per cent of Morningside's females were 'common whores'. Who were they? Did their vicious lives drive them to madness, or did participation in the 'oldest profession' reflect inherent mental and moral weakness? Did they have venereal disease? How did their treatment differ from that of other inmates?

Table 12:2 *Proportion of General Paralysis in Scottish Asylums*

Name of Establishment	*Average Annual Proportion of Deaths of Pauper Patients in Establishments Per 1,000 Pauper Patients resident, in which General Paralysis was present either as a Principal or Contributing cause*		
	Males	*Females*	*Total*
1 Edinburgh Royal Asylum	56.4	26.1	41.0
2 Kirklands Asylum	49.1	11.3	30.9
3 Govan District Asylum	49.4	6.7	30.0
4 Edinburgh District Asylum	35.2	16.3	25.5
5 Glasgow District Asylums	35.9	8.4	22.9
6 Ayr District Asylum	34.5	7.8	21.4
7 Stirling District Asylum	31.3	8.1	20.9
8 Aberdeen District Asylum	24.6	6.8	16.2
9 Paisley District Asylum	22.2	3.8	12.4
10 Dundee District Asylum	20.7	3.7	11.8
11 Lanark District Asylum	18.5	3.2	11.4
12 Fife District Asylum	17.1	4.3	10.4
13 Greenock Parochial Asylum	12.9	7.4	10.4
14 Renfrew District Asylum	17.1	2.9	10.1
15 Perth District Asylum	18.1	2.1	10.0
16 Midlothian District Asylum	18.8	3.7	9.8
17 Banff District Asylum	10.7	7.2	9.0
18 Roxburgh District Asylum	12.2	2.5	7.4
19 Montrose Royal Asylum	10.6	3.4	6.8
20 Dumfries Royal Asylum	10.0	3.3	6.4
21 Aberdeen Royal Asylum	8.6	3.8	6.0
22 Elgin District Asylum	5.9	4.2	4.9
23 Argyll District Asylum	7.9	—	4.0
24 Haddington District Asylum	8.9	—	3.9
25 Inverness District Asylum	4.0	1.0	2.3
Average	24.5	6.3	15.5

Source: *Fifty-fifth Report of Commissioners of Lunacy for Scotland* (1912), p. lxxv.

Table 12:3 *Deaths from General Paralysis in Scottish Asylums, 1865–1911*

	Year	Deaths from General Paralysis per 1,000 Patients Resident		
		Males	*Females*	*Both Sexes*
Quinquenniads	1870–74	14.6	3.7	8.9
Quinquenniads	1875–79	15.8	2.5	8.8
Quinquenniads	1880–84	13.5	2.8	7.9
Quinquenniads	1885–89	14.9	3.6	9.1
Quinquenniads	1890–94	20.0	3.8	11.6
Quinquenniads	1895–99	20.1	3.8	11.6
Quinquenniads	1900–04	20.4	4.8	12.4
	1907	23.9	6.2	15.0
	1908	24.1	3.3	13.6
	1909	22.9	5.1	13.9
	1910	19.4	5.2	12.2
	1911	21.3	5.6	13.5
	Average of 5 years	20.1	5.1	12.5
	1912	21.1	5.2	13.1

Source: *Fifty-fifth Report of Commissioners in Lunacy for Scotland* (1912), p. lxvi.

Prostitutes were treated differently from other women inmates at Morningside. Six were single, one was married. Most were young – the youngest was 19, referred from the Magdalen Home. Her distraught mother claimed that she was totally 'out of control'. The eldest was a woman in her 30s. One was a puerperal case, rushed from Simpson Memorial Hospital after delivery. All were paupers.

As a group prostitutes drank more than other women. Three out of seven were heavy drinkers. Two had syphilis. One was a syphilitic-alcoholic. One neither drank, nor was syphilitic. None was suicidal, but three were labelled as 'dangerous'. Four were discharged 'recovered' in a surprisingly short time. Their average length of stay was two months as opposed to thirty-six months for other West House women. One died and the remainder were transferred back to their local parish poorhouse.

It is clear that this small group of 'deviant' women were dispatched out of Morningside as quickly as possible. The question remains, where did they get care after discharge? The answer is not yet clear. Edinburgh's Lock Hospital had a short life due to lack of funding and was only viable between 1835 and 1847.[72] It would appear from our small sample of prostitutes that when they fell ill and were destitute the poorhouse was the final resting place for 'fallen women'.

Clouston was acutely conscious of a profound social revolution towards the century's end and acknowledged that women had increased potential to 'evolve' and have more choices. American women had, he believed, most freedom.[73] Yet such reasoning applied only to middle- and upper-class women – and contradicted his own notions and the reality of his experience of the pernicious effects of social class on pauper women.

It is clear that psychiatry is a complex social artefact, as has recently been argued by historians.[74] Different social and cultural conditions produced diverse manifestations of mental anguish. Many fashionable contemporary diagnoses were not prevalent in Scotland. 'Hysteria' and neurasthenia were examples. Instead, frustration, rage, and anger in both sexes manifested themselves in what we might now label reactive depression. Yet Clouston paid little attention to the endemic depression that pervaded Scottish society. Indeed, he argued that depression was the form of madness that most closely resembled the normal state.[75] In a way his detachment is remarkable and perhaps it was actually beneficial.

It is obvious that we need to scrutinize the impact of social class as well as gender, marital status, and age when studying asylum inmates, to understand public policy, the asylum's admission policy, local legal and bureaucratic structure and leadership. It is a mistake to think of nineteenth-century psychiatrists as omnipotent. In Scotland they had to comply with the law which gave paupers priority admission rights – a host of bureaucrats, inspectors of poor, Lunacy Commissioners, families, and friends. Moreover, patients were far from being submissive and compliant. Nor were they expected to be.

Towards the end of his tenure Clouston had nagging anxieties about the future of psychiatry. In spite of better nutrition, improved asylum facilities and sanitary conditions, and interesting compelling 'amusements' for all inmates, he believed that the numbers of 'cures' were diminishing. In addition, he was faced with contemporaneous concerns over increased alcohol abuse, syphilis, numbers of pauper insane and their increasing age.

Clouston, like many Scottish psychiatrists, was unperturbed about the alleged increase in insanity. He maintained that community tolerance for the mad had diminished as the century progressed. He reiterated the theme and described cases which he considered harmless yet whom he was forced by Poor Law authorities and families to commit, and complained about the ever-increasing number of aged, dependent inmates. He preferred to accept suicidal or dangerous inmates. Moreover, Clouston was determined to prevent Morningside from degenerating into a 'museum of madness'.[76] Yet, since he primarily dealt with a deprived urban population, 'incurability' was a given fact. He sought to solve the problem by boarding out 'harmless, incurable' inmates in private homes in the country or to return them to their parish poorhouse when it became evident that they were incurable, a system which he called 'movement of the population'. Impoverished middle-class individuals devastated by the economic crunch of paying for prolonged asylum care were always his main concern.

At the century's end there were three inherent paradoxes in perception and reality about insanity that confounded Scots. First, psychiatrists were proud of their system of mental health care, which had improved considerably since the 1857 Lunacy Act. Paradoxically, there was increased distress in the perceived rise in numbers of the insane. Second, Presbyterianism and the idea of personal responsibility for behaviour caught psychiatrists in another dilemma. Society mandated that psychiatrists accept responsibility for the insane, but it condemned dissipated inmates as unworthy individuals. The third paradox had complicated treatment of the mad all along. Prejudice against the insane remained profound and deep. It mirrored the distaste and contempt with which Lock Hospitals were viewed and the stigma attached to venereal disease. The power of the sexual taboo was also evident in the harsh treatment of unwed mothers that led to the largely undocumented crime of infanticide, yet to be investigated.

Presbyterianism imposed upon all Scots high expectations about conformity in behaviour in age, gender, and class roles. Scottish society did not tolerate swearing and was extremely punitive of promiscuous sexuality. Paradoxically, there was general acceptance of high levels of alcohol consumption.

The rise of science and the doctor competed with the determinism of Presbyterianism. Yet the conflict failed to liberate individuals from Victorian piety and respectability. Instead psychiatrists substituted secular for divine determinism – heredity, 'periodicity'. Dissipation could be combated with 'mental hygiene'. Questions of madness were now seen to be determined by nature or nurture.

But the most frightening change in these years was the rise in numbers of cases of general paralysis and, with the discovery of the spirochete for syphilis, an end of innocence about its cause. Clouston was caught up in distinguishing appropriate age, gender, and class roles. He represents the new professional élite which has its own rules and norms. Belatedly, Clouston was compelled to deal with the social reality of syphilis, which came as an unpleasant shock to a man who had been raised in the heyday of Victorian prudery. Clouston personifies the dichotomy represented by the two sides of the Scottish character. The one kind, decent, sentimental, and compassionate. The other darker, ominous, censorious, and forbidding. They suggest the conflict and ambivalence of the psychiatrist caught in the frustrating reality of his place, culture, and time. As such, Clouston remains an enigmatic, contradictory, and maddening figure.

Yet, for a man whose aim had always been to discover 'cause' and 'cure' for insanity, the result must have been disappointing. The result was yet more bitter because the medicalization of madness had earlier appeared to offer a promising solution while remaining in constant tension with the moral model. For a time the result had worked beautifully, but with the discovery of the spirochete Clouston had to move on to other ways of coping with reality. One answer was to build Craig House in 1894, an 'asylum-home' for the pampered wealthy. Another was renewed vigour in pursuit of 'mental hygiene'.

Before I Wed (1915) was a polemic aimed at an audience of young men which warned of the irrevocable relationship between sexuality and madness. Clouston stressed the importance of idealized, pure womanhood, sanctified monogamous sexual relationships, ideas which he considered timely, appropriate, and 'modern' in virtuous, continent marriage. If, he warned, men masturbated, inevitably the habit would lead to drunkenness, the trip down the primrose path towards liaisons with prostitutes then syphilis, and ultimate insanity. Burns provided an example of a profligate who treated love and women cruelly. Given the poet's love affairs and numerous bastard children, the allegation held a kernel of truth. Ironically, Burns did not go mad – a fact which the tract ignored.

It is unclear if Clouston had become a eugenicist when he wrote *Before I Wed*. The timing of his intellectual progress is still unclear, although it follows that after thirty-five years of observing the results of dissipation, alcoholism, syphilis, and general paralysis, when his prescription for *Hygiene of Mind* was prudent self-control and the ideal of mechanistic harmony, the horror of syphilis must have been devastating.

Clouston's successors seem to have been embarrassed at *Before I Wed*. The book is not available in Morningside's library nor in the Royal College of Physicians' Library. Nor is it mentioned in the lengthy obituary in the *Journal of Mental Science*.[77] Yet, Clouston's reaction to the discovery of the aetiology of tertiary syphilis can be interpreted as that of the honest physician who chose to join the new wave of mental hygienists.[78] Clouston's anxiety mirrored concern early in the twentieth century in America by doctors for improved sex education for young people, 'purity crusades', and the movement to raise the age of sexual consent for young women and girls.[79] Ironically, there is a grain of truth in Clouston's message against self-destructive behaviour which has come full circle in the current hysteria against the sexually transmitted disease AIDS.

In these actions we see psychiatry assuming a new role that suggests the expanding power of medicine, while complying with prevailing social norms. Craig House was created in an optimistic spirit of convincing the public of the legitimacy of psychiatry's medical integrity and claims.

Nevertheless, the wages of sin and dissipated behaviour were not Clouston's only concerns. He recognized that poor married women were the most exploited in society and was at his best with these cases. He was less tolerant of women of his own class, especially those who were deviant in behaviour, ambitious, and remained oblivious to their endemic depression. Women remained difficult, contradictory creatures.

As the enigma surrounding general paralysis was resolved the 'guns of August' blasted Britain's youth. Young men classified as 'biologically unfit' were systematically excluded from the fray. The cream of Britain's young manhood would die and many of those who returned would have new, different mental disorders. Shell-shock was only one. Clouston, now an old man, did not recognize the cataclysm of the First World War, nor did he live to see its consequences.

Clouston was caught in a medical and moral dilemma of a man whose society would see venereal disease as just punishment for promiscuous sexuality and a metaphor for social decay. His response was renewed vigour in 'mental hygiene'. Yet, for a freely chosen act of an individual to be seen as powerful and impersonal as natural law, bespeaks a sexual horror more profound than scientists could comprehend. His cosmic hope that 'no more stigma should attach in the public mind to the incidence of an attack of mania than to an attack of measles', would never be fulfilled.[80] The suggestion of the new young Turks of the psychiatric profession in Clouston's obituary that his work was already dated suggests the ultimate paradox. The irony remains that the psychiatric profession has even now failed to achieve the 'scientific' legitimacy it so desperately wishes to obtain. And the same allegation would in turn, be levelled at their own innovative theories.

Notes

1 J. Edward Chamberlin and Sander L. Gilman (eds) (1985) *Degeneration: The Dark Side of Progress*, New York: Columbia University Press; Elaine Showalter (1985) *The Female Malady: Women, Madness, and English Culture, 1830–1980*, New York: Pantheon Books, chapter 4; Ian Dowbiggin (1985) 'Degeneration and hereditarianism in French mental medicine, 1840–1890: psychiatric theory as ideological adaptation', in W.F. Bynum, Roy Porter, and Michael Shepherd (eds), *The Anatomy of Madness: Essays in the History of Psychiatry*, London: Tavistock, vol. I; Charles Rosenberg (1976) 'The bitter fruit: heredity, disease and social thought in nineteenth-century America', in C. Rosenberg, *No Other Gods: On Science and American Social Thought*, Baltimore: Johns Hopkins University Press.

2 Thomas Smith Clouston (1884) *Clinical Lectures on Mental Diseases*, Philadelphia: Henry C. Lea's Son & Co. For the purpose of this chapter the 1884 American edition was used. Other titles by Thomas Smith Clouston are (1879) *The Study of Mental Disease*; (1879) *An Asylum or Hospital Home for 200 Patients*, Boston; (1882) *Female Education from a Medical Point of View*; (1890) *The Neuroses of Development*; (1906) *The Hygiene of Mind* (the edition used in this chapter was published in 1912); (1911) *Unsoundness of Mind*; (1915) *Before I Wed*.

3 Lunacy (Scotland) Act, 1857, 20 & 21 Victoria, Cap. 71.

4 William Ll. Parry-Jones (1981) 'The model of the Gheel Lunatic Colony and its influence on the nineteenth-century asylum system in Britain', in A. Scull, *Madhouses, Mad-doctors and Madmen*, London: Athlone, pp. 201–7.

5 Nancy Tomes (1984) *A Generous Confidence: Thomas Story Kirkbride and the Art of Asylum-Keeping, 1840–1883*, Cambridge: Cambridge University Press. Clouston shared Kirkbride's passion for architecture and interior design.

6 Showalter, *The Female Malady*, p. 122. Clouston was no 'psychiatric Darwinist', as this chapter will argue, and it is a mistake to pair him with the English psychiatrist Henry Maudsley.

7 Thomas Smith Clouston (1912) *The Hygiene of Mind*, London: Methuen.

8 Margaret S. Thompson (forthcoming, 1988) 'The problem with women: women inmates in the Royal Edinburgh Asylum, 1874–94', in Malcolm Nicolson (ed.),

Scottish Health Care in the Ninettenth Century, London: Routledge.
9 K.M. Boyd (1980) *Scottish Church Attitudes to Sex, Marriage and the Family*, Edinburgh: John Donald, pp. 174–85, and part 2, chapters 11–15.
10 ibid., p. 9.
11 ibid., pp. 27–40.
12 R.K. Marshall (1981) *Virgins and Viragos*, Chicago: Academy Press, pp. 268–74; Lawrence Stone (1977) *The Family, Sex and Marriage in England, 1500–1800*, New York: Harper & Row, pp. 675–6.
13 Malcolm B. MacGregor [n.d. but *c.* 1947] *Towards Soctland's Social Good: A Hundred Years of Temperance Work in the Church of Scotland*, London: Gilmour & Dean, pp. 9–45.
14 Boyd, *Sex, Marriage and the Family*, pp. 17, 28, 74, 129, 133.
15 MacGregor, *Towards Scotland's Social Good*, p. 21.
16 W. Paton (1979) 'Drink and the Temperance Movement in Scotland'. Edinburgh University PhD dissertation, p. 179; Brian Harrison (1971) *Drink and the Victorians: The Temperance Question in England 1815–1872*, London: Faber. Harrison discusses the Scottish Temperance Movement on pp. 96–7, 104–5 and 314.
17 Paton, 'Drink and the Temperance Movement', p. 45.
18 Clouston, *Clinical Lectures*, p. 312. Clouston made no comment on a work by Dr Benedict Augustin Morel (1809–73) (1857) *Traité des Dégénérescences de L'Espèce Physiques, Intellectuelles et Morales de l'Espèce Humaine* or Dr J.J. Moreau de Tours (1959) *La Psychologie Morbide dans ses Rapports avec la Philosophie de l'Histoire*; E.H. Ackerknecht (1968) *Short History of Psychiatry*, trans. S. Wolff, New York: Hafner, chapter VII.
19 Departmental Committee on Habitual Offenders, Inebriates, &c. (Scotland) (1895) *Report from the Departmental Committee on Habitual Offenders, Vagrants, Beggars, Inebriates and Juvenile Delinquents* (London: HMSO), pp. 101–6. See too Eric T. Carlson (1985) 'Medicine and degeneration: theory and praxis', in Chamberlin and Gilman (eds), *Degeneration*, pp. 121–44. Carlson explicates Morel's position on alcoholism and the rise and fall of the degeneration theory.
20 Clouston, *Clinical Lectures*, p. 312.
21 ibid.
22 Clouston, *Clinical Lectures*, pp. 312–18.
23 A.B. Sclare (1981) 'John Carswell: a pioneer in Scottish psychiatry', *Scottish Medical Journal* 26: 265–70.
24 Letter to Clouston from the administrator of St Cuthbert's Parish Poorhouse, Edinburgh.
25 ibid.
26 Clouston, *Clinical Lectures*, p. 317.
27 Report ... on Habitual Offenders, Vagrants, Beggars, Inebriates and Juvenile Delinquents.
28 Clouston, *Clinical Lectures*, p. 316.
29 ibid.
30 Report ... on Habitual Offenders, Vagrants, Beggars, Inebriates and Juvenile Delinquents, pp. 101–6.
31 Physician's Annual Report (1894), p. 11. Clouston, *Hygiene of Mind*, pp. 207–8. See too Roy Porter (1982) 'Shutting people up', *Social Studies of Science* 12: 467–76; Roger Smith (1981) *Trial By Medicine: Insanity and Responsibility in Victorian Trials*, Edinburgh: Edinburgh University Press. Clouston used the

same logic as psychiatrists described by Smith who excused women who were guilty of infanticide because of 'insanity'.

32 Report ... on Habitual Offenders, Vagrants, Beggars, Inebriates and Juvenile Delinquents.

33 George Rosen (1968) *Madness in Society: Chapters in the Historical Sociology of Mental Illness*, New York: Harper Torchbooks, pp. 248–58; Allan M. Brandt (1987) *No Magic Bullet: A Social History of Venereal Disease in the United States since 1880*, expanded edn Oxford: Oxford University Press, p. 9; Roger L. Williams (1980) *The Horror of Life*, Chicago: Chicago University Press; R.A. Hunter and I. Macalpine (1974) *Psychiatry for the Poor*, London: Dawsons, pp. 207–11.

34 Boyd, *Sex, Marriage and the Family*, pp. 205–53.

35 William Tait (1841) *Magdalenism: An Inquiry into the Extent, Causes and Consequences of Prostitution*, Edinburgh: P. Rickard, pp. 145–56.

36 ibid., pp. 5–9.

37 ibid., p. 112; Barbara Hobson (1981) 'Sex in the marketplace: prostitution in an American Victorian city', Boston University PhD dissertation, p. 97–8.

38 ibid., p. 235–9. Tait's work followed hard on the heels of A.J.B. Parent-Duchatelet's study (1836) *De la Prostitution dans la ville de Paris* which pointed out the fluid social structure of prostitution in France and claimed that it was a phase through which young women passed relatively unscathed.

39 Boyd, *Sex, Marriage and the Family*, pp. 188–9; Judith Walkowitz (1980) *Prostitution and Victorian Society: Women, Class and the State*, Cambridge: Cambridge University Press, pp. 44–7.

40 Walkowitz, *Prostitution and Victorian Society*, pp. 69–147; Boyd, *Sex, Marriage and the Family*, p. 194; Brandt, *No Magic Bullet*, chapter 1.

41 Clouston, *Clinical Lectures*, lecture XII, pp. 301–11. Contrast Clouston's theory of syphilis with that of organic brain disease and of general paralysis, lecture X, pp. 260–76.

42 Clouston, *Clinical Lectures*, p. 302.

43 ibid., p. 303.

44 ibid., p. 304.

45 ibid. See too J.J. Brown (July 1875) *Journal of Mental Science*.

46 Clouston, *Clinical Lectures*, lecture X, pp. 260–76.

47 ibid., p. 260.

48 Physician's annual report (1892), p. 14.

49 Clouston, *Clinical Lectures*, pp. 260–76.

50 ibid., p. 276.

51 Physician's annual report (1887), p. 12.

52 Physician's annual report (1892), p. 14.

53 Rolf Fjelde (1982) *Henrik Ibsen: The Complete Major Prose Plays*, New York: Farrar, Strauss, Giroux, p. 2; Simon Williams (1985) 'Theater and degeneration: subversion and sexuality', in Chamberlain and Gilman (eds), *Degeneration*, pp. 241–62. Williams analyses contemporary plays depicting sexuality. See too Barbara Gutmann Rosenkrantz (1979) 'Damaged goods: dilemmas of responsibility for risk', *Health and Society* 57: 1–37. Brieux's play made its Broadway debut in 1915. See too Brandt, *No Magic Bullet*, pp. 47–9.

54 Boyd, *Sex, Marriage and the Family*, pp. 163, 177, 188, 192, 241, 245 and 354.

55 Brandt, *No Magic Bullet*, p. 21.

56 ibid., pp. 32–44.

57 Philippe Ricord (1838) *Traité Pratique des Maladies Vénériennes ou Recherches*

Critiques et Experimentales sur l'Inoculation Appliquée a l'étude de ces Maladies, Paris; Rouvier; William Allen Pusey (1933) *The History and Epidemiology of Syphilis*, Springfield, Ill: University of Illinois Press, pp. 53–61.

58 Alfred Fournier (1880) [*Syphilis et Marriage*] *Syphilis and Marriage* trans. by Prince A. Morrow, New York; L. Duncan Bulkey (1894) *Syphilis in the Innocent*, New York.

59 Brandt, *No Magic Bullet*, pp. 14–21.

60 Carl Miller (1976) *Cockburn's Millenium*, Cambridge, Mass.: Harvard University Press, p. 175.

61 Physician's annual report (1892), p. 34.

62 Clouston, *Clinical Lectures* (1884 edn), p. 301; Thomas Stretch Dowse (1879) *Syphilis of the Brain and Spinal Cord*, London: reviewed (1881) in the *Journal of Mental Science* XXVII: 74–80.

63 David Kennedy Henderson (1964) *Evolution of Psychiatry in Scotland*, Edinburgh: E. & S. Livingstone, pp. 123–7.

64 ibid. See too Ludwik Fleck ([1935] 1979) *Genesis and Development of a Scientific Fact*, trans. Trenn, Chicago: pp. 340–2; Isador Rosen and Nathan Sobel (1950) 'Fifty years' progress in the treatment of syphilis', *New York Surgical and Medical Journal* 50: 2694–6.

65 Fifty-Fifth report of the General Board of Commissioners in Lunacy for Scotland, VIII, pp. lxv–lxxvii.

66 ibid.

67 Walkowitz, *Prostitution and Victorian Society*, p. 256. Walkowitz argues that in England doctors hid the diagnosis of venereal disease from wives of victims.

68 Guenter Risse (1986) *Hospital Life in Enlightenment Scotland: Care and Teaching at the Royal Infirmary of Edinburgh*, Cambridge: Cambridge University Press, pp. 126–7. Risse points out that venereally diseased inmates were admitted to Edinburgh's Royal Infirmary – a policy that was not followed in contemporary English institutions.

69 Brandt, *No Magic Bullet*, pp. 23–31.

70 Walkowitz, *Prostitution and Victorian Society*, chapter 10, pp. 192–213.

71 ibid., pp. 11–21.

72 David Hamilton (1981) *The Healers: A History of Medicine in Scotland*, Edinburgh: Canongate Press, p. 21.

73 Clouston, *Hygiene of Mind*, p. 213.

74 Klaus Doerner (1981) *Madmen and the Bourgeoisie: A Social History of Insanity and Psychiatry*, trans. Joachim Neugroschel and Jean Steinberg, Oxford: Basil Blackwell; Mark Finnane (1981) *Insanity and the Insane in Post-Famine Ireland*, London: Croom Helm.

75 Clouston, *Clinical Lectures*, p. 54.

76 A. Scull (1979) *Museums of Madness*, London: Allen Lane; A. Scull (ed.) (1981) *Madhouses, Mad-doctors, and Madmen: The Social History of Psychiatry in the Victorian Era* , London: Athlone.

77 (1915) *Journal of Mental Science* LXI: 332–8.

78 Rosenkrantz, 'Damaged goods', 19 and 21.

79 Mary Odem (20 June 1987) 'Protecting girlhood chastity: the age of consent campaign in the United States', paper presented at the Seventh Berkshire Conference on the History of Women, Wellesley College, Mass.

80 (1915) *Journal of Mental Science* LXI: 332–8.

Name Index

Subject Index